Neonatal Nursing

What ceaseless dread a mother's breast alarms whilst her lov'd offspring fills another's arms!

La Balia (The Nurse)
Tansillo, 1569

Neonatal Nursing

A Practical Guide

Edited by

Anne Marie Dazé, R.N., B.S.N.
Columbia Hospital for Women

John W. Scanlon, M.D.
Georgetown University School of Medicine

University Park Press · Baltimore

University Park Press
International Publishers in Medicine and Allied Health
300 North Charles Street
Baltimore, Maryland 21201

Production editor: Megan Barnard Shelton
Cover and text design by: Caliber Design Planning, Inc.

Typeset by: Bi-Comp, Incorporated
Manufactured in the United States of America by: Halliday Lithograph

Library of Congress Cataloging in Publication Data
Main entry under title:

Neonatal nursing.

  Includes bibliographies and index.
  1. Infants (Newborn)—Diseases—Nursing. I. Dazé,
Anne, Marie. II. Scanlon, John W., 1939–
[DNLM: 1. Infant, Newborn, Diseases—nursing.
2. Pediatric Nursing. WY 159 N439]
RJ253.N44 1984   610.73′62   84-17400
ISBN 0-8391-1875-9

This book is dedicated to M.D.S., a nurse, who was a very early and enduring model of the very best nursing can offer to mankind,

and

to E.K.D. and D.J.D., whose love for infants inspired a life commitment to their care.

Contents

Contributors

Parveen Chowdhry, M.D.
Neonatology Division
Columbia Hospital for Women
2425 L Street, N.W.
Washington, D.C. 20037
    and
Assistant Professor of Pediatrics
Georgetown University School of Medicine
Washington, D.C. 20007

Carmel Anne Cunningham, R.N., B.S.N.
Pediatric Surgery Nurse Coordinator
University of Maryland Hospital
22 South Greene Street
Baltimore, MD 21201

Anne Marie Dazé, R.N., B.S.N.
Coordinator, NICU Education
Columbia Hospital for Women
2425 L Street, N.W.
Washington, D.C. 20037

Betty Lou Glass, R.N.
Staff Nurse, NICU
Columbia Hospital for Women
2425 L Street, N.W.
Washington, D.C. 20037

Kenneth L. Harkavy, M.D.
Neonatology Division
Columbia Hospital for Women
2425 L Street, N.W.
Washington, D.C. 20037
    and
Assistant Professor of Pediatrics
Georgetown University School of Medicine
Washington, D.C. 20007

Patricia E. Ionides, M.S.W.
Director, Social Work Service
Columbia Hospital for Women
2425 L Street, N.W.
Washington, D.C. 20037

Doris Johnson, R.N., B.S.N.
Coordinator, NICU
Columbia Hospital for Women
2425 L Street, N.W.
Washington, D.C. 20037

Mary T. Maholchic, R.N., M.S.N., C.P.N.P.
Sinai Hospital
Baltimore, MD

Linda G. Matthews, R.N.
Supervisor, NICU
Columbia Hospital for Women
2425 L Street, N.W.
Washington, D.C. 20037

John W. Scanlon, M.D.
Director of Neonatology
Columbia Hospital for Women
2425 L Street, N.W.
Washington, D.C. 20037
    and
Department of Pediatrics
Georgetown University School of Medicine
Washington, D.C. 20007

Kathleen B. Scanlon, R.N., M.S.N.
Clinical Coordinator
Infant Developmental Evaluation Clinic
Columbia Hospital for Women
2425 L Street, N.W.
Washington, D.C. 20037
    and
Research Associate
Department of Pediatrics
Georgetown University School of Medicine
Washington, D.C. 20007

Johannah L. Williams, R.N., M.S.N.
Clinical Instructor
American University School of Nursing
Washington, D.C. 20016

Preface

When we first conceived this book, we thought to describe a collection of nursing care plans. On reflection, however, we realized there were too many shortcomings to this approach. First, there is always more than one way to deliver nursing care to sick neonates. A simple collection of care plans could not do justice to this variety of approaches. Second, from our observation, one common cause of error among neonatal health care providers is inadequate understanding of those principles that guide interventions. This led us to attempt to combine theory with a day-by-day approach to the care of ill newborns. Thus we have tried to consolidate many scattered pages of neonatal intensive care nursing strategies and make them consonant with theory.

Each chapter contains discussions about psychosocial theory, physiology, and pathophysiology as they specifically apply to intensive care nursing. We hope such discussions illuminate the "whys" behind care and stimulate further reading. We also hope our book can be used in the clinical setting as a guide. To this end each chapter contains numerous appendices that describe specific practical protocols or approaches to common basic problems and tasks confronted daily by the NICU nurse. We have also included numerous tables that list drugs and doses, equipment, normal values, or certain salient points about neonatal assessment, prognosis, and treatment. Since our approach emphasizes the experiential, case studies plus real clinical examples have been used to highlight the basic discussion.

This book was written by clinicians. These, our friends and colleagues, have repeatedly demonstrated their crib-side skills and enthusiasm for neonatal care. Clearly, there are other approaches to care and practical suggestions or techniques about which we are unaware. We would sincerely appreciate feedback (written or verbal) from you. Worthwhile suggestions or additions will be considered (and acknowledged) for subsequent editions.

Thank you for your interest in our approach to newborn care. Most of all, thanks for persisting in your care of the most small and fragile human—the sick neonate.

Anne Marie Dazé
John W. Scanlon

Suggested Reading

Chess S: Mothers are always the problem; or are they? Pediatrics 71:976, 1983.

Cutter M: Maternal Deprivation Reassessed, 2nd ed. Penguin Books, Middlesex, England, 1981.

Klaus M, Kennel J: Maternal-Infant Bonding, 2nd ed. Mosby, St. Louis, 1981.

Lamb ME: Early contact and maternal-infant bonding. Pediatrics 70:763, 1982.

Marhsall RE, Kasman C, Cape LS: Coping with Caring For Sick Newborns. Saunders, Philadelphia, 1983.

Stinson R, Stinson P: The Long Dying of Baby Andrew. Little, Brown, Boston, 1983.

Acknowledgments

The editors acknowledge the secretarial help of Ms. Carrie Grose and Ms. Charlene Andrews. We also thank Mr. Albert Belskie for his support, encouragement, and patience.

1

Strategies for Stress Management
Nursing Organization and Intervention with Parents

Linda G. Matthews
Patricia E. Ionides

Stressful situations are so common to all newborn intensive care situations that coping strategies must be addressed along with physical health care issues if total family care is to be given. Stresses are also faced daily by the staff in the form of practical, ethical, environmental, and psychosocial dilemmas. This chapter addresses two sides of this problem. First we discuss what can be done by nursing management to minimize stress, keep staff morale as high as possible, and avoid "burn out." Then we outline major problems confronted by parents of sick infants and strategies to help them cope successfully.

Organizational Considerations

Staffing

In a study by Astbury and Yu (1) physicians and nurses rated overwork and understaffing as problems associated with the highest level of stress. Overwork and understaffing have historically been accepted as part of nursing, but they need not be accepted as inevitable. Nursing management can cut down considerably on chronic work overload. The nurse manager can act as a nurse advocate by convincing the hospital administrators and budget committees that caring for sick newborns is a complex task, not just a matter of feeding babies. This requires documentation of the scope of nursing care that sick infants need. The use of a patient classification tool with a clearly outlined system for determining nurse/patient ratios is employed by many hospitals. Appendix 1.1 depicts the tool we have developed at the Columbia Hospital for Women for this purpose. Data systematically collected with such a tool can be

1

used to document caretaking needs in the neonatal intensive care unit (NICU). With the daily use of a patient classification system, the need for extra staff and their extra expense can be exactly defined and defended. By using this format we have been able to provide flexible staffing according to changing nursing care needs of the infant.

Lobbying to increase budgeted positions is only the beginning of the work to ensure adequate staffing. Nurse managers nationally face the twin problems of inadequate numbers of available nurses and high staff turnover. Resources we employ to alleviate this problem are temporary nurses, float pools, and per diem staff. These help to alleviate excessive overtime and overwork by the full-time intensive care nursery staff when all-too-frequent peaks in patient load occur. We have been most satisfied with using a per diem pool that the hospital controls because we are able to interview applicants and ensure that they are skilled in NICU care before they report for duty. This is a luxury not afforded by temporary agencies.

Education

Ideally, any newly hired nurse would already possess the required knowledge and skills to work with critically sick newborns. Unfortunately, this is usually not the case in practice. Therefore, we have developed a 6-week training program for all inexperienced new employees. This is not just an orientation period. Theoretical considerations are presented along with, and integrated into, the clinical experience. This 6-week training program for NICU includes 40 hours of theoretical background, lab experience, and clinical work under the supervision of the NICU nurse educator. The ability to understand what is being done (and why) plus familiarity with the clinical and technical aspects of care is extremely important for quality nursing care and equally important for developing heightened self-esteem. It is stressful and frightening for a nurse to feel inadequately prepared to care for tiny patients. Therefore, we feel that an initial training program and ongoing education are essential to ensure that the entire staff feels confident and motivated to continue to learn.

Continuing education programs serve to enhance and increase the experienced staff nurses' expertise. The NICU nurse educator is responsible for coordinating biweekly continuing education classes, periodic workshops, and an annual seminar for staff members. The budget is structured to permit paid educational leave so that vacation time does not need to be used for outside conferences and seminars. Tuition reimbursement for nurses who attend courses is also a benefit that helps attract new personnel. Additionally, this demonstrates the hospitals's interest in and commitment to staff motivation and growth. The involvement of individuals in unit projects, research, and teaching can be encouraged by giving educational leave to increase knowledge about those special projects.

Scheduling

Scheduling can also be viewed as an area of controllable stress. Obvious problems like chronic sleep deprivation from "switch backs" between evening and day shift, or from split days off with night shift, can be prevented. Loss of control is often cited as a stressor, so granting leave requests as often as possible gives staff more control over their own lives.

One creative approach to schedule-induced stress is the use of alternative scheduling patterns. In our unit we have successfully used the 10-hour shift. It is popular with our staff because it is not an excessively long day and creates a 4-day work week. Overlapping shifts can be used to advantage depending on unit needs and routine. Peak periods of the day, such as when babies return from surgery, feeding times, parent or staff education classes, or unit meetings, can be staffed by overlapping personnel since there may be as many as six "extra" nurses on duty. We have also found that the need for overtime can be reduced from one complete 8-hour shift to only part of one shift when "overlapping" nurses are deployed. Occasionally overtime can be eliminated completely.

Many hospitals have been moving away from the traditional 5-day, 40-hour work week and are experimenting with a variety of alternate shifts (2). It is important that the nursing management consider alternatives for nurses who cannot, or will not, work the traditional 8-hour, 5-day-per-week schedule. Providing alternative scheduling may increase the number of nurses per shift at the same time that morale is boosted. Not everyone in our unit must work 10-hour shifts, but it is an option for each staff member to consider. Sometimes increased expense incurred by nontraditional staffing patterns can be defended because of other measurable benefits to the institution. Increased recruitment and retention of nurses have been significant in our nursery since we introduced flexible and alternative scheduling.

Delivery of Care

Once organizational problems have been handled, one must examine the nursing goals for the unit and how they can be best achieved. Then a nursing care system must be developed so these can be met. Certainly few things can be more frustrating than not being able to reach one's goals. Goals of nursing in the NICU include optimal physical growth and development, prevention of complications, the development of a nurturing parent-infant relationship, and successful resolution of the parental crisis of having a sick newborn. We believe a primary system of nursing care is the most effective way for nursing to contribute to these goals.

Primary care nursing is defined as individualized, total care by the same nurse from the time of the newborn's admission until discharge. It provides personalized, specific, comprehensive care with continuity. Primary care can be beneficial both for parents and staff. Parents will express an increased sense of security after they develop a trusting relationship with the person who is taking care of their baby. They will have one consistent person to turn to with concerns and questions. Nurses also express greater professional satisfaction and a sense of accomplishment because of the professional relationship they develop with families through primary care nursing.

In an intensive care nursery, the primary care nurse has several roles. Obviously two essential tasks are those of being the primary caregiver to the baby and a central resource to his parents. This latter role involves being a support person during a time of crisis and a teacher as the crisis resolves. By caring for the baby from admission through discharge, the primary care nurse becomes immediately aware of problems and special needs of the infant or his parents as they present themselves. Because of this, the primary care nurse takes on another important role as communicator to other professionals. The primary care nurse may initiate or participate in group conferences with physicians, social workers, and other nurses. She also contributes to therapeutic decision making and ongoing care. Discharge planning and teaching become her responsibility as well. These tasks are accomplished gradually throughout the baby's hospitalization.

There are always problems in implementing anything new to an established unit. Many personnel are wary of change. It is important to obtain the staff's input and opinions about benefits and problems of primary care nursing in order to decrease resistance. Because of these concerns we discuss below some problems and possible solutions found when implementing primary care nursing.

1. ***Assignments*** These can be made by the charge nurse if any infant does not acquire a primary care nurse within 24 hours of birth. Each new admission can be assigned on a rotating basis. Posting names of primary care nurses in the NICU makes it clear which nurse has what primary care patient and who will be assigned to the next admission. This system does not prevent a nurse from requesting a particular baby.
2. ***Long-Term-Care Babies*** Ideally, a nurse will care for her primary care patient every time she is on duty. Since some babies may be hospitalized for 6 months or more, however, such consistency may not always be possible or realistic. Although the primary care nurse need not be the daily caregiver, she must keep the care plan current. She remains responsible for parent contact and teaching.
3. ***Rotating to the Night Shift*** This has been seen as a stumbling block to primary care nursing. It need not be because parental contact can be continued by telephone. Furthermore, input to day shift can be provided through the head nurse or an associate primary nurse as an intermediary.
4. ***Patient Load*** The number of primary care patients assigned to one nurse depends on the number of registered nurses on the unit. It should probably not exceed 2 per nurse, particularly if one baby is acutely sick or has a lengthy problem list.

Primary care nursing in a neonatal intensive care setting does have problems in implementation and maintenance. However, if it is seen to be valuable by the staff and has the support of the head nurse and nursing administration, it can be made to work to the benefit of staff, patients, and parents. The primary care nurse's role comprises:

1. Accepting a primary care patient and making a commitment to the patient, family, and staff.
2. Keeping informed about all areas of the baby's disease, prognosis, history, and needs, as well as the doctors' plans; keeping informed about family status and problems; communicating to other professionals while preserving confidentiality.
3. Writing, keeping current, and implementing and evaluating a care plan with a clear problem list and dates of their resolution.
4. Recording any problem noted about family and parental visiting patterns and the degree of their involvement with baby care; again, communicating this knowledge.
5. Giving care while on duty unless it is made known that a change is requested.

If the intensive care nursery (ICN) is part of a hospital that transports infants long distances, primary care nursing becomes especially valuable. Parents may be able to only infrequently visit and participate in the care of their baby. With the added stress of such separation, knowledge that there is one person who is the primary caregiver and source of information and support can be especially comforting.

When going on a transport, the potential primary care nurse should visit with the parents, and have them see and, if possible, hold their baby. She may visit the mother while she is in the hospital or keep her informed through phone calls. The primary care nurse should also keep the referring hospital nursery staff informed through phone calls. Polaroid pictures are a particularly warm way to keep parents updated and involved in their infants's changing condition.

A secondary, or associate, nurse works well in a primary care system. Often she is a nurse from a shift (particularly nights) who does not have enough direct contact with parents to be the primary care nurse. She should identify herself and her involvement to parents and staff and be the caregiver when the primary care nurse is off duty. She should be well informed and be able to make systematic nursing decisions as well as be a backup support person for the primary nurse.

Preparing the Family for Discharge

Discharge planning is an ongoing process that should be started early in the infant's hospitalization once survival becomes probable. Teaching needs for home care should be delinated and included in the care plan by the primary care nurse. Transition from the ICN to home is often stressful for parents even if their infant's stay was short and uneventful. Discharge planning and teaching for parents whose baby requires long-term, specialized care at home is mandatory. This requires input from all disciplines involved in the infant's care. Regular meetings should be held with physicians, nurses, and social workers to discuss medical follow-up, home care, visiting nurse requirements, or special programs for specific chronic problems.

Some hospitals have a full-time discharge-planning nurse (3). The advantage is that one person ensures that the task of planning has been completed. It is not necessary to omit primary care nursing if the discharge-planning nurse acts as coordinator for community and hospital resources. No matter who carries out discharge planning, a written plan and teaching tools should be established with goals and needs clearly outlined as well as the level of parent understanding documented. This maximizes communication between personnel about parents' progress and the baby's current needs. In this way consistent, nonrepetitive teaching is provided. The list of topics and skills needed can be very long because parents need to be familiar with their infant's special needs as well as knowledgeable about basic "well baby" care.

Frequency of rehospitalization is increased for very low birth weight babies. Reasons for some readmissions are respiratory tract infections, other acute illness, or chronic problems originating from their preterm birth. Parents of such infants should be made familiar with signs and symptoms of infection, thermal regulation, visiting recommendations, and travel restrictions. There are parents who prefer to have their babies at home rather than continuing their convalescence in hospital, even if their baby requires cardiorespiratory monitors or oxygen therapy. These parents must be taught to use (and demonstrate that they understand) the equipment their babies require. Such parents must clearly know who to contact about acute problems. The health care facility that provides follow-up may not provide emergency services. Be sure that parents have all appropriate phone numbers and know who to call for specific problems.

Some units have rooming-in for parents when the child requires special care during the convalescent period. Overnight or daily care becomes their responsibility in the hospital, but they are able to receive support and help from the staff. As an alternative to rooming-in before discharge, a home pass system has been found helpful (3) for the discharge process of infants who have complex care needs or who have been hospitalized for a long time. Infants can be taken home for periods from 4 to 24 hours and then returned. A nurse, ideally the primary care nurse, can accompany them for the first one or two times. Passes can be given as often as necessary. Through the support and encouragement given by the hospital staff in the home, anxiety or social upheaval caused by care transition can be lessened.

Sibling Visitation and Counseling

If family-centered care is to be given in the NICU, the siblings of sick newborns must be considered. Most ICNs have open visiting for parents. Now many also allow grandparents or "significant others" to visit for a limited time during the day. However, few units allow small children to visit sick newborn siblings except under very unusual circumstances. There are two reasons for this restriction: one is the real chance of spreading infection; the other is potential psychological shock. Some authorities believe that a small child may be emotionally traumatized by exposure to an intensive care setting. An alternate belief is that, by not seeing the infant, the sibling fantasizes an unkown, faceless being who has taken up his parent's time, concern, and love. Thus, early on, feelings of rivalry and resentment are established. There is no consensus for either viewpoint.

Each hospital should consider the notion of sibling visitation, its advantages and disadvantages. As a minimum, an enclosed area with windows onto the unit should be available for siblings of any age to view the nursery and their "own" baby. For nursery admittance, most units require that the sibling has no infectious disease and is afebrile, and that the parents feel such a visit would be beneficial. Usually a limited time can be allowed, perhaps 10 minutes once a week for visiting. No increased rate of infection has been documented in our unit with such a policy.

Hospitals have various ways to aid a small child's understanding during this time. We use a coloring book called "The Frog Family Has a Baby" for children in the 2- to 6-year age group. This was designed by Jerri Oehler at Duke University Medical Center. While telling the story to the sibling, parents put in their names and the name of the baby to make the story pertinent to them and their experience.

Crisis Intervention

As professionals how can we assist parents through the crisis of having a sick newborn? All parents experience stress when they have a sick newborn, and many will experience a crisis. By applying crisis theory when assessing parents' stress levels, appropriate interventions and referrals can be made. In this section we address how parents in crisis may act and propose some interventions for the NICU setting. Appendix 1.2 lists books, information sources, and resource groups for parents.

Crisis Theory and Individual Response

There are varying, but related, models of crisis theory. Described in the most simplistic way, a crisis is an "upset in a steady state" (4), or an unanticipated state of emotional disequilibrium. To understand this concept and apply the principles of crisis intervention, it is important to first recognize the signs and symptoms of an individual's response to a crisis. Determining the level of crisis helps determine the extent of intervention needed.

From the parents' viewpoint, admission of their baby to an NICU almost always signifies a threat to his life or future health. One generalized response to this is depression. However, individuals also experience fear and anxiety during the early stages of crisis. Fear may persist if previously used coping techniques are inadequate for handling the threat of death or permanent disability. Anxiety may continue if a person's defense mechanisms are not able to control the intrapsychic conflict, or repressed thoughts lying near consciousness. As Eaton et al. (5) pointed out, "fear warns of an external danger; anxiety of an internal danger. To the extent that each is a warning, though unpleasant, it is useful. . . ."

Both anxiety and fear may be thought of as unsuccessful attempts to restore a previous state of equilibrium. This leaves the individual vulnerable and feeling threatened. As you may have already experienced in your work, some parents have heightened defense reactions. Anxiety will be experienced until a defense mechanism for coping with the new situation is either adaptively reinstated or learned. Fear may persist unless that individual establishes adequate methods of coping with the threat, the threat resolves, or they choose the flight alternative of the "fight or flight" impulse as a mechanism until equilibrium is reestablished.

Principles of Crisis Resolution

At this juncture it is important to look at principles of crisis intervention as well as which techniques or methods might be employed to encourage healthy resolution. This should be one goal for the professional who deals with a parent in crisis. The long-term effects of an unresolved crisis usually go unseen, but are believed to be detrimental to the quality of the mother-infant relationship as well as decreasing the mother's ability to ensure a positive developmental process for her child. In essence, once the crisis is resolved the mother becomes "freed up" and able to care for her child.

Rappoport (4) described the following stages of response necessary for healthy crisis resolution: 1) correct cognitive perception of the situation, which is furthered by seeking new knowledge and by keeping the problem in consciousness; 2) management of affect through awareness of feelings and appropriate verbalization leading toward tension discharge and mastery; and 3) development of patterns of seeking and using help with tasks and feelings by using available interpersonal and institutional resources.

Being one of the first to interact with the parents, the baby's nurse has an opportunity to help begin the process of healthy crisis resolution. Purposefully focused efforts early on may serve more meaningfully than extensive help at another later, more critical period. This is because of the individual's emotional accessibility at the start of a crisis. Successful early resolution may also serve as a model for learning how to cope with future crisis.

Methods used in guiding parents toward healthy resolution are not complicated. First, to help them get a correct cognitive perception, clarify the problem their infant is experiencing in understandable terms. They probably do not understand much medical jargon. Ask them to repeat back what they have heard. If you detect that they are very anxious or that it is difficult for them to assimilate information, use drawings to describe the baby's problem and use expressions or terms commonly understood. Speak to them with words and use ideas that are easily recognized in a lay person's vocabularly or experience. Be sure to acknowledge that what is happening *is* overwhelming and that it takes time to understand the total picture. Suggest that they can begin to decrease their sense of feeling overwhelmed by compartmentalizing each separate problem involved in the whole crisis. In other words, take one thing and one day at a time. Help them focus on understanding what the baby's condition may be like for the next 24 hours, rather than 5 years from now.

A professional needs to learn to accept irrational attitudes or negative responses by parents. Guard against communicating shock or rejecting negative feelings, ideas, or behavior that parents may express. This may be difficult, but it is important neither to increase the parents' fear and anxiety nor to create a sense of isolation. Being able to express even negative ideas allows parents an opportunity to address their own feelings without judgment or inhibitions. It also helps parents to achieve the second step of crisis resolution (i.e., tension discharge and mastering of feelings). At some time you may become the target of displaced anger caused by parents' inability to control a life-threatening situation. It may be helpful to remember that fear is always the base of such anger. This reaction to fear, while unfair to you, is an expression of their inability to rid themselves of such feelings.

Negative or painful responses by parents may be more subtle than an angry response. It is not uncommon to see a mother flinching as though it were she getting the IV or having her heel stuck for blood. When such behavior is excessive or continuously expressed it may indicate some symbiotic or narcissistic pathology that needs further psychiatric evaluation. Expressed to a lesser degree, which is more common, such personalization indicates the attachment process that began in utero and seems to be a prerequisite for maternal-infant interaction later on. A pathological response would be that of a mother who, over time, is continually unable to distinguish boundaries between herself and her baby. In such a case, it would be helpful that she not observe particularly intrusive procedures and that she be encouraged to leave the nursery for periods of rest during the baby's acute illness. This might be accomplished by gentle suggestions from the baby's nurse or through the encouragement of another support person. If these interventions are successful, this stage should be completed with the parents' ability to verbalize their fears in a rational context. An indication of success is the parent's ability to realistically appreciate special needs or problems their infant has.

Finally, the parent(s) must be assisted to mobilize energy and reach out to other support resources, both familial and social. In most hospitals this is accomplished by referral to a social service worker who has more mobility and access to such support systems as well as more time to be with the parents. This final aid in the resolution process can be considered as the mobilization of institutional, community, and personal resources.

Denial and Pathological Coping Responses

The way an individual responds and behaves during crisis is an attempt to cope or to assimilate this terrifying experience as part of life and to maintain a positive feeling about himself. This is both instinctual and learned. Extremes in behavior, such as withdrawal or verbosity, are chacteristics of denial. One example is the quiet mother who appears resistant to visiting her baby and seems not to be integrating significant information. Another may be the parent who avoids talking to her baby's nurse and seems preoccupied with looking at other babies in the nursery. The other extreme is the parent who repeatedly asks the same questions or is continually talking with the baby's nurse or other nurses about unrelated events or superficial topics of discussion. Another variant is the parent who asks incessant questions about technical minutiae. These very dissimilar behaviors are all attempts to fend off fear and internal anxiety. Each type of response is an attempt to maintain equilibrium. By recognizing specific patterns the nurse can individualize her support and approaches to intervention.

Not everyone will respond to a crisis with denial. Some parents who are anxious have physical signs such as crying, hand wringing, or an obviously distressed appearance (i.e., distorted facial movements or ticks, possibly a disheveled appearance). Such persons may be responding in a more appropriate, healthy, and effective way through experiences learned in an earlier crisis. They may be able to silently verbalize, think through, and then deal with feelings, good or bad, and yet not feel totally devastated.

An outwardly emotive response is neither right nor wrong. Its value is based on whether it is a healthy or a pathological coping mechanism. The goal is to help the parents feel supported no matter how they respond. This allows them to transfer positive feelings from their experience with accepting adults to their interactions with their baby. They may have absent or abnormal translation of feelings if their coping mechanisms are unhealthy. This may be evidenced by an inability to establish attachment with the baby, suggested by infrequent or erratic visiting patterns, persistently angry and/or ambivalent responses, or a lack or preoccupation with their baby when they visit. Such behavior strongly suggests the need for further evaluation and appropriate intervention.

When responding to parents' state of crisis it is important to remember that the parent who is responding in a way you consider "inappropriate" may not have developed coping strategies from earlier crisis. Do not expect them to act as you would wish, or in a manner that represents your own personal coping strategy. Talking with them about how they feel about their baby, further explanations, or just silence are all mechanisms to encourage an expression of their feelings. All are supportive. An individual may be more comfortable with silence if he has limited ego strengths and little self-trust, or has had no positive past experience upon which to base a belief that he will be able to regain control or feel better. Furthermore, he may lack sufficient internal resources, or ego strength, to believe that he will ever function "normally" again.

The significant message for the NICU nursing and medical staff is that many times parents need to be "parented." They may need to know that someone will provide comfort and understanding even if their worst fears come true. They need to know that the control they fear losing, or may have lost, is a manifestation of a need to feel emotionally stable. Crisis intervention assists validation of their response.

The delivery of any premature, sick, or malformed baby, by itself, may be a crisis simply because it is unanticipated and undesirable. In applying what has already been discussed about principles of intervention, it is important first to assess whether coping seems within the parents' ability and whether or not usual means will lead to a healthy resolution. This will help you determine the best approach to take with them as well as plan for continued intervention. Keep in mind, however, that reassessment will need to be done as time goes on and the situation changes.

Death in the NICU

Death is a permanent separation, the effects of which are individual to each parent. Shock, depression, grief, anger, guilt, and feelings of acute loss or emptiness are all part of a grieving reaction. As Klaus and Kennell (6) stated, "Whether the baby lives one hour or two weeks, whether the baby is nonviable or weighs 4000 grams and whether or not the mother has had physical contact with the baby; clearly identified mourning will be present." By recognizing grieving reactions, the NICU staff can offer understanding and compassion where it is needed and will be able to recognize the parents whose grief is such that more extensive, skilled help and guidance is needed.

Bowlby (7), discussing factors that contribute to a heathly outcome of the mourning process, suggested that models of available, responsive, and helpful individuals with whom the parents have been associated during childhood positively influence their ability to form loving and trusting later relationships. Bowlby also noted that the individual may grieve deeply and, on occasion, be intensely angry. Provided that the causes and circumstances of the death were not especially adverse, however, the person is likely to be spared experiences that cause mourning to become unbearable, unproductive, or both.

Bowlby (7) described four phases of mourning that are not peculiar to any one type of affectional bond (e.g., spouse to spouse, child to parents):

1. *Numbing,* which usually lasts from hours to a week and may be interrupted by outbursts of extremely intense distress and/or anger.

2. *Yearning*, searching for the lost figure, which lasts months and sometimes years.
3. *Disorganization* in personal activities and despair in the emotional content of relationships and self-esteem.
4. Greater or lesser degree of *reorganization* and *resolution* of grief response.

He noted that these stages are not clear-cut, but represent parts of an overall sequence that has been observed in individuals responding to the loss of a close relative. Any individual response may oscillate for a time between any two of the phases. Kubler-Ross (8) also developed a model that divides grief into the following stages of response: anger, bargaining, depression, and final acceptance. This model was developed from studies of people coping with their own impending death.

It must be remembered that it is *normal* to grieve. It is also important that this loss eventually be accepted by parents and integrated as a realistic part of their family's experience with a life crisis. As noted before, many elements of the grief reaction are found in the crisis response involved in the birth of a sick, premature, or malformed baby. Encouraging frequent nursery visits for contact with the critically sick or dying baby helps initiate the process of acceptance and a lasting identification of the infant. Forming a concrete identity of, and relationship with, the deceased infant is the first step of resolving the loss of the infant.

If death follows soon after birth the baby should be shown to the parents, and they should be encouraged to hold their infant. Preferably they should have the opportunity to do this in privacy. A room adjacent to or nearby the nursery is optimal. Using a screen in the nursery may be acceptable. It is additionally important to remark to parents that you realize they may want to fondle, touch, and simply examine their baby together as parents. Details such as sex, gestational age, weight, the likely cause of death, or other specific information should be provided at an appropriate time following their private moments with the baby and with each other. If the parents cannot be present when the baby dies, they should be informed immediately and have the above information presented later.

As Nance (9) pointed out, when discussing parental grief reactions, "Despite separate reactions by two partners, mothers and fathers are usually grateful to learn about an infant's death together. The silent support of knowing that someone else is enduring the same crisis seems to lessen despair." Bowlby (7) placed value on helping parents grieve together. This grief begins with the birth of a sick infant and is enhanced by concerted efforts to have both parents together during significant discussions regarding the baby's status. The content of such discussion should be shared with other appropriate caretakers, physicians, social workers, chaplains, etc.

An opportunity to talk with the staff members who have cared for their baby as well as a physician's verbal report should be available to the grieving parents. This can be done before they are to spend private time with the baby so that they may be able to more clearly focus on the baby rather than on the primary questions they may have regarding the initiating cause of death.

Special Considerations When the Infant is Malformed

The birth of a malformed child often stimulates a deep sense of loss and pain similar to that with neonatal death. With death there is a finality and a promise that there will be an end to such intense feelings of grief; that these feelings will assuredly become lessened and there will no longer be a daily confrontation with the source of the pain. A malformed but viable infant presents a lifelong reminder of the loss of the expected healthy infant. This is, in a sense, protracted grief. Thus it is appropriate to discuss techniques that help parents cope with such a tragedy.

Despite the initial emotional responses of parents, it is wise to assume that parental attachment to the baby has begun in pregnancy. Preparatory developments for attachment include the mother developing what Solnit and Stark (10) described as a composite of herself and her individual love objects (i.e., mother, father, husband, and sibling) into a perceived image of the expected baby. Using this idea as part of the theoretical approach to work with mourning parents, it is important to understand that love objects take an idealized image. Solnit and Stark further stated that one of motherhood's normal developmental tasks for establishing a healthy mother-child relationship is working out discrepancies between the wished-for love object and the actual child. When a baby is born malformed this discrepancy is exaggerated to an extent where compromise between the two may, at least temporarily, become impossible.

It is not uncommon to view denial or guilt as the parents' primary response as they attempt to cope with this situation. This may be evidenced by an apparent calmness and/or lack of inquisitiveness about the baby's physical status or malformation and its feared effects on growth and neurological development. The need to deny reflects the parents' acute inability to bridge the gap between their wished-for, or "ideal," baby and the reality of delivering a malformed baby. It is *not* an unhealthy sign. Often it denotes a healthy defense technique for ego preservation.

Initially, denial may be an effective coping mechanism that helps prevent severe depression. In fact, denial of the malformation may be a positive force enhancing attachment. However, denial that blocks the developmental task of recognizing a baby's special needs for follow-up care becomes maladaptive and ineffective for longer term healthy coping. Indications that parents have begun grieving and eventually will be able to focus on their baby's special needs ideally should occur prior to discharge. This is not always the case. Many individuals either need the privacy of familiar surroundings or the reality of providing day-to-day special care before they are able to assimilate the malformed baby into their psyches and lives. In either situation contact with a comprehensive service follow-up agency should be initiated prior to discharge.

Helping parents accept their malformed baby can be accomplished by clarifying the baby's condition and special needs. Perhaps the baby's suck is poor or delayed. This provides an opportunity for the nurse to appropriately note this to the parents as a symptom of the malformation and elaborate that this is one of the problems requiring special attention. Parents need reassurance that they can learn required skills to meet such needs.

When attempting to measure the parents' progressive readiness to accept the baby before discharge, keep in mind that, as you clarify the baby's special care needs, you must do so without questioning the parents' awareness of these needs. This approach may enhance their acceptance by giving them a sense of dignity and control over their baby's situation. In an innocuous way your own acceptance of the baby's malformation may also deemphasize whatever self-esteem injury the parents feel. As Solnit and Stark (10) said, "When a person is mourning, their ability to recognize, evaluate and adapt to reality is often significantly impaired." Using a presumptive basis for intervention with parents also relieves them of the burden of having to be the first to acknowledge and accept the malformation.

A hypothetical sequence of parental reactions to a malformed infant's birth and the process of parental attachment has been described by Drotar, et al. (11), and is outlined below. Note how similar this scheme is to the previously described grief reaction for neonatal death.

1. ***First stage: shock*** Characterized by crying, feelings of disappointment, helplessness and an urge to flee.

2. ***Second stage: denial***   The intensity of the emotional response often varies with the visibility of the malformation.
3. ***Third stage: sadness, anger, and/or anxiety***   Often characterized by hesitancy in attachment.
4. ***Fourth stage: adaption***   A gradual lessening of the anxiety and intense emotional reaction. Increased comfort with interactions and confidence in their ability to start caring for their baby.
5. ***Fifth stage: reorganization***   Parents begin assuming their responsibility to care for the baby's problems. The mourning process, and related complex issues of interpersonal relationships begin to be discussed. Ideally, this should occur around the time of discharge.

This can be a clinically useful framework for nursing intervention. In its practical application, this framework is designed to emphasize the adaptive aspects of parental attachment as well as parental responses. Note, too, that the parents' emphasis on a baby's strengths and normal attributes are healthy adaptations rather than denial.

This stage scheme can be used to guide your understanding about the normal process involved in parents' accepting a malformed baby. Similar to the previously noted stages of the grief process defined by Kubler-Ross (8), it is neither a rigid nor a fixed process that every parent experiences. Nor does each parent travel the same successive channels of response. The process is best viewed as a mixture of responses, all needing to be addressed with an equal level of importance and sensitivity. All have the possibility of being present independently of the others.

Applications to the Clinical Setting

Many times staff ask what they should do immediately after a malformed infant is born. There are no absolute rules to guide care, but follow-up discussions with parents years after the birth of a malformed child are revealing. Parents describe feeling very sensitive to nonverbal messages that caretakers give. Minimizing the extent of the infant's defect was often interpreted as an unkindness, just as was overdramatization of the defect. Parents reported being most helped by those capable of both factually describing the defect and pointing out what was normal. This has clear implications for how parents should be informed of the defect.

Parents also reported feeling intense pain during the time between being informed about the defect and the time they saw the infant. Delay hurts! Whenever possible, parents should see their infant, defect and all, in the delivery room. One mother with an infant who had gastroschisis thought the baby's abdomen had been covered because it was so horrible that she would not love the baby if she saw it. When she saw the defect she did not find it terrifying. She then expressed anger at the staff, who probably were just trying to protect her.

In general, show the baby to both parents as soon as possible. Examine the infant's normal and abnormal findings together. Even grossly defective infants, such as anencephalics, have normal characteristics and some "competencies" like urinating, breathing, or startling. These should be pointed out to the parents. If the mother or baby is seriously sick, a Polaroid snapshot of the baby substitutes for hands-on examination.

Once initial contact has been made, parents have the complex task of resolving their grief at the same time they attempt attachment to the child. These are conflicting emotional tasks; the former requires letting go, the latter requires increasing one's emotional intimacy. Keeping this ongoing conflict in mind will help staff understand some contradictory behaviors parents exhibit. Not until parents have resolved grief and moved into the fifth stage of reorganization can their attachment be completed. This may take days or months depending on the parent's *perception* of the defect. It does not necessarily depend on the objective, clinical severity of the problem. Even if delayed, a satisfactory parent-infant relationship can be achieved.

Initially parents may blame themselves or others for the defective child. It is very normal for parents to connect their malformed child with some negative personal or family characteristic, as long as the parents also identify the infant with positive characteristics. One sign that parental attachment and acceptance is occurring is a growing perception by the parents that the child is a positive part of their identity and a member of their family. Awareness of this unfolding perception can help those working with the family determine if the parent-child reciprocity is developing and if it will lead to a positive nuturing relationship. One way to enhance a positive relationship is to reflect with the parents about the attractive and socially acceptable traits the infant possesses. Facilitating the parents' learning to care for their child also helps the infant become a source of pride and comfort rather than pain. Families who exclusively connect their infant with negative personal or familial characteristics may need special psychological evaluation and help.

References

1. Astbury J, Yu VY: Determinants of stress for staff in a neonatal intensive care unit. Arch Dis Child 57:108–111, 1982.
2. Price E: The demise of the traditional 5–40 workweek. Am J Nurs 81:1138–1141, 1981.
3. Lund C, Lefrank L: Discharge planning for infants in the intensive care nursery. Pediatr Nurse 2:49–58, 1982.
4. Rappoport L: The State of Crisis: Some Theoretical Considerations Crisis Intervention: Selected Readings. Family Service Association of America, New York, 1980.
5. Eaton MT, Peterson NM, Davis JA: Psychiatry. Medical Examination, Garden City, NY, 1976.
6. Klaus MH, Kennell JH: Parent-Infant Bonding. Mosby, St. Louis, 1982.
7. Bowlby J: Attachment and Loss, Vol III, Loss: Sadness and Depression. Basic Books, New York, 1980.
8. Kubler-Ross E: On Death and Dying. Macmillan, New York, 1969.
9. Nance S: Premature Babies: A Handbook For Parents. Arbor House, New York, 1982.
10. Solnit J, Stark MS: Mourning and the birth of a defective child. Psychoanal Study Child 16:523, 1961.
11. Drotar D, Backiewics A, Irvin N, et al.: The adaption of parents to the birth of an infant with a congenital malformation: A hypothetical model. Pediatrics 56:712–715, 1975.

Suggested Reading

Brown BJ (ed): Perspectives in Primary Nursing. Aspen, Rockville, MD
Horan ML: Parental reaction to the birth of an infant with a defect. An attributional approach. Adv Nurs Sci 5:3, 57–68, 1982.
Valentin LDE: The problems of grief and separation in the special care nursery. Nurs Times 77:1942–1944, 1981.
Wooden B: Death of an infant. Am J Maternal Child Nurs 6:257–260, 1981.

Appendices

Appendix 1.1
Task Classification in NICU[1]

Procedure	Time (min)	Procedure	Time (min)
Minimal care (each 8-hour shift); includes:	36	Medication:	
Skin care		PO	5
Diaper change		IM	5
Linen change, clean isolette, weigh, tubing and suction change		IV	
		Slow push	20
		Fast push	6
Parent phone calls and visits			
		Respiratory care:	
		O_2 check (per shift)	12
TPR	3	Care of nasal prongs (per shift)	15
BP cuff	6	Suction OP/NP	3
BP central (set up)	10	Vibration drainage	20
Monitor (per shift)	5	Mist treatment	12
Abdominal girth/head circumference	1½	ET tube check (per shift)	20
Surface cultures	2	Ventilator check	2
Positioning	3	Intubation	15
		Humidifier check	9
Urine:		ET culture	6
Weigh diaper I & O	2	ET cytology	9
Specific gravity	2	Calibration $TcpO_2$; monitor and site change	15
Clinitest	2		
Multitest	1		
		Chest tubes:	
Stool:		Insertion	20
Guaiac	3	Maintenance (milk, etc.)	20
pH	1½		
Reducing substance	1½	Lumbar puncture	15
		X-ray	12
Feeding:		Isolation technique	20
Oral	30	Assist with circumcision	20
Gavage	15	Exchange transfusion	120
Continous (per shift)	60	Terminal cleaning of isolette	30

[1] Abbreviations used: BP, blood pressure; CPR, cardiopulmonary resuscitation; ET, endotracheal; IM, intramuscular; I & O, intake and output; IV, intravenous; OP/NP, oral pharyngeal/nasal pharyngeal; PO, per os (by mouth); $TcpO_2$, transcutaneous partial pressure of oxygen; TPR, temperature-pulse-respiration.

Procedure	Time (min)	Procedure	Time (min)
Eye care	1½	Teaching, demonstration of:	
Mouth care	1½	Bath	30
Umbilical care	2	Diapering, skin care	9
		Assist with breastfeeding	20
Lab work:		Breast pump use	15
Dextrostix	2	Administering medica-	
Blood gases:		tions	20
Capillary	6	CPR	45

Score Interpretation:[2]

Nurse/patient ratio	Total time (min)
1 : 1	560–420
1 : 1.5	420–345
1 : 2	345–200
1 : 3	200–150
1 : 4	150–90
1 : 5	90–36

Procedure	Time (min)
Umbilical	3
Radial	12
IV:	
Mixing IV	12
IV check (per shift)	15
Start IV	15
Tubing change	6
Umbilical catheter	20
Intralipid	9
Blood transfusion	20

Total score: 8 hours _____

[2] Score system adjusted to Columbia Hospital for Women NICU equipment and layout.

Appendix 1.2
Resources for Parents

Books for Parents

Badger E: Infant/Toddler: Introducing Your Child to the Joy of Learning. Instructo/McGraw-Hill, New York, 1981.

Brazelton TB: Infants and Mothers. Delta, New York, 1969.

Caplan F: The First Twelve Months of Life. Bantam Books, New York, 1978.

Chess S, Thomas A, Birch HG: Your Child is a Person. Penguin Books, New York, 1980.

Harrison H: The Premature Baby Book. St. Martin's Press, New York, 1983.

Johnson and Johnson Baby Products Company: The First Wondrous Year: You and Your Baby. Macmillan Publishers, New York, 1978.

Nance S: Premature Babies. Harbor House, New York, 1982.

Stern D: The First Relationship. Harvard University Press, Cambridge, MA, 1980.

Information for Parents

Learning Together: A Guide for Families with Genetic Disorders, by Debra Haffner, National Clearinghouse for Human Genetic Diseases, P.O. Box 28612, Washington, DC 20005; 1980, 24 pp, free.

Genetic Counseling, March of Dimes Birth Defects Foundation, available from the national office or from local chapters.

Autosomal Chromosome Abnormality: A Cause of Birth Defects, by Diane Plumridge, Genetics Clinic, Crippled Children's Division, University of Oregon Health Sciences Center, P.O. Box 574, Portland, OR 97207; 1980, 126 pp, $5.00.

A Reader's Guide for Parents of Children with Mental, Physical or Emotional Disabilities, by Coralie B. More and Kathryn G. Morton, National Clearinghouse for Human Genetic Diseases, P.O. Box 28612, Washington, DC 20005; 1979, 144 pp, free.

Amniocentesis for Prenatal Chromosomal Diagnosis, National Clearinghouse for Human Genetic Diseases, P.O. Box 28612, Washington, DC 20005; 1980, 40 pp, free.

When Pregnancy Fails: Families Coping with Miscarriage, Stillbirth, and Infant Death, by S. Borg and J. Lasker, Beacon Press, 25 Beacon Street, Boston, MA 02108; 1981, 252 pp, $6.95.

When Hello Means Goodbye: A Guide for Parents Whose Child Dies at Birth or Shortly Thereafter, by P. Schweibert and P. Kirk, University of Oregon Health Sciences Center, Department of Obstetrics and Gynecology, 3181 S.W. Sam Jackson Park Road, Portland, OR 97201; 1981, 32 pp.

Support Organization for Trisomy 18/13 Newsletter, edited by Kris Holladay, 478 Terrace Lane, Tooele, UT 84074; free.

Parent Resource Groups

Support Organization for Trisomy 18/13 (Soft 18/13)
c/o Kris and Hal Holladay
478 Terrace Lane
Tooele, UT 84074
(801) 882–6635

The Compassionate Friends
P.O. Box 1347
Oak Brook, IL 60521

The Association for Retarded Citizens (ARC)
2709 Avenue E East
Arlington, TX 76011

March of Dimes Birth Defects Foundation
1275 Mamroneck Avenue
White Plains, NY 10605
(914) 428–7100

Closer Look
P.O. Box 1492
Washington, DC 20013

National Clearinghouse for Human Genetic Diseases (NCHGD)
P.O. Box 28612
Washington, DC 20005
(202) 842–7610

Mothers of Twins
5402 Amberwood Lane
Rockville, MD
(301) 460–9108

The Parent Network
c/o Pat Korber
553 North Pennsylvania Street
Indianapolis, IN 46220

Parents Helping Parents
47 Marco Drive
San Jose, CA 95127
(408) 272–4774

Parents-helping-parents groups can be identified by contacting either of the two last-mentioned organizations. They will give you information about the support groups available in your region.

2

Assessment and Stabilization of the Newborn

Johannah L. Williams

This chapter provides a guideline toward a logical progression of nursing care for the immediate delivery and postdelivery period. The focus is on the assessment and stabilization of the newborn. In assessing the adaptability of the neonate, it should be determined prior to delivery whether a normal term infant is expected (one who will undergo the stress of birth optimally) or whether the infant has a reduced capacity to adapt, i.e. is at risk. This determination permits appropriate preparation to assist the infant through this life-determining transition.

The normal term infant falls within 38 and 42 weeks gestation, weighs 2700–4000 grams, and has head and chest measurements of 33–35.5 cm and 30.5–33 cm, respectively, with the relationship of head to chest equal or the head no more than 4 cm larger than the chest (1). The baby should exhibit no gross anomalies and be able to successfully make the transition from a passive intrauterine to an active extrauterine life.

The risk assessment is directed mainly at recognizing alterations in the placenta and/or fetus that have potential to endanger the newborn. Important prenatal risk factors are shown in Table 2.1. Table 2.2 lists some important labor and delivery processes that increase the infant's risk. If it is determined that the infant is high risk, preparation for emergency resuscitative maneuvers during the labor and delivery process is indicated. The importance of all personnel who care for newborns being skilled in infant cardiopulmonary resuscitation methods and theory cannot be overemphasized. We recommend that NICU nurses, and delivery room nurses in particular, annually review these techniques so that prompt care can be initiated for asphyxiated newborns. For detailed information on care of the infant at risk, see Dazé and Scanlon (2).

The First Twenty-four Hours

The first 24 hours are critical for the newborn since extensive respiratory and circulatory changes take place during this period. Failure in transition can occur rapidly and

Table 2.1 Prenatal High Risk Factors

1. Maternal history
2. Parental age: mother under 16, or primipara over 35 years of age; father over 40 years of age
3. Hereditary diseases or abnormalities: inborn diseases of metabolism, inherited anomaly patterns, sickle cell anemia, and others
4. History of obstetrical complications
5. Uterine abnormalities
6. Maternal size: prepregnant weight 20% over (obesity) or under standard normal for height
7. Grand multiparity
8. Maternal disease: toxemia, hypertension, malignancy, endocrine disease (diabetes, thyroid disorder), heart disease, renal disease, hemoglobinopathy
9. Maternal infection
10. Maternal disorders associated with pregnancy: hyperemesis gravidarum, toxemia, placental abnormalities (placenta previa, abruptio placenta), diabetes
11. Socioeconomic problems: malnutrition, inadequate prenatal care, severe poverty
12. Abnormal fetal size: small or large for gestational age (as determined by serial fetal sonograms, etc.)
13. Polyhdramnios or oligohydramnios
14. Uterine accidents
15. Isoimmunization: ABO or Rh blood incompatabilities
16. Maternal addiction: narcotics, alcohol, barbiturates, amphetamines, hallucinogens
17. Maternal exposure to teratogenic agents/medications
18. Maternal surgical procedures
19. Multiple gestation

with little warning. There is a higher incidence of neonatal death during the initial 24 hours than during the following 28-day period.

The First 2 Hours

The most profound physiological change the infant must make in its extrauterine adaptation is the successful onset of respiration with transition from fetal to neonatal circulation (see Chapter 5). External stimuli as well as chemical factors trigger the respiratory center, causing the first breath. With exposure to the external environment, the onset of respirations occurs.

Measures for assessment and stabilization of any newborn at birth should include the following:

1. Apgar scoring at 1 and 5 minutes (normal score, 7–10) (see Table 2.3).
2. Silverman scoring for respiratory effort and quality (3) (see Table 2.4).
3. Assessment of respiratory rate and the newborn's ability to keep his airway clear.
4. Thorough drying of the infant, placing him in a warm environment.
5. Examination of the infant for gross congenital abnormalities; examination also for any evidence of trauma such as bruises, abrasions, asymmetrical limb movement, cephalohematoma.

Table 2.2 Intrapartum Risk Factors

1. Multiple gestation
2. Maternal fever
3. Premature onset of labor
4. Premature or prolonged rupture of membranes
5. Abnormal labor and/or delivery
6. Vaginal bleeding
7. Excessive maternal analgesia and/or anesthesia

Table 2.3 Apgar Newborn Scoring System

	Score		
	0	1	2
Heart rate	Absent	<100	>100
Respiration	Absent	Irregular or gasping	Regular sustained
Tone	Limp, flaccid	Some flexion of extremities	Good flexion and tone
Reflex (response to suction)	No response	Weak grimace	Cough, sneeze, or cry
Color	Blue or pale	Lips pink but blue extremities	Pink all over

Adapted from Apgar V: The newborn (Apgar) scoring system. Pediatr Clin North Am 13:645, 1966.

6. Prophylactic administration of silver nitrate (or erythromycin) to each eye; may be delayed up to 1 hour (see Appendix 2.1). (Erythromycin 0.5% ointment is an acceptable substitute for silver nitrate for eye prophylaxis; see Appendix 2.2.)
7. Determination of temperature, heart, and respiratory rates: should be taken and recorded every 15–20 minutes while the infant is in the delivery or recovery area with his mother. Ensure that the airway is cleared using gravity drainage by lowering the head 10–15°. Use a bulb syringe to clear first the mouth and then the nares of mucus. The infant may be placed head down to facilitate gravitational drainage and should be closely observed while in this position. Catheter suction is the most efficient way to clear the airway and should be used for the infant having difficulty clearing his secretions. Monitor the heart rate whenever suctioning and stop if bradycardia occurs. Dry the infant immediately and maintain a neutral thermal environment by wrapping him in a prewarmed blanket or placing him under a radiant heater (see section on "Thermoregulation," below). A healthy term infant can be kept warm by placing him next to his mother and covering his head with a stocking cap to reduce heat loss. Infants lying on heated tables should be left naked, but the sides of the bed should be up to reduce heat loss by convection.

The need for additional resuscitation can be measured by the Apgar score. An Apgar score of 7 with spontaneous undistressed respirations after 5 minutes indicates successfully proceeding transition. If the infant is stable at this time, mother-

Table 2.4 Assessing Respiratory Effort in the Newborn

	Silverman score[a]		
	0	1	2
Nasal flaring	Absent	Slight	Wide flaring with each breath
Xyphoid retractions	Absent	Retractions limited to xyphoid process	Retractions involving whole lower costal border
Intercostal retractions	Absent	Slight	Involving entire length of rib
Grunt[b]	Absent	Heard only with a stethoscope	Audible with ear
Abdominal/thoracic synchronization	Synchronized movement of chest and abdomen	Lag between abdomen and chest movements	"Seesaw" movement of chest and abdomen

[a] Adapted from Silverman and Anderson (3).

[b] The presence of a grunt can never be considered normal.

Table 2.5 Criteria for Admission of Infant to Intensive Care Nursery

The following situations make admission to the ICN mandatory:

1. Ventilatory support requirements of any kind, including supplemental oxygen
2. IV and/or arterial infusion
3. Prematurity; weight less than 1.8 kg
4. Requirement of vital signs or other nursing observations more frequently than every 4 hours
5. Requirement of electronic heart rate or respiratory monitoring
6. Requirement of the availability of a neonatologist for anticipated problems (as judged by the responsible pediatrician or nurse)
7. Rupture of membranes more than 24 hours before birth
8. History of maternal diabetes
9. One-minute or 5-minute Apgar score of 6 or lower

infant interaction can begin. Place the infant in the mother's arms. Allow them privacy for eye-to-eye contact before prophylactic eye treatment. Begin breastfeeding, if desired, and if the infant's condition permits.

The infant must be identified before leaving the delivery room. Matching bands with identical numbers for mother and infant, attached to the infant's wrist and ankle as well as the mother's wrist, is a standard method. Footprinting is still recognized as a method for identification.

Once stabilization is complete, identification is ascertained, and the parents have had an opportunity to see, touch, and begin interacting with their infant, the infant may be put in a warmed transporter and transferred to the nursery. Upon arrival in the nursery, it is essential that a clear picture of what occurred during the intrapartum and immediate postpartum period be communicated to the nursery staff so that appropriate on-going care can be provided.

At the end of the first 2 hours of life, most newborns will have stabilized. The infant with difficulty during the transition period should either be sent to an intensive or intermediate care unit or transferred to an appropriate facility. Table 2.5 lists criteria for admission to the intensive care area at Columbia Hospital for Women.

The Next 22 Hours

The newborn infant is transported to the nursery in a sterilized, warmed portable incubator by designated delivery room personnel. Immediately upon his arrival, the infant is identified by comparing delivery records with identification bands on his wrist and ankle. On receipt to the normal nursery, it is essential for the receiving nurse to assess the infant's respiratory status by counting breathing rate and observing for grunting, retractions, flaring of nares, and skin color. This is a second check that the infant has made a satisfactory transition to neonatal status. If there is any doubt, the infant should be rerouted; otherwise, the infant is admitted. (See Appendix 2.3 for admission procedures for cesarean or large babies.) The admitting nursery nurse, having previously washed her hands, receives the infant and immediately weighs him if this has not been done in the delivery room. Nursing care and continued assessment, and stabilization of the newborn in the normal nursery, should follow.

Upon Admission

1. Weigh the infant, wrapped in a previously weighed warmed blanket, on a clean, balanced scale. Subtract the weight of the blanket from the total weight and record the resulting weight on the infant's record.

2. Immediately place the infant in a prewarmed isolette (warmed blankets and clean, warm isolettes should be ready at all times for admission of infants to the nursery so there will be no delay in providing a neutral thermal environment).
3. Administer vitamin K IM (1 mg for term infants) to prevent hemorrhagic disease of the newborn.
4. Obtain routine lab tests if required, such as Dextrostix (see Appendix 2.4) or hematocrit.
5. Notify pediatrician of the infant's admission, time of birth, sex, birth weight, and general condition. The initial physical examination should be performed within 24 hours.

Newborn Assessment

The neonate can best be assessed by determining his adaptive capabilities and by being alert to any potential difficulties. The physical examination is very helpful in such endeavors. The reader is referred to Scanlon et al.'s text about the neonatal physical exam, which discusses common variations and signs of potential problems (4).

After determination of gestational age by physical exam and/or by reviewing the records for the estimated date of confinement, the infant is classified by gestational age and weight. If the gestational age is less than 37 weeks, the infant is preterm; if 37–42 weeks, the infant is term; and if greater than 42 weeks, the infant is postdates or postmature. After the gestational age is determined, the infant's weight can be plotted against an intrauterine growth curve to determine if the infant is small, appropriate, or large for dates. There are standard charts and tables available for plotting length, weight, and head circumference (1).

Categorization below the 10th or above the 90th percentiles in length or weight should alert nursing staff to observe the infant for potential morbidity and to provide necessary care. For an excellent review of assessment of weight and gestational age and their implications for care of the newborn, see Lubchenco (1).

Cardiorespiratory Assessment   Check the infant's respiratory effort every 15 minutes for the first hour. (Vital signs taken in the labor-delivery area may already have covered this period.) Also, evaluate respiratory effort by use of Silverman scoring (see Table 2.4). If stable, check respiratory rate and effort hourly four times. If stable, then check only every 8 hours. The infant is normally a nose breather, that is, he sleeps with a closed mouth and is able to eat without interruption for breathing. Observe for any abnormal sounds during inspiration and expiration. Note the infant's ability to sneeze and swallow to maintain a clear airway. Observe for color changes during feeding. Continue to observe the infant closely for the first 24 hours, since problems can occur during this time. Resuscitation equipment must be available in any nursery area (2).

Assess the infant's color. A pink color over the head, trunk, and mucous membranes indicates adequate oxygenation. Feet and hands may remain slightly cyanotic for 24 hours, especially when cold. It is never normal for the lips or face to be cyanotic. Assess vital signs, especially the heart rate (rhythm, regularity, and any changes with activity), and the presence or absence of murmurs. Blood pressure should be taken each day; in general, the normal term baby's systolic blood pressure ranges between 40 and 70 mm Hg (see Table 2.6 and Appendices 2.5, 2.6, and 2.7).

Neurological Assessment   Examine the head by checking fontanelles for bulging or depression. Overriding sutures are normal, and if there is significant molding, the posterior fontanelle may not be palpable. Observe the level of alertness

Table 2.6 Normal Vital Signs

Temperature: 36.5°–37°C (97.7°–98.6°F)

Heart rate: 110–160 beats/minute

Respiratory rate: 30–60 breaths/minute

Blood pressure (first 12 hours of life)[a]:
  Infant >4000 g: systolic 55–80, diastolic 30–50; mean, 42–60 mm Hg
  Infant >3000 g: systolic 42–66, diastolic 25–48; mean, 36–58 mm Hg
  Infant >2000 g: systolic 42–66, diastolic 22–42; mean, 30–50 mm Hg
  Infant >1000 g: systolic 36–58, diastolic 17–38; mean, 24–45 mm Hg
  Infant >600 g: systolic 35–55, diastolic 14–35; mean, 10–28 mm Hg

[a] Adapted from Versnold HT, Killerman Phibbs RH, Gregory GA, Tooley WH: Aortic blood pressures during the first twelve hours of life in infants with birth weights 610–4220 grams. Pediatrics 67:607–612, 1981.

and whether the baby smoothly changes to different alert or sleep states. Discrete states of alertness are a sign of health. Check overall muscle tone and reflex reaction. There are a number of neurological and behavioral tests that can be used, in part or in total, to assess the integrity of the nervous system and its integrative functioning (4). During the first 24 hours, assessment of neurological status in conjunction with physical examination will provide a picture of the infant's prognosis for successful transition through the 28-day neonatal period. Once the baby is stable, parents will benefit from seeing their infant's neurobehavioral abilities. This demonstration can be important in helping parents to care for their infant since it will increase their knowledge and awareness of their own baby.

Assessment of Elimination   Usually the first meconium stool is passed at birth or within the first 24 hours. If a meconium stool has not been recorded during the first 24-hour period, ask the mother if she has changed the infant's diaper and if she noted any black tarry stool. If not, contact the pediatrician and continue to observe the infant. Specifically measure the abdomen at birth, listen for bowel sounds, palpate the abdomen for the presence of any mass, and check for anal patency.

Transitional stools vary with the method of feeding. In general, bottle-fed infants have more formed stools. Breast-fed infants have looser and possibly more frequent stools. Stool frequency among bottle-fed infants may range from several times daily to once every day or two. Stool frequency for breastfed infants may vary from once or twice daily to every feeding time or more. The important thing is to observe for stooling patterns and the presence of mucus, fat, reducing substances, and/or blood, which are abnormal.

Voiding may be noted at delivery. Urination should occur within the first 24 hours. If not, check with the mother and other staff in case a voiding has not been charted. Notify the pediatrician if urination does not occur within 24 hours of age.

Protection from Infection and Trauma

Handwashing before and after handling each infant cannot be overstressed. This is the most effective means for preventing contamination of infants. Hospital staff, parents, and visitors must be scrupulous in washing their hands before touching any infant. Another infection control technique is the administration of prophylactic eye medication into the conjunctival sac to prevent ophthalmia neonatorum. Teach the mother to observe for discharge from the infant's eyes, and explain the reason for chemical conjuctivitis caused by silver nitrate (this conjunctivitis should resolve by

48 hours of age). Check the eyes for persistent purulent discharge. This indicates the presence of infection despite prophylactic treatment.

The umbilical cord is a primary entry site for infection. On admission, first observe the umbilical stump, making certain the clamp is intact and that no oozing of blood is noted. Then swab the stump with Triple Dye to prevent infection. Keep the umbilical stump clean and dry, using alcohol as needed, and fasten diapers below the stump to facilitate drying and prevent irritation. Observe the cord for proper drying, checking for oozing, odor, and/or redness of the surrounding skin, which may indicate infection. Teach mothers how to care for the cord.

The initial bath should be administered after vital signs have stabilized and the infant's axillary temperature is 36.5°C (97.7°F) for 2 consecutive hours. Initially, the term infant should be bathed with pHisoHex in the warm admission isolette or under a radiant heater to prevent excessive heat loss. The bath should be administered with skill and rapidity (see Appendix 2.8). After being bathed, the infant should remain in an incubator or on a radiant heated table until the axillary temperature normalizes. Guard against overheating the infant.

Facilitating Mother-Infant Interaction

The first 24 hours are a period of stabilization for both infant and mother. The infant may not be alert, may suffer from chemical conjunctivitis, and may cause concern to the mother by his apparent lack of interest. The mother is also undergoing physiological and psychological changes that put demands on her. The nurse can be helpful by coordinating moments of infant alertness with the mother's routine. Providing an optimum environment (i.e., quiet and private) for the mother, infant, and father will give them time to get to know each other. For an in-depth discussion of this subject, see Klaus and Kennell (5) and Brazelton (6).

The Next 27 Days

The period after the first 24 hours is one of continued stabilization and adaptation to an extrauterine environment. Depending on the type of delivery, the first 2 to 5 days may be spent in the hospital. This time can be used by the nursing staff for continued assessment and observed stabilization. This is also an excellent time to teach the parents about their new child. It allows them to acquire and polish skills under the supervision of knowledgeable personnel. The hospital can also be a very stressful environment with arbitrary routines and "mandatory" medical care. Attunement to the needs of the mother and infant can greatly enhance their transition from gravid woman with fetus to mother and baby.

Newborn Assessment

Cardiorespiratory Assessment and Intervention

The respiratory rate is usually 40–60 breaths per minute while awake. Breathing should be relatively regular, varying with states of alertness. Mothers should be taught to observe for changes in their infants' alert states. As the infant begins to attend to stimuli longer, respirations usually slow and become more quiet. Knowing this helps a mother to become attuned to her infant's ability to respond and socialize. There should be no grunting or nasal flaring. Feedings should take place without color change or major changes in breathing rate, and the infant should not have to take "rests" while feeding. Mothers should be taught to observe for these signs to help them to be aware of subtle clues of distress.

With the exception of prolonged crying, which may briefly cause a heart rate of greater than 160, there should be no extreme or abrupt increases or decreases in heart rate. By 24 hours the skin color should have become uniform, with minimal, if any, cyanosis of hands and feet. Circumoral cyanosis during feedings or while crying indicates a cardiovascular problem. Murmurs, which can be normal during the first 24 hours of life, are suspicious when they persist beyond this time.

Neurological Assessment

Neurological assessments should continue with appreciation for central nervous system (CNS) development. Neurological disorders may present during this period of adaptation and development (see Chapter 4). The mother should be taught to observe her baby's states of sleep/wake activity, and lengthening periods of alertness and attention spans. (See Chapter 4 for information on infants at risk for developmental delay.)

Assessment of Elimination

The infant should now be beginning to establish a stooling pattern of his own. The color and consistency should be recorded, as well as frequency. Parent teaching should include descriptions of the normal patterns of stooling for the type of feedings an infant is receiving. In addition to appreciating normal patterns of elimination, parents should be taught how to carefully clean the genital area and to check diapers for soiling at regular intervals. The infant's skin can be protected by keeping the diaper area dry and clean.

A normal voiding pattern should be documented before discharge. Many breastfeeding mothers ask, "How do I know my baby is getting enough?" Point out that an infant who is getting sufficient milk will soak his diaper about as many times as he is fed. Suggest to breastfeeding mothers that if their infant is not frequently wetting his diaper, the baby may be offered 10–15 cc of sterile water post-breastfeeding or midway between feedings. This will not fill the baby or reduce the demand for breast milk. This simple point can reduce anxiety about breastfeeding and, at the same time, help prevent dehydration.

Protection from Infection

The umbilical stump is a cause of concern for many parents. Teaching proper care and cleanliness to promote drying is important. Parents should also be taught to observe for signs of possible infection such as redness, discharge, odor, or tenderness. After at least 24 hours, and after checking for proper drying, the clamp should be removed by nursery personnel. It should be removed prior to hospital discharge except under very special circumstances, such as early discharge, and then parents should be given careful instruction for its removal and subsequent cord care.

Eye drainage from silver nitrate should have completely subsided by the third day after delivery. If continued discharge is noted, alert the pediatrician and obtain a culture. Parents should be taught proper eye care using sterile cotton balls and water. Stress prevention of cross-contamination by handwashing and using clean cotton balls for each eye.

A normal phenomenon is erythema toxicum, a discrete pustular rash. However, the nurse must observe for certain skin infections that are also pustular, such as those that are staphylococcal in origin. They may present in the inguinal area or near the umbilical cord stump. This type of infection is transmitted by hand; therefore, handwashing technique cannot be overemphasized. If such skin infections are suspected, the pediatrician should be notified immediately and all precautions taken as dictated by hospital policy. Parents should be taught to observe for rashes and to be careful to wash their hands, especially after handling pets, soil, or trash or using the bathroom. Parents with chronic viral infections, such as herpes or hepatitis, will need to be especially meticulous about handwashing.

Nutrition

It is normal for infants to lose weight during the first 5–7 days of life. The infant's weight should be checked on the second day and then at least every other day until discharge. Weight loss greater than 10% of the birth weight is considered excessive and requires notifying the pediatrician.

The term infant should be observed for jitteriness during the first day of life. This may suggest hypoglycemia, among other things. A Dextrostix or Chemstrip test for blood glucose is a simple procedure you can do to rule out hypoglycemia or suggest further laboratory evaluation. Any blood sugar result ≤25 mg/dl should be immediately reported to the pediatrician or nurse practitioner and a serum glucose promptly obtained.

The frequency of feedings should be recorded in addition to the amount taken. Quality of sucking should also be noted as well as any reflux or regurgitation. Feeding also provides an excellent opportunity for the nurse to assess how the mother is progressing with infant care, how she handles and approaches her infant.

It is important to stress to the formula-feeding mother not to overfeed. Recent findings about obesity in adults suggest a possible relationship between infant feeding practices and a predisposition to obesity. Infants should not be fed more often than every 2 hours since it takes about that long to empty the stomach. It must also be stressed that infants up to 9 months of age need infant formulas for adequate nutrition; unaltered cow's milk is not recommended.

By hospital discharge, the nursing mother may not yet be confident about breastfeeding her baby. In addition to providing assistance in methods to get the infant to take the breast, the nurse can refer the new mother to community resources such as the La Leche League and other support groups to help her in the early, sometimes difficult period. An excellent text by Lawrence (7) describes in detail how to teach breastfeeding.

Discharge of Infant (see Appendix 2.9)

Prior to discharge, assessment and stabilization of the newborn should be documented in the permanent medical record. The infant should have been examined by a pediatrician or pediatric nurse practitioner within 24 hours after admission and prior to discharge. Ideally, the parents will have chosen a pediatrician, general practitioner, or well baby clinic for their newborn before delivery. If not, referral to a conveniently located service is appropriate. Stress the need for all infants to be seen regularly throughout the first years of life. Phenylketonuria and thyroxine screening tests should be obtained at 72 hours of life, or prior to discharge after adequate milk intake has been established. Follow-up testing should be arranged.

Any complications from a circumcision should be documented. Healing progress should be noted, and parents should be taught proper care. Parents should be told to alert their pediatrician or general practitioner if the infant stops voiding, develops excessive swelling or frank bleeding, or becomes febrile, or if pus is seen around the circumcision wound. All teaching contacts with parents should be documented.

Identification papers should be on the chart. Just prior to discharge, infant and mother should be identified by ID bands with matching numbers, the procedure being done by one of the nursery personnel. Mother and infant should be accompanied to the car.

There has been much recent emphasis on the importance of using an infant automobile restraint. Although it is not a law in every state, findings suggest infant restraints may greatly reduce infant morbidity and mortality. We support such use.

Thermoregulation

A critical component of the basic care of a newborn is to provide for his thermal stability. Whenever caring for an infant one must consider maintaining an environment that is thermally neutral for the infant so he does not become heat or cold stressed. Thermal neutrality refers to an environment in which the individual performs minimal metabolic work while maintaining a normal core temperature. The larger his body mass and the more mature his nervous system, the better a baby will conserve heat when cold stressed and eliminate heat when overheated. An adult has a wide neutral thermal environment but a newborn infant has a very narrow range within which to maintain a normal core temperature without expending excessive energy.

Neonates are unique in their method of increasing body temperature when stressed. Unlike adults, who can shiver, infants utilize specialized fat deposits, called brown fat, that they rapidly metabolize to produce heat. This process is called chemical thermogenesis. Heat produced in brown fat is carried via the circulation to warm the rest of the body. Brown fat is vascularly rich and each cell has many mitochondria, giving it the capacity for rapid metabolism. Because brown fat stores are small, all newborns are restricted in their ability to produce heat by this method. Small-for-gestational-age (SGA) and preterm infants are especially limited in their capacity for chemical thermogenesis because brown fat is derived from maternal calorie supplies. An SGA infant has been deprived of maternal nutrition, and a preterm infant has missed at least part of the third trimester, during which fat storage is a major task.

There are problems associated with chemical thermogenesis that pose an immediate risk to an infant. First, oxygen utilization increases as brown fat is metabolized. Brown fat metabolism consumes 20 times more oxygen than does white fat (8). Thus, cold stress, the stimulus for brown fat metabolism, dramatically increases an infant's oxygen requirement. If oxygenation is diminished, brown fat metabolism ceases and cold injury occurs at a more rapid rate. The infant with compromised respiratory function or asphyxia will lose body heat more rapidly than a healthy infant under a comparable cold-stressing environment. Even well-oxygenated infants can have cold-induced respiratory problems as they increase their respiratory rate in an effort to increase oxygen intake.

Two other consequences of chemical thermogenesis in infants are the risks of hypoglycemia and metabolic acidosis. As the metabolism of brown fat increases, serum glucose levels fall and serum organic acid levels rise. The latter is a reflection of rising serum ketones, free fatty acids (FFAs), and lactic acid. Brown fat metabolism is the source of FFAs and ketones. Lactic acid is produced secondary to diminished tissue oxygenation. In fact, the presence of unexplained metabolic acidosis and/or hypoglycemia may be the earliest clinical evidence of significant cold stress. Both compounds are easily measured in the lab. Blood gases and Dextrostix should be obtained when an infant is found to have a significant fall in core temperature.

Considering such profound effects, it is no wonder that early in the history of modern neonatal care it was found that maintaining a normal core temperature was associated with improved survival (9). However, this basic knowledge is not enough. One must also be able to safely manage an infant's thermal environment, and, when necessary, treat the cold- or heat-stressed infant.

Managing the Thermal Environment

Table 2.7 illustrates how mechanisms for heat exchange operate in a clinical setting. Sources of heat loss—evaporation, conduction, convection, and radiation—must be reduced as much as possible. Simple examples of preventing heat loss are drying an infant immediately after delivery, keeping the baby on dry linen, insulating nursery windows, eliminating drafts, and closing cuffs on isolette portholes.

The next step in managing an infant's thermal environment is to help the infant conserve heat already produced by normal metabolism. Stockinette caps are commonly used in nurseries and delivery rooms. They insulate approximately 20% of the infant's body surface area from heat loss. Dressing the infant in a shirt and diaper is also effective in preventing heat loss. Thin plastic tents placed just over an infant have advantages in heat conservation by reducing convective losses. When an infant is kept on a radiant heated table, he should be undressed, since clothing insulates the infant from receiving heat as well as from losing it.

Once extrinsic heat loss is eliminated and methods of heat conservation have been employed, extra heat sources should be considered. Healthy term infants usually do not require any additional heat source once their temperatures are normal and they have been dried and dressed. Preterm or sick newborns, as well as newborns kept nude for observation, must be provided an external source of heat.

Table 2.7 Heat Exchange in Neonatal Care

Mechanism of heat exchange	Source of cold stress	Source of heat gain
Conduction	1. Unwarmed blankets 2. Cold scale 3. Cold mattress	1. K-pad 2. Warmed water mattress 3. Prewarmed blankets and mattress 4. Warm tub bath
Convection	1. Air conditioning unit 2. Open isolette portholes 3. Sides down on heated table 4. Unwarmed oxygen flow	1. Isolettes
Radiation	1. Single-thickness wall exterior	1. Radiant heated table
Evaporation	1. Radiant heated tables 2. Sponge baths 3. Lying on open wet diaper 4. Amniotic fluid	None

Isolettes and radiant heated tables are most commonly employed. Most often, one heat source will be enough, but sometimes a second is necessary. Whenever possible, heat sources should be added one at a time. For example, when an infant has a low temperature, increase the isolette temperature. If after an hour there is no rise in the infant's temperature, then add a K-pad. When more than one source is used, the number of variables involved makes it difficult to keep the environment stable. It becomes easier to either over- or underheat the infant. Be certain to check frequently for overheating.

Radiant Heated Tables

Radiant heated tables currently available are servo-controlled. In other words, a heat-sensing probe is placed on the infant's skin and the heater goes on when the infant's skin cools below a preset value. It turns off when the skin temperature exceeds this pre-set range. A skin probe is more sensitive than a rectal probe since core temperature remains normal even as heat is being lost through the skin. Servo-control prevents overheating an infant. No infant should be left on a heated table without a probe in place. After the probe has been put on the infant, care must be taken that it does not come loose or fall off. If the probe is no longer firmly attached, a falsely low temperature is sensed and the infant will get more heat than necessary. This can result in severe hyperthermia.

When an infant is receiving radiant heat, it is still possible for him to lose heat by the other three mechanisms of heat exchange. Convection and evaporation are the most significant means of heat loss for an infant on an open radiant heated table. Evaporation of water through the skin doubles when an infant is under a radiant heat source (10). As water evaporates from the skin, heat is lost. Unfortunately, little can be done to prevent heat loss by evaporation under these circumstances. Thin plastic wrap tents over the infant may reduce evaporation losses. Convection also occurs whenever an open radiant table is used. Adjustable sides and thin plastic wrap tents also reduce such losses, but it is nearly impossible to totally eliminate all drafts in a busy NICU.

Experiments by Silverman and Agate (11) indicated that servo-control of an infant's skin temperature at 36.5°C (97.7°F) results in minimal oxygen consumption. Darnal and Ariagno (12) showed that infants warmed using a servo-control between 36.1° and 36.8°C (97–98.2°F) had oxygen consumption values similar to those of infants warmed by isolette-control. A good general rule of thumb is that if all extraneous sources of heat loss have been eliminated then the skin temperature will be approximately 0.5°C *cooler* than the core.

When the skin is more than 0.5°C warmer than the core:

1. Evaluate whether the servo point is too high and the infant is gaining heat too rapidly through the skin. This produces excessive evaporation and heat stress.
2. Check the probe placement: if the infant is lying directly on the probe, it will be insulated from heat loss. If so, the skin temperature will reflect only the temperature under the probe and will not represent the infant's body temperature.

When the skin temperature is more than 0.5°C cooler than the core:

1. Make sure the probe is taped securely to the skin since it may be reading air temperature.
2. Observe for signs of circulatory collapse; the cooler skin may be due to poor skin perfusion.

We routinely admit infants requiring intubation to a heated table since they allow maximal access to the infant. Once an infant has stabilized, usually after the umbilical artery catheter can be removed, we move them to isolettes. The advantages of decreasing evaporative water losses become greater than the inconvenience of caring for an intubated infant in an isolette.

Isolettes

Isolettes use the principle of convection to warm infants. Warm filtered air is circulated over the infant. The environment in the isolette can either be kept at a constant temperature or a servo-probe can be attached to the infant's skin. When employing servo-control for isolettes, skin-core temperature ratios should be maintained similar to those obtained with radiant warmers. There are risks to watch for when using servo-probes. If the probe becomes loose, the heater will turn on unnecessarily. Or, if the probe site is insulated from the heat loss that the rest of the skin is experiencing, (for example, if the infant is lying on the probe) the probe will sense a warmer skin temperature than is the infant's true temperature and not enough heat will be delivered. Also, the problem of detecting an unstable temperature as a symptom of sepsis or some other systemic problem is masked by using servo-control mechanisms.

One of the advantages to a servo-control mechanism in isolettes is that, if the skin cools, there will be an immediate increase in environmental heat to offset the loss. Marks et al. (13) found that weight gain increased by almost 50% in babies of 28–31 weeks gestation who were both servo-controlled and dressed in an isolette. A combination of servo-controlling and dressing was found to be significantly effective for reducing cold-related metabolic work.

As mentioned above, as an alternative to the servo-control, the isolette temperature may be kept at a constant. Table 2.8 lists the recommended temperature

Table 2.8 Neutral Thermal Environmental Temperatures[a]

Age and weight	Starting temperature (°C)	Range of temperature (°C)
0–6 hours		
Under 1200 g	35.0	34.0–35.4
1200–1500 g	34.1	33.9–34.4
1501–2500 g	33.4	32.8–33.8
Over 2500 g (and >36 weeks)	32.9	32.0–33.8
6–12 hours		
Under 1200 g	35.0	34.0–35.4
1200–1500 g	34.0	33.5–34.4
1501–2500 g	33.1	32.2–33.8
Over 2500 g (and >36 weeks)	32.8	31.4–33.8
12–24 hours		
Under 1200 g	34.0	34.0–35.4
1200–1500 g	33.8	33.3–34.3
1501–2500 g	32.8	31.8–33.8
Over 2500 g (and >36 weeks)	32.4	
24–36 hours		
Under 1200 g	34.0	34.0–35.0
1200–1500 g	33.6	33.1–34.2
1501–2500 g	32.6	31.6–33.6
Over 2500 g (and >36 weeks)	32.1	30.7–33.5

continued

Table 2.8 *continued*

Age and weight	Starting temperature (°C)	Range of temperature (°C)
36–48 hours		
Under 1200 g	34.0	34.0–35.0
1200–1500 g	33.5	33.0–34.1
1501–2500 g	32.5	31.4–33.5
Over 2500 g (and >36 weeks)	31.9	30.5–33.3
48–72 hours		
Under 1200 g	34.0	34.0–35.0
1200–1500 g	33.5	33.0–34.0
1501–2500 g	32.3	31.2–33.4
Over 2500 g (and >36 weeks)	31.7	30.1–33.2
72–96 hours		
Under 1200 g	34.0	34.0–35.0
1200–1500 g	33.5	33.0–34.0
1501–2500 g	32.2	31.1–33.2
Over 2500 g (and >36 weeks)	31.3	29.8–32.8
4–12 days		
Under 1500 g	33.5	33.0–34.0
1501–2500 g	32.1	31.0–33.2
Over 2500 g (and >36 weeks)		
4–5 days	31.0	29.5–32.6
5–6 days	30.9	29.4–32.3
6–8 days	30.6	29.0–32.2
8–10 days	30.3	29.0–31.8
10–12 days	30.1	29.0–31.4
12–14 days		
Under 1500 g	33.5	32.6–34.0
1501–2500 g	32.1	31.0–33.2
Over 2500 g (and >36 weeks)	29.8	29.0–30.8
2–3 weeks		
Under 1500 g	33.1	32.2–34.0
1501–2500 g	31.7	30.5–33.0
3–4 weeks		
Under 1500 g	32.6	31.6–33.6
1501–2500 g	31.4	30.0–32.7
4–5 weeks		
Under 1500 g	32.0	31.2–33.0
1501–2500 g	30.9	29.5–32.2
5–6 weeks		
Under 1500	31.4	30.6–32.3
1501–2500 g	30.4	29.0–31.8

Reprinted with permission from Klaus M, Fanaroff A. Care of the High-Risk Neonate. Mosby, St. Louis, 1979.

[a] Adapted from Scopes J, Ahmed I: Range of critical temperatures in sick and premature newborn babies. Arch Dis Child 41:417–419, 1966. For their table, the walls of the incubator were 1°–2° warmer than the ambient air temperatures. Generally speaking, the smaller infants in each weight group will require a temperature in the higher portion of the temperature range. Within each time range, the younger the infant the higher the temperature required.

Table 2.9 Summary of Management of the Thermal Environment

1. Eliminate all sources of heat loss:
   a. Dry the baby
   b. Protect from drafts
   c. Prewarm surfaces
   d. Dress infant as much as possible
   e. Warm oxygen
2. Provide a calorie source to support internal heat production:
   a. Early feedings within 2 hours with breast milk or formula for well newborns
   b. IV glucose if infant is unstable to receive gastric feedings

If insufficient then:

3. Provide a primary heat source:
   a. Radiant heated table
   b. Isolette

If insufficient then:

4. Provide a second source of heat:
   a. K-pad
   b. Radiant lights

settings for the isolette depending on the infant's weight and age. An infant who is kept in an isolette at the recommended temperature should maintain a constant normal core temperature with minimal metabolic work. Nurseries who use this method should keep this chart of recommended isolette temperatures prominently posted since it is much too long to memorize.

Infants in isolettes gain heat by convection but lose heat by evaporation, conduction, and radiation. Double-walled isolettes were developed to reduce radiant losses by cool isolette walls, but a recent study (14) could find no net gain in heat conservation by the double wall. Evaporative water losses increase as the isolette temperature increases, and conductive heat loss to an unheated mattress is constant. In addition, whenever portholes are opened, cooler nursery air is sucked in over the infant and warm air escapes. This increases convective loss. Cuffs around the portholes that fit around caretaker's arms while working with the baby help reduce this problem. Probably the safest and simplest means of reducing heat loss is to dress the infant. Even infants who cannot be fully dressed because they must be observed or because of apparatus can be partially dressed. Hats, booties, diapers, and thin plastic tents help to insulate the infant against heat loss. Table 2.9 summarizes the management of an infant's thermal environment.

Rewarming the Cold Infant

The infant whose core temperature has fallen below 36.5°C (97.7°F) is losing heat more rapidly than he is producing it. This can occur:

1. When the environment overwhelms the infant's brown fat, glucose, and oxygen supplies.
2. When the infant is hypoxemic and cannot effectively increase metabolic work.
3. When the infant is hypoglycemic and cannot increase metabolism in response to the environment.
4. When an infant has a systemic infection (sepsis).

No matter what the cause of cold stress, similar steps should be taken. The infant should quickly be assessed for signs of additional distress by obtaining:

1. Dextrostix
2. Silverman Score and respiratory rate
3. Blood gases if the respiratory rate is above 60 and/or grunting is present

Interventions include:

1. Placing the infant in a neutral thermal environment (isolette or radiant heated table).
2. Removing sources of heat loss (e.g., wet linen, unwarmed oxygen).
3. Administering a source of calories (do not nipple feed if the infant has respiratory distress).
4. Administering oxygen symptomatically if the infant is hypoxemic.

The core temperature will rise 0.5°C hourly if the interventions have been adequate.

When an infant is placed in a servo-controlled unit (radiant heated table or isolette), the neutral thermal environment is obtained by setting the control point at 1.5°C warmer than the abdominal skin temperature (15). Oxygen consumption is lowest in this range. Placing the infant in a constant, thermally neutral environment as described in Table 2.8 is recommended when a constant isolette temperature is used. Probably the most common mistake made when rewarming a cool infant is to proceed too quickly. Rebound hyperthermia and excess oxygen consumption often occur when an infant is too rapidly rewarmed. Additionally, the cold infant needs both a heat source and and a calorie source to be successfully rewarmed. Because hypoglycemia can be caused by cold stress, blood sugar should be followed closely until the infant's temperature is normal. The temperature will rise about 0.5°C hourly if proper rewarming measures have been taken. If the infant's temperature does not rise, recheck for sources of heat loss, add another heat source (e.g., K-pad or heat lamp) and make sure adequate calories are being given.

Parent Education

The healthy infant should be able to maintain a normal axillary temperature while normally dressed and covered with blankets. The risk of cold stress is reduced as the CNS develops, metabolic processes mature, and the infant feeds more effectively. Emphasize to parents to be alert to heat loss, especially when bathing, during cold weather, and in air conditioned rooms.

Overheating is as important as cold stress. A good rule of thumb is that the baby will be comfortable in whatever number of garment layers you are comfortable. Temperature need not be routinely checked by the mother unless the infant exhibits signs of possible infection, but instruction in taking temperatures should be provided prior to discharge from the hospital.

References

1. Lubchenco LO: Assessment of weight and gestational age. In GB Avery (ed), Neonatology: Pathophysiology and Management of the Newborn, 2nd ed, pp 205–224. Lippincott, Philadelphia, 1981.
2. Dazé AM, Scanlon JW (eds): Code Pink: A Practical System for Neonatal/Perinatal Resuscitation. University Park Press, Baltimore, 1981.
3. Silverman WA, Anderson DH: Criteria for evaluating respiratory distress. Pediatrics 17:1, 1956.
4. Scanlon JW, Grylack LG, Nelson T, Smith YF: A System for Newborn Physical Examination. University Park Press, Baltimore, 1979.

5. Klaus M, Kennell J: Maternal-Infant Bonding: The Impact of Early Separation or Loss on Family Development. Mosby, St. Louis, 1976.

6. Brazelton TB: Infants and Mothers. Dell, New York, 1969.

7. Lawrence RA: Breast Feeding: A Guide for the Medical Profession. Mosby, St. Louis, 1980.

8. Dawkins M, Hull D: Brown adipose tissue and the response of newborn rabbits to cold. J Physiol 172:216–237, 1964.

9. Budin P: The Nursling. Caxton, London, 1907.

10. Williams PR, Oh W: Effects of radiant warmers on insensible water loss in newborn animals. Am J Dis Child 128:511–514, 1974.

11. Silverman W, Agate F: Variations in cold resistance among small newborn animals. Biol Neonates 6:113, 1964.

12. Darnal RA, Ariagno RL: Minimal oxygen consumption in infants cared for under overhead radiant warmers compared to conventional incubators. J Pediatr 93:283–287, 1978.

13. Marks KH, Uhrman SB, Friedman Z, Maisels MH: The effect of clothing on the growth of very low birth weight infants. Pediatr Res 11:537–539, 1977.

14. Bell EF, Rios GR: A double-walled incubator alters the partition of body heat loss of premature infants. Pediatr Res 17:135–140, 1983.

15. Adamson K, Gandy G, James L: The influence of thermal factors upon oxygen consumption of one newborn human infant. J Pediatr 66:495–507, 1965.

Suggested Reading

Schwartz RH, Hey EN, Baum JD: Management of the newborn's thermal environment. In JC Sinclair (ed), Temperature Regulation and Fuel Energy Metabolism in the Newborn, pp 205–225. Grune & Stratton, New York, 1979.

Whaley LF, Wong DL: The normal neonate. In LF Whaley, DL Wong (ed), Nursing Care of Infants and Children. Mosby, St. Louis, 1979.

Appendices

Appendix 2.1
Procedure for Silver Nitrate Instillation in the Newborn

Purpose

To prevent ophthalmia neonatorum (gonorrhea infection of the conjunctiva of the neonate).

Equipment

Sterile 4 × 4 gauze   1% silver nitrate ampule
Sterile water   Sterile needle

Procedure

1. Wipe eyelid with sterile gauze and water to remove excess vernix, allowing for easier opening of lid (use separate sterile gauze for each eye to prevent cross-contamination).
2. Puncture wax ampule of 1% silver nitrate with sterile needle.
3. Open infant's eye by using thumb and index finger, applying gentle pressure in opposite directions.
4. Drop two drops of silver nitrate into the eye. The lids should be separated and elevated away from the eyeball so a lake of silver nitrate may lie for a half minute or longer between them, coming in contact with every portion of the conjunctival sac.
5. Wipe off excess with sterile gauze.
6. Repeat steps 1 through 5 in opposite eye.
7. Record on chart that procedure was done.

NOTE   Discoloration of the liquid in silver nitrate ampules indicates that a chemical reaction has taken place and the ampule should not be used.

Appendix 2.2
Guidelines for Administration of Erythromycin Ophthalmic Ointment as an Alternative to Silver Nitrate

Purpose:

To provide prophylaxis for ophthalmia neonatorum due to *Neisseria gonorrhoeae.* Alternative eye prophylaxis (i.e., other than silver nitrate) must be ordered by a physician. Erythromycin has been accepted as an alternative to silver nitrate by the Centers for Disease Control and the American Academy of Pediatricians.

Procedure

1. Obtain 0.5% erythromycin ointment from the pharmacy (individual tubes must be used for each neonate).
2. Instill a ribbon of ointment approximately 0.5–1 cm in length into each conjunctival sac.
3. Do not flush ointment from eyes.
4. Document administration of erythromycin on chart.

References

American Academy of Pediatrics: Prophylaxis and treatment of neonatal gonococcal infections. Pediatrics 65:1047, 1980.

Hammerschlag MR, et al.: Erythromycin ointment for ocular prophylaxis of neonatal chlamydial infection. JAMA 244:2291, 1980.

Appendix 2.3
Admission Care of Cesarean Section and Large Babies

Purpose

To provide guidelines for the care of infants delivered by cesarean section and large babies admitted to the normal nursery.

Recommendations

1. All newborns delivered by elective cesarean section will be admitted directly to the regular nursery unless the newborn has a specific indication for high risk or ICN status.
2. All babies weighing >4000 g will be admitted to the normal nursery using the following admission procedure.

General Instructions

Upon newborn admission to the regular nursery, the following should be performed after the routine admission procedures:

1. Observe baby in isolette for 4 hours.
2. Take and record hourly temperature, heart rate, and respiratory rate for 4 hours; then per routine, once a shift.
3. Obtain Dextrostix—hourly times 2. (NOTE: Notify the private physician if the Dextrostix reading is less than 45 mg/dl. Call the doctor immediately if Dextrostix reading is below 25 mg/dl and obtain a STAT blood sugar.)
4. Take blood pressure on admission.
5. Begin feeding as per routine for vaginal delivery when vital signs are stable and no sign of distress is noted.

Call physician if:

1. Respirations are more than 80/minute, *or* more than 60/minute on two separate occasions.
2. Heart rate is persistently above 180/minute or below 120/minute.
3. Any flaring, retracting, or grunting is noted.
4. Any cyanosis (except acrocyanosis) is noted.
5. Any unusual behavior or activity such as jitteriness or floppiness is noted.
6. Temperature is below 35.8°C (96.5°F) *or* 2 recordings are below 36.1°C (97°F); record isolette temperature when recording infant's temperature.
7. Blood pressure is less than 45/25 for infants 2–3 kg or 50/30 for infants greater than 3 kg; repeat blood pressure 1 hour later.

Appendix 2.4
Obtaining Dextrostix Reading

Purpose

To obtain an approximate percentage of blood sugar concentration.

Policy

1. Report to physician if Dextrostix reading is below 45 mg/dl, or over 130 mg/dl.
2. Obtain a STAT blood glucose reading and call the doctor immediately if the Dextrostix reads 25 mg/dl or less.
   a. Feed the infant immediately after the blood glucose is obtained. *DO NOT FEED* if the infant is in respiratory distress. Call the physician STAT.
   b. Formula or breast milk is the preferred feeding for hypoglycemia; glucose water is acceptable if ordered by the physician.
   c. Repeat the Dextrostix ½ hour after feeding to document response to the feeding and notify the pediatrician of the results.

General Instructions

Dextrostix is to be taken:

1. On large babies (above 4200 g) or infants of diabetic mothers—hourly times 2.
2. On cesarean section babies—hourly times 2.
3. If the baby seems jittery or has any other symptoms of hypoglycemia.
4. On high risk or intensive care status babies—hourly times 4.
5. When the infant has been cold stressed [temperature of 36.1°C (97°F) or below].
6. When an infant is on IV fluids—every 8 hours (every 4 hours when on parenteral nutrition).

Procedure

1. Cleanse baby's heel with alcohol.
2. Puncture heel with sterile lancet.
3. Freely apply a large drop of blood to paper side of Dextrostix strip.
4. Wait for 60 seconds. (Apply Band-Aid while waiting.)
5. Wash off blood from Dextrostix with sharp stream of cool water.
6. Read strip by comparing to color chart on Dextrostix bottle.
7. Document the results on nurses' notes.

Appendix 2.5
Blood Pressure—Use of Ultrasonic Doppler Flow Detector

Purpose

To obtain an accurate reading of the systolic arterial pressure.

Equipment

1. Ultrasonic Doppler flow detector
2. Properly fitting blood pressure cuff with manometer (the cuff should cover two-thirds of the upper extremity)
3. Contact gel (Aquasonic 100)
4. Alcohol swab

Procedure

Select a limb with a readily palpable pulse and take blood pressure as follows:

1. Apply the blood pressure cuff in the usual manner.
2. Apply a small amount of gel to the indented side of the clear plastic probe.
3. Place the probe over an artery below the cuff. (NOTE: if the probe is under the cuff, an erroneously high blood pressure may be taken.)
4. Turn on Doppler. Listen for the hissing pulse sound, then inflate the cuff until this sound stops. Lower the pressure slowly until you hear the pulse sound reappear. This is the systolic pressure reading on the manometer.
5. Do not inflate the cuff to a pressure greater than 80 cm unless the pulse sound is still audible. For greater accuracy, the cuff pressure should not be pumped more than 20 mm Hg higher than the systolic pressure.
6. Cleanse probe with alcohol swab and replace Doppler to storage position.
7. Record results next to the pressure, and record which extremity was used (e.g., right leg, left arm).

The Doppler flow detector can also be used as a heart rate monitor by placing the flow probe over the apical or brachial pulse.

Blood Pressure Limits

Infants 2–3 kg: 45/25 to 70/40
Infants 3 kg: 50/30 to 80/40

NOTE   *Recharging the Doppler Battery:* Plug the charging unit into the inlet marked on the Doppler and then into a wall electrical outlet. Disconnect the probe from the Doppler while it is recharging. *Do not leave the charger plugged in for longer than 12 hours.* Prolonged use of charger will damage the battery.

Appendix 2.6
Blood Pressure—Use of the Sentry
ASD 400 P

Purpose

To obtain an accurate reading of the systolic and diastolic blood pressure.

Equipment

1. Sentry Machine ASD 400 P
2. Disposable blood pressure cuff

Procedure

1. Plug power cable into electrical outlet.
2. Attach correct size cuff for limb to be used (to cover two-thirds of upper part of extremity): size 10 for infants 1800 g or less, size 20 for those over 1800 g.
3. Turn on power. Beeper will sound for several seconds. All readouts will display 8's to show that all segments are functional.
4. Squeeze air out of cuff and install it snugly, but not constrictively, around limb (upper arm is usually best position). Keep limb as still as possible.
5. Depress "Man" button to start measuring process in manual mode. Sentry will make one measurement and display values.
6. For automatic operation:
   a. Turn on
   b. Push "1," "2," "3" (to unlock computer)
   c. Enter three numbers for frequency of blood pressure e.g., for 15 minutes, enter "0," "1," "5"; for 20 minutes, enter "0," "2," "0"
   d. Depress cycle time
   e. Push "cycle time" button
   f. Push "set" button and "lock" button
   g. Push "cycle time," "recall" to see if desired limit was obtained.
7. Remove cuff, keep at infant's bedside for next blood pressure reading. Turn sentry off before unplugging to move to next infant.
8. Record blood pressure on data sheet and chart pertinent observations. Indicate next to blood pressure results which extremity was used.

Appendix 2.7
Continuous Arterial Pressure Monitoring

Purpose

To maintain direct observation of arterial pressures.

Equipment

1. Transducer with cord
2. Sterile plastic dome and pressure tubing
3. Syringe with ordered IV solution (any dextrose concentration of to dextrose (10%) in water is acceptable for pressure monitoring)
4. Tektronix monitoring
5. Harvard pump

Procedure

1. Screw dome onto transducer and plug cord into back of monitor into outlet marked "Pressure Transducer Input."
2. Open dome stopcock. Close patient end of stopcock. Fill dome with IV solution, holding stopcock upright, so all the air escapes through the stopcock. (NOTE: Flush red tab must be pulled out while filling dome or tubing.)
3. Close dome stopcock and open system stopcock. Fill the tubing with IV solution, making sure no air remains in the tubing. Pull flush tab out as when filling dome. (NOTE: Even a small amount of air in the line or dome will dampen the pressure transmitted to the transducer.)
4. Close patient stopcock, open dome stopcock. Hold dome at patient's mid-apical level with dome stopcock *open to air.* Push "Zero Readout" button until −0 or +0 appears on the screen. Release zero button, and push "0–125" button, then hold in the "100 mm CHK" button until 98–102 shows on the readout screen. The monitor is now calibrated. Close dome stopcock and tape transducer at mid-apical level.
5. The pressure tubing is now ready for connection to patient arterial line.
6. Set Harvard pump at ordered rate per minute (3 cc/hour is usually sufficient to maintain a patent line unless arterial pressures are unusually high).
7. If air or blood enter the line at any time, they must be flushed out before a reading can take place.
8. Tubing and dome should be changed every day, at which time the zero should again be recalibrated.
9. When disassembling the setup, discard all tubing in the dome. The head of the transducer must be handled very carefully. Clean with Tergisyl between patients, and cover transducer with dome before placing it into the storage box.

Appendix 2.8
Admission Bath of the Newborn

Purpose

1. To cleanse the infant.
2. To promote comfort.
3. To provide an opportunity for observing condition of skin and mobility of extremities, and to note any unusual condition.

General Instructions

1. Prior to bath, infant's axillary temperature should be 36.5°C (97.7°F) for 2 consecutive hours.
2. Collect all equipment before beginning procedure.
3. Bathe infant in isolette; shampoo over sink.

Equipment and Supplies

1. Infant basin kit, which includes:
   a. Plastic basin
   b. Disposable washcloths
   c. Cotton balls
   d. Q-tips
   e. Two safety pins
   f. Measuring tape
   g. Brush
2. pHisoHex (not to be used on premature infants; use only castile soap)
3. Vaseline
4. Cloth diapers and shirt
5. Two blankets—one to be used as bath blanket

Procedure

1. Wash hands thoroughly.
2. Assemble equipment.
3. Remove diaper, if infant is wearing one.
4. Cleanse infant's eyes using cotton balls moistened with clear water. Cleanse eyes from inner to outer aspect. Use a separate cotton ball for each eye.
5. Wash face with clear water, starting at forehead and cleansing down over the nose, cheeks, external ears, and neck creases. Pat dry with clean blanket.
6. Fill basin with warm tepid water (use elbow for testing, because fingertips are less sensitive to temperature) and pHisoHex.
7. Moisten disposable washcloth with solution. Wash upper extremities and chest down to umbilicus, rinse with warm, wet diaper, and pat dry with clean diaper. (NOTE: Be sure to dry well between fingers.)
8. Turn infant on abdomen and wash back; rinse and pat dry.
9. Wash lower abdomen and legs; rinse and pat dry. (NOTE: Be sure to dry well between toes.)
10. Wash genitalia last, cleansing the area and drying it well.
11. Wash cord with alcohol after initial bath. Apply Triple Dye.

12. Dress infant in shirt and diaper.
13. Wrap infant in bath blanket. Remove from isolette. Hold over sink to wash scalp. Fill admission basin with fresh warm water. Dampen scalp and apply small amount of pHisoHex to area. Using brush, wash gently, removing dried blood and vernix from scalp. Rinse thoroughly with water in basin and dry with clean diaper.
14. Return to isolette after shampoo and take temperature within 1 hour. When the temperature is 36.5°C (97.7°F) the infant can be placed in an open crib.

NOTE   Following the admission bath, baths are given as needed, using only castile soap and tap water.

Appendix 2.9
Infant Discharge Criteria

The following must be done prior to discharge for *all* infants:

1. Silver nitrate or antibiotic prophylaxis for eyes (1 hour after birth).
2. AquaMEPHYTON intramuscularly.
3. Physical exam by a pediatrician within 24 hours of discharge.
4. Metabolic screen (thyroxine and phenylketonuria) required on the third day of life.
5. Footprinting.
6. Identification of mother and infant.

Normal Nursery

Normal Term Infant (more than 2500 g)

May be discharged no sooner than 8 hours postpartum and/or at the time the infant's mother is discharged postpartum. Under individual circumstances, discharge may be made to an individual other than the mother with the mother's consent and proper identification.

Discharge Criteria

Minimum of two physical exams, an uneventful course, and a discharge order from an M.D.

High Risk Status

Discharge (or transfer to normal nursery) criteria

1. Infant able to maintain normal temperature in open unheated crib.
2. Infant taking an adequate fluid and caloric intake.
3. Family prepared to care for infant.
4. Resolution of complications necessitating high risk status.

Infant Requiring Continued Specialized Therapy

Criteria for discharge and placement of the infant who continues to require specialized care (e.g., medication, oxygen therapy, gastrostomy care) will be established on a case-by-case basis. In each case, community and family resources will be evaluated and referral made as indicated (e.g., sleep-apnea evaluation clinic).

Criteria for Transfer from Neonatology/Intensive Care Status to Private Pediatrician

1. Birth weight greater than 1800 g.
2. Condition no longer requires cardiorespiratory monitor.
3. Condition no longer requires IV.
4. Condition no longer requires oxygen supplementation or ventilatory assistance.
5. Available private pediatrician.

3

Fluids, Electrolytes, and Nutrition for Neonates

Kenneth L. Harkavy

The goals of water and nutrient therapy are threefold. The first, most basic, is maintenance of normal cellular function. The second is provision for growth. The third, and least understood, is the support of optimal neurodevelopment. This review presents theoretical and clinical guidelines for fluid, electrolytes, and nutrition, and describes how adjustments are made for differences in patients' size, age, and environment.

Principles of Fluids Replacement

Water requirements are determined by the balance between 1) changes in body composition, 2) gastrointestinal losses, 3) obligatory urine flow, 4) abnormal losses, and 5) insensible water loss (IWL) (1).

From the late second trimester until term, the fetus deposits more and more water-free fat cells. Total body-water (TBW) falls from 84% to about 75% of body weight. In the first few days of life TBW, as a percentage of body weight, may actually rise because of fat and carbohydrate catabolism. TBW remains stable through the first 3 days, but between the second week and sixth month of life there is a steady fall in TBW to adult levels.

A diet high in protein and mineral content can postpone the change in TBW at least until 28 days. Contraction of TBW occurs slowly and this is probably reflected to some degree in the postnatal weight curves discussed below (see "Assessment of Fluid Balance"). The physiological changes in TBW are so much smaller than other components of daily fluid maintenance requirements that these changes need not be considered when calculating water needs. However, these changes, along with the gradual shift of body water from extra- to intracellular, are important when estimating the distribution of electrolytes.

Gastrointestinal (GI) losses are usually 10% of oral intake, up to a maximum of 10 ml/kg/day. Many sick infants have no stools, and therefore have no GI water losses for several days after birth. In feeding infants, water formed during cellular metabolism (~10 ml/100 kcal) balances that lost by the GI tract.

Required urine flow depends on the amount of solute that must be excreted and the ability of the kidney to concentrate these solutes. Growing infants excrete between 7 and 16 mOsm/kg/day. The renal solute load depends on the rate of growth and the amount of protein and "ash" (e.g., Na^+, K^+, PO_4^{2-}, CL^-) in the formula. Some of the newer special formulas for premature infants have increased amounts of protein and minerals. They may be inappropriate for the infant in a catabolic state. At a conservative 300 mOsm/kg H_2O, calculated urine flow must be 25–50 ml/kg/day. These figures are consistent with urine volumes recorded in infants with varying birth weights and gestational ages (2). Ninety percent of infants who were thirsted for 6 to 12 hours, voided 12 to 120 cc/kg/day. Osmolalities ranged from 75 to 300 mOsm/L. Urine volumes and concentrations were independent of gestational age. Thus hourly urine output will normally range from 0.5 to 5 cc, with 24-hour losses of 12 to 120 cc/kg. An average figure might be 50 ml/kg/day of urine production.

Abnormal losses of water usually can be measured and then replaced in equal amounts. Such losses might include ileostomy drainage, diarrhea, pleural effusions, or external cerebrospinal fluid drains. Third space loss is defined as loss into body cavities, which cannot be measured and is not reflected in body weight changes. This is a real problem! An example is the intraluminal bowel fluid in the ileus associated with necrotizing enterocolitis. In such cases estimates of replacement volumes must be made from physical examination, vital signs, and laboratory tests such as serum/urine electrolytes, hematocrit, and total protein. In those few babies with damage to the tubular concentrating mechanism, urine flow may be excessive and may constitute an abnormal loss requiring replacement.

The last component of water balance, insensible water loss (IWL), is the most difficult to predict and the most difficult to measure. Losses via the respiratory tract are a small part of IWL. They range from 0 to 10 ml/kg/day depending on the humidity of inspired gases and the respiratory rate. Cutaneous losses are the most prominent source. IWL is determined primarily by the permeability of the skin, ambient radiant energy, local convection, and environmental humidity. Larger, more mature infants have the lowest IWL. The small-for-gestational-age (SGA) infant may lose less than his more premature peer. By about 3 weeks of life, premature and term infants have similar IWL values. Table 3.1 lists representative IWLs for babies of various weights and ages.

If newer double-walled incubators or single-walled incubators with a heat

Table 3.1 Estimated Water Losses[a]

Route	Amount lost (ml/kg/24 hours)		
	<1500 g BW	1500–2000 g BW	>2000 g BW ("term")
Stool	0–10 (10% of oral intake)		
Urine	48 (range, 12–120)		
IWL[b] from single-wall incubator			
1 week old	57–83	20–33	13–41
2 weeks old	50	30–36	NA
3 weeks old	41	30	NA
4 weeks old	38	30	NA

Abbreviations: BW, birth weight; NA, not available.

[a] Figures provided are mean values obtained from the literature. Standard deviations for group measurements are wide. Therefore, the range of values for an individual baby is wide, as much as 50% in either direction. Required fluids up to 200 ml/kg/day have been reported in the <750-g birth weight group.

[b] The impact of IWL on fluid balance may be minimal, as for a term infant in an incubator, or overwhelming, as for a 650-g infant kept on a radiant heated table and treated with phototherapy.

shield are used as standards, IWL will be increased in the usual single-walled incubators, under radiant heated tables (infrared lamps more than quartz rods), and under phototherapy lights. IWL may be reduced with the use of dermally applied waxes, transparent thermal blankets, or thin plastic films (e.g., Saran Wrap). The latter may be effective because they create a micro-climate of higher humidity and less air turbulance, thus reducing convective water loss. Rigid plastic body hoods do not reduce IWL from radiant heaters, and cause uneven heating of covered (trunk) and uncovered (head) parts of the body. Newer evidence suggests that double-walled incubators may not decrease IWL (and oxygen consumption) but simply shift it from radiant to convective loss (3). Table 3.2 lists differences in IWL in various environments.

Of great importance is the wide variability noted in values for water loss and replacement volumes. It is imperative that the individual infant be evaluated to determine the appropriateness of the prescribed therapy (see "Assessment of Fluid Balance," below) and modifications be made promptly when required. Published values only serve as guidelines for groups of infants.

In summary, from the above discussion:

Water needs = IWL + renal flow + GI loss − water of combustion (+ abnormal losses)

In simplest terms

Water needs = IWL + 50 ml/kg/day (+ abnormal losses)

Infusion volumes can be estimated from the values for IWL in Table 3.1. When calculating fluid intake, include colloid infusion into these calculations because its protein is rapidly catabolized, allowing the water to distribute throughout the body.

Table 3.2 Differences in IWL for Various Environmental Conditions[a]

Conditions	Percentage change in IWL vs. single-walled incubator		
	<1500 g BW	1500–2000 g BW	>2000 g BW ("term")
SGA vs. AGA (all weights)		49	
Double-walled incubator	0–30	0–30	NA
Hard plastic heat shield	40	—	17
Phototherapy	30	33	24
High NTE vs. mid-NTE	70	50	NA
Sub-NTE	9	9	NA
Radiant heater			
Heat shield (IMI)	18	14	NA
Infrared (KDC)	47	34	NA
Quartz-nichrome (air shield)	22	18	29
Quartz plus phototherapy	27	34	NA
Quartz plus plastic film			
vs. quartz alone	43	NA	NA

Abbreviations: AGA, apropriate for gestational age; BW, birth weight; NA, not available; NTE, neutral thermal environment; ↑, increased; ↓, decreased; —, unchanged.

[a] The figures provided are mean values obtained from the literature. Standard deviations for group measurements are wide. Therefore, the range of values for an individual baby is wide, as much as 50% in either direction. Required fluids up to 200 ml/kg/day have been reported in the <750-g birth weight group.

Principles of Electrolyte Replacement

Prescriptions for electrolytes (Na^+, K^+, Cl^-, HCO_3^- equivalent) will be determined by the requirements for growth and any concurrent losses. During periods of catabolism, K^+, HPO_4^{2-}, and to a lesser degree Na^+ and Cl^- will be released from cells. Anabolic requirements, based on intrauterine retention rates for these minerals, are 1–2 mEq/kg/day. However, because some Na^+ and K^+ are lost in the urine as buffers to organic acids, daily requirements of these cations during growth are 2–3 mEq/kg/day. Cutaneous and GI losses are usually 0.4 mEq/100 cal of K^+, Na^+, and Cl^-. In unusual circumstances (cystic fibrosis, adrenal insufficiency) cutaneous losses can be much higher. In general, if stools are watery their electrolyte concentrations are high. These values should be measured in a stool sample and replaced.

Renal processing of sodium is quite dependent on gestational age. The number of juxtamedullary nephrons, which are the ones most able to reabsorb Na^+, continues to increase throughout the last trimester. In infants <30 weeks (<1250 g) fractional sodium excretion (FeNa)[1] averages 5% but may be as much as 10%. The deficiencies are in both the proximal and distal tubules (4). This suggests that the kidney cannot compensate for agents that affect either type of tubule. Renal actions of furosemide (distal tubule) and theophylline (proximal tubule) are exaggerated (compared to older infants), resulting in greater losses of K^+ and Na^+. By 34 weeks of conceptual age most kidney function is the same as at term (5).

An important determinant of sodium excretion for very low birth weight (VLBW) infants is fluid intake. High IV rates (and probably oral intakes) are associated with a significant increase in sodium excretion. Because of tubular immaturity and large feedings, hyponatremia is a common finding in preterm infants 1 to 4 weeks of age.

A mild form of tubular acidosis has long been noted in neonates. Term infants have serum bicarbonate levels 5 mM/L below adult values. Preterm levels are still another 5 mM/L lower. Similar to HCO_3^- reabsorption, tubular reabsorption of phosphate tends to improve at 34 weeks from 85% to 95%. Renal processing of K^+ and Cl^- in preterm infants has not been completely evaluated, but urine losses are ordinarily quite low. Potassium loss may increase in the presence of hyponatremia (aldosterone effect) or during diuretic therapy. Calcium reabsorption is under the complex control of vitamin D, parathyroid hormone, and calcitonin [see Tsang et al. (6) and Steichen et al. (7) for a complete discussion]. It is not possible to always predict what electrolyte losses will be. Therefore it may be clinically necessary to measure serum levels frequently and measure renal excretion of electrolyte components when serum components reach the limits of normal.

Maintenance electrolytes are usually withheld during the first 24 hours because serum K^+ is relatively high, renal function is uncertain, and Na^+ often accompanies medications or blood products. When maternal therapy is likely to have altered normal fetal fluid and electrolyte balance (for example, with tocolysis or long-term dependence on IV infusion), neonatal serum electrolyte values may indicate the need for early supplementation. Hypocalcemia is common in sick preterm infants, especially if they receive $NaHCO_3$. This may be prevented by the early use of IV calcium (0.5 mEq/kg/day), or the use of 1,25-$(OH)_2$-D_3 (vitamin D; 1 μg/day by 8–12 hours of life. After 24 hours, Na^+ (2–3 mEq/kg/day), K^+ (1–3 mEq/kg/day), and Ca^{2+}

---

[1] FeNa is the percentage of glomerularly filtered sodium not reabsorbed in the tubule. It is calculated as:

$$\frac{(\text{serum creatinine}) \times (\text{urine Na})}{(\text{urine creatinine}) \times (\text{serum Na})} \times 100$$

(0.5–1.0 mEq/kg/day) are added to IV fluids if serum electrolytes are normal. The choice of anion (Cl⁻, acetate, bicarbonate) is based on the acid-base value in blood and urine. Maintenance requirements may be increased by drugs or decreased by oliguria.

Assessment of Fluid Balance

The adequacy of fluid and electrolyte prescription should be assessed in a number of ways. Table 3.3 suggests several bedside observations for hydration status. Table 3.4 lists some suggested measurements for further assessment in the VLBW infant. The "ideal" pattern of postnatal weight change in preterm infants is still quite controversial, since prematurity is a decidely nonphysiological event. The weight curves developed by Dancis et al. (8) seem appropriate. They were derived from "healthy" infants, and are consistent with calculations of the consumption of carbohydrate and fat stores for energy. Infants who follow these curves have lower morbidity (9). The frequency of vital signs, clinical signs, and laboratory determinations depends on the size of the patient, the nature of the illness, and the ease with which the measurement is made. The tiny premature infant receiving mechanical ventilation may need hourly blood sugar estimates and weights two to three times daily, but only daily hematocrits. Interpretation of these measurements must be made with great care. No result can be considered in isolation. For example, hypertonic urine and oliguria may result from several diseases, including cardiac failure, inappropriate antidiuretic hormone secretion, and dehydration. The clinician must also remember that serum electrolyte concentrations do not measure the total body burden of mineral. Excess water as well as depletion of sodium body stores can cause hyponatremia. Measurement of urine electrolytes may help the interpretation of serum electrolytes, but primary renal disease must be excluded and the kidney's priority of response to electrolyte derangements must be considered. In the above example of hyponatremia, the kidney will retain Na⁺ in response to the hyponatremia rather than respond to the excess body burden of salt with a naturesis. Excess salt will be retained until the excess water is excreted or the serum becomes isotonic. Drug side effects on renal function must be remembered too. Theophyllin, given for apnea, will cause naturesis and confuse interpretation.

Table 3.3 Observations for Hydration Status

Parameter	Fluid overload	Dehydration
Urine volume	Often increased (>3–5 cc/kg/h)	<0.5 cc/kg/h
Urine specific gravity	<1.005	>1.015
Skin	Edema; dependant or pitting	Dry mucous membranes; poor turgor
Eyes	Orbital edema	Sunken eyes
Fontanelles	May be bulging	Depressed
Liver size	Increased (a sign of heart failure)	—
Respiratory tract	Thin secretions, rales, increased pCO₂, increased FiO₂ᵃ	Thick endotracheal secretions
Weight	2–3% above expected weight *or* gain 2% of previous day's weight	>3–4% below expected weight or loss 3–4% of previous day's weight

Fluid imbalance is a syndrome that affects all body tissues. If fluid imbalance is present more than one sign will be present on exam.

ᵃ pCO₂, Carbon dioxide pressure; FiO₂, fractional inspired oxygen.

Table 3.4 Assessment of Fluid and Electrolyte Balance in the VLBW Infant

Indicators	Frequency observation	Optimal value
Weight change	every 8–12 hours	Loss of 1.5–3.5%/day if 72 hours old; 10–15% loss in the first week of life
Vascular volume		
Hematocrit	every day or as required	Changes consistent with blood loss or transfusion
Blood pressure	every 1–2 hours	Gestational and postnatal age standards (*see* Table 2.6)
Skin perfusion	every 1–2 hours	Capillary filling time ≤3 sec
Time to void	continuously	95% of all infants within 24 hours if no IV; within 1–2 hours with IV
Serum		
Osmolarity	as required	285–295 mOsm/L
Electrolytes	every 8–12 hours	Na^+ between 130 and 150; K^+ between 2.5 and 5.0
Urine		
Specific gravity	each void	1.004–1.010
Osmolality	each void	Varies with serum values
Electrolytes	every 8–12 hours	Varies with clinical circumstances
pH	each void	Varies with blood pH

Complications of parenteral fluid therapy are common and quite varied, especially in the smaller infants (Table 3.5 outlines some of these). In addition these smaller infants also develop complications related to the amount of water they receive. An increased incidence of necrotizing enterocolitis, bronchopulmonary dysplasia, and patent ductus arteriosus (PDA) has been suggested to be associated with high water intake. Available evidence suggests that a positive water balance is more important than the infusion rate. Fluid restriction to prevent PDA can result in serious dehydration. The high incidence of hypernatremia found in VLBW infants (40%) has been related to inadvertant fluid restriction. As many as three-fourths of patients with oliguria and azotemia respond promptly to a fluid challenge (20 ml/kg of 10% dextrose in 0.2% saline over 1–2 hours) and do not suffer renal failure.

Table 3.5 Potential Complications of Fluid Therapy

	Too little	Too much
Water	Dehydration and hypertonicity	Edema PDA Necrotizing enterocolitis Bronchopulmonary dysplasia
Electrolytes	Electrical impulse conduction defects in nerves and muscles (including heart) Seizures Rickets (with chronic deficiency) Central pontine myelinosis[a]	Electrical impulse conduction defects Brain hemorrhage

[a] Described in adults after correction of hyponatremia.

PROBLEM   What are the estimated fluid requirements of a 3-day-old infant, birt'
who is on a ventilator and receiving IV therapy? The patient is under intra.
lights.

SOLUTION   A. Water requirements:

Urine	=	50 ml/day
Stool	=	0
IWL	=	85 (±40) ml/day
(Respiration)	=	−10 ml/day
Water of combustion	=	0

125 (±40) ml/day, or 5 (±1.7) ml/hour

B. Additives
Glucose: ≥4 mg/kg/min = 5.76 g/day (5% at 125 cc/day)
Na^+: 3–4 mEq/day
K^+: 2–3 mEq/day (as Cl^-)
Ca^{2+}: 0.5 mEq/day

NOTES   1. Water of combustion is ignored because of the low caloric intake.
2. There are no significant respiratory water losses in patients who breathe humidified gases.
3. It is important to recognize the wide range for estimated IWL.
4. Glucose tolerance may have progressed significantly over the previous two days. Values up to 8–10 g/kg/day may be tolerated.

Parenteral Nutrition

Parenteral nutrition (PN) begins any time IV solutions are used to provide part of the fluid needs of the neonate. In its simplest form PN consists of IV dextrose used to sustain infants during temporary periods of food prohibition. (See Appendices 3.1 and 3.2 for information on IV therapy.) Heird and Anderson (10) have estimated that survival of infants of 1, 2, or 3 kg birth weight is increased by 7, 18, and 50 days, respectively, by the administration of 7.5 g/kg/day of glucose. This is 150 ml of 5% dextrose or 75 ml of 10% solution. An increase in calories and the addition of protein can sustain growth of 5 to 20 g/day. There are many approaches to PN. This section contains suggestions for providing PN, some risks, and precautions.

Infants have an endogenous glucose turnover of 6 mg/kg/minute (8.6 g/kg/day), and glucose infusion at this rate is usually well tolerated. The most tiny infant may assimilate only 4.5 mg/kg/minute. If tolerated, 9–10 g/kg/day glucose is desirable because it will minimize negative nitrogen balance. As discussed above, electrolytes (Na^+, K^+, Cl^-) and calcium are added as appropriate at the correct time. Further nutrients may be unnecessary for larger infants, in whom adequate caloric reserves are found *and* in whom feedings may be anticipated in a reasonable time. For example, dextrose may be sufficient for the 35-week, 2.2-kg infant whose hyaline membrane disease should resolve in 4 to 6 days. The 28-week, 1-kg infant on mechanical ventilation may not tolerate full enteral feeding for several weeks, so PN should be started and advanced early. When gastrointestinal illness occurs or surgery is required, PN must begin.

Parenteral nutrition, if needed, should begin when the patient's fluid requirements are relatively stable. If multiple changes in electrolyte doses or IV infusion are anticipated, PN should be deferred. Stability of fluid needs usually occurs after the acute phase of the illness has resolved. At this point maintenance doses of macrominerals, trace elements, and vitamins may be started. Table 3.6 outlines various nutritional and electrolyte requirements.

Table 3.6 Comparison of Formula and Breast Milk Content to Minimum Daily Requirement of Various Nutrients

Nutrient	"MDR" for prematures (per kg/day)[a]	Typical premature formula (per 100 kcal)[b]	"Preterm" breast milk (per 100 kcal)[c]
Energy content (kcal/dl)	—	80	51–73
Energy (kcal)	100–120*	—	—
Carbohydrate (g/dl)	—	11	6–7
Percentage of kcal	35–65	42	32
Protein (g)	2.2–<4.*	2.7–3.0	2.7–4.7
Percentage of kcal	7–16	12	15
Fat (g)	—	5.5	3–6
Percentage of kcal	30–55	48	53
Linoleic acid (mg)	300	1100	450
Percentage of kcal	1–4	10	(5–7)
Vitamins			
A (IU)	200	312–679	(300)
D (IU)	100–?*	62.5–148	(3)
E (IU)	≥25*	<4	(0.3)
K (μg)	4	10	(2)
C (mg)	25–100*	8–37	(7.8)
B_6 (μg)	15/g protein*	60–250	(15)
B_{12} (μg)	1–3	<0.6	(0.15)
Thiamine (μg)	40–50	80–250	(25)
Riboflavin (μg)	80–100	90–620	(60)
Niacin (mg)	1–1.25	1.25–4.9	(0.25)
Folic acid (μg)	5	35	(4)
Pantothenic acid (μg)	250–500	500–1850	(300)
Minerals			
Na (mEq)	>0.9*	1.8	1.5–10.5
K (mEq)	2.1	3.0	2.5
Ca (mg)	132*	117–178	35
P (mg)	65–80*	59–89	20
Mg (mg)	6*	11	4.0
Fe (mg)	2–4 (>2 mo. old)*	0.16–0.37	0.2
Zn (μg)	0.7*	1.0–1.48	0.075–1.9
Cu (μg)	100*	90–250	100
Cr (μg)	0.2	—	0.9–2.7
I (μg)	4–5	7.9–18.5	6–12
Se (μg)	0.4	—	(>1.0)
Mn (μg)	5	0.025	0.6–1.2
Co (μg)	7	—	
Mb (μg)	0.3	—	—
F (μg)	250 per day	0	3.7
Potential renal solute (mOsm)	<15	27	(11.3)

[a] MDR, or minimum daily requirement, is based mostly on studies of term infants fed human milk. Those values marked with an asterisk have been modified based on estimates in preterm infants. The MDR of Ca^{2+}, PO_4^{2-} and vitamin D has not been established.

[b] Where values between Enfamil Premature Formula and Ross Special Care Formula are similar, an average value is given; otherwise a range is provided. Consult the product literature for details.

[c] The exact composition of breast milk obtained from mothers who deliver prematurely depends on the time of day, days postpartum, days postconception, and technique of collection. Values in parentheses are from "term" milk. Diet greatly influences the type of fatty acids and sodium content in human milk. A caloric density of 67 cal/dl is assumed for the calculation of content per 100 kcal.

Protein is gradually added in increments of 0.5 g/kg/day in the form of crystalline amino acids. The maximum dose, 2.5–3.0 g/kg/day, was chosen because it is associated with good growth, has a low incidence of side effects, and meets the estimated minimum daily requirement of 2.2 g/kg. Protein intake of 2.7–3.5 g/kg/day is associated with fetal accretion rates of nitrogen when given with at least 70 kcal/kg/day (11). Weight gain and absolute nitrogen retention are related to protein intake, but body length is not affected. Slightly larger doses of amino acids may be appropriate in larger infants after surgical procedures to facilitate healing. Protein intakes greater than 4 g/kg/day produce azotemia, anorexia, metabolic acidosis, and GI symptoms. Very often acetate, as the sodium or potassium salt, in a dose of 0.5 mEq for each gram of protein, is needed to maintain a normal serum bicarbonate level.

In adults essential amino acids are isoleucin, leucine, lysine, methionine, tryptophan, valine, phenylalanine, and threonine. Synthesis of cysteine (from methionine), taurine, and perhaps tyrosine is reduced in premature infants (12), thus increasing the list of essential amino acids for preterm infants. At this time hyperalimentation amino acid formulations reflect adult requirements. The impact of using adult amino acid formulas for preterm infants has not been fully explored.

At the same time that amino acid intake is increased, glucose infusions are increased as long as serum glucose levels remain normal. Daily increases are made until the solution is 10% dextrose and reaches a maximum of 20 g/kg/day (if no lipids are used) or 12–14 g/kg/day (if lipids are being simultaneously administered). In fact, if only 1.0 g/kg/day of protein and 60 cal/kg/day are given to a stable premature infant, growth (about 5 g/day) can be achieved. Insulin administration is rarely indicated as a means of increasing glucose tolerance because alternate sources of calories are available. Administration of small insulin doses is subject to error, with hypoglycemia as a serious, potentially lethal, side effect.

Since the advent of safe, stable lipid emulsions, IV alcohol is no longer used as a source of calories. (See Appendix 3.3 for information on parenteral lipid administration.) Lipid emulsions contain soybean or safflower oil stabilized with egg lecithin and glycerol. The particle size is comparable to natural chylomicra and clearance is thought to be similar for the two. Solutions used are either 10% or 20% emulsions with a density of 1.1 or 2.2 cal/cc. The content of linoleic acid is 54 mg/cc (soybean; Intralipid) or 77 mg/ccl (safflower; Liposyn).

Administration of lipids serves two purposes (13). One purpose is prevention of essential fatty acid (EFA) deficiency. In this case 3–6 ml/kg/day will provide minimal maintenance doses of linoleic acid. Although EFA deficiency has been documented in a few very small premature infants as early as 4 days of life, there is no proof that early use of linoleic acid is beneficial, and there is some question whether it might alter normal prostaglandin production. The second purpose of administration of lipids is as a calorie supplement. The 10% emulsion is isotonic and provides a high density of calories without fluid overload or associated venous thrombosis. Studies suggest that 0.5 g/kg of lipids given over 4 hours will be cleared efficiently in appropriate-for-gestational-age infants. SGA infants may occasionally have elevated levels of triglycerides and free fatty acids (FFAs) at this dose. Higher infusion rates (2.0 g/kg/4 hour) in preterm infants produce marked elevation in FFAs, glucose, and insulin levels; also FFA/albumin molar ratios approach the potential risk value (see "Complications of Total Parenteral Nutrition," below). The 0.5 g/kg/4 hour rate can be maintained as the incremental dose is increased from 0.5 up to 3.0 g/kg/day (33 cal/kg/day). Infusions may be continuous over 24 hours to maintain the desired hourly rate. Infants ≤32 weeks may have trouble clearing lipids because of low lipoprotein lipase activity. The addition of heparin (1 U/ml) to the fluid will improve this activity. Anticoagulant activity at these doses is minimal (14). The use of carnitine has also been tried to help transport FFA into cells. Inability to metabolize the administered lipid dose can be detected by measuring serum triglyceride levels daily.

Vitamins and minerals are added to PN solutions to meet estimated daily requirements (see Table 3.6). Vitamins may be provided in multivitamin supplements or as separate injections. Requirements for trace elements can only be estimated and deficiencies are noted only after extended periods of PN. Solutions of trace elements are available commercially. Current recommendations are shown but several deserve special comment.

Phosphate (PO_4^{2-}) is a major buffer for the renal excretion of H^+. PO_4^{2-}, along with Ca^{2+}, is required for the mineralization of the skeleton. Vitamin D in the active form [$1,25$-$(OH)_2$-D_3 or 1,25-dihydroxycholecalciferol] prevents hypocalcemia by increasing intestinal absorption of calcium and enhancing renal reabsorption of Ca^{2+} and PO_4^{2-}, and by bone calcium mobilization. Conversion of vitamin D_3 (the usual form of supplemented vitamin) to 25-OH-D_3 is reduced in the premature infant. However, conversion of 25-OH-D_3 to $1,25$-$(OH)_2$-D_3 appears to be normal.

The daily doses of Ca^{2+}, PO_4^{2-}, and vitamin D are uncertain in the VLBW infant. Rickets has been noted relatively often with many different vitamin D regimens but is most often seen after long-term PN, especially if the vitamin D daily dose is below 400 IU. Personal observations suggest that early administration of maintenance PO_4^{2-} and Ca^{2+} along with 400 IU vitamin D and early introduction of enteral feedings result in a low incidence of rickets. Given the bone-mobilizing effect of vitamin D, perhaps large doses should be reserved for infants on oral feedings.

Caution should be exercised when Ca^{2+} and PO_4^{2-} are used in the same bottle of IV fluid. If the product of their concentrations approaches 15 $(mEq/L)^2$, precipitation is likely, especially if the fluid has an alkaline pH. If large amounts of Ca^{2+} and PO_4^{2-} are required, an alternative approach is to make two separate solutions with similar composition (one of Ca^{2+} and one of PO_4^{2-}) and run the bottles consecutively.

Complications of Total Parenteral Nutrition (TPN)

Caution should be exercised in the use of TPN (see guidelines in Appendix 3.4). The optimal distribution of calories should be 7–16% protein and 35–65% carbohydrate, with the remainder fats. A high intake of calories without adequate protein will predispose to marasmus. Adjustments in infusion rates must be made with extreme caution. The daily dose of each nutrient must be calculated as the amount per kilogram of that day's body weight, not in solution strength (for example, 12 g/kg/day of glucose, not 10% glucose).

The potential side effects of PN are legion. Imbalances of each of the nutrients have been reported, including water, salts, and glucose. Hypoglycemia is the most common problem and usually occurs with sudden removal of the IV (infiltration, for example). Hyperglycemia may also herald infection or general deterioration in medical status. Excessive amounts of amino acids may cause uremia. Symptoms may include fever and irritability. Hyperammonemia is found much less often with the use of crystalline amino acids than with protein hydrolysates, but PN should be considered a cause if serum ammonia is elevated. Such infants look "septic" and have seizures.

Amino acid levels in the neonate, while not routinely measured, are often quite different from normal adult values. In newborn animals isolated amino acids such as glutamate, methionine, and tyrosine have caused neurotoxicity. No evidence has been found in humans that IV amino acids produce neurotoxicity. However, tissue damage is a serious risk if concentrated solutions are inadvertently injected.

Intravenous fats are processed into triglycerides, then FFAs. Clearance of either may be delayed. Hypertriglyceridemia (triglyceride value >200 mg/dl) may interfere with laboratory biochemical determination and may be a potential factor in the subsequent development of atherosclerosis. In addition, FFA is bound to albumin and may compete with bilirubin binding; however, this is controversial. A few observed cases suggest that a molar ratio of FFA to albumin of less than 6 is safe, but the impact of lipid infusions on bilirubin toxicity is not well defined. As a result lipids may be witheld from neonates with significant jaundice.

A few infants who received lipid infusions have been found to have had intrapulmonary fat emboli. This suggests that babies with acute pulmonary disease and marginal pulmonary reserve should receive lower than normal doses of lipids. Lipid emulsion particles are cleared partly via the reticuloendothelial system. These same cells clear bacteria from the blood; therefore, sepsis may contraindicate IV lipids. Inadvertant subcutaneous infusion of lipids appears to have no long-term effect (15, 16). There are no known contraindications to abrupt discontinuance of either amino acids or IV lipids.

A worrisome complication of PN is cholestatic jaundice. This syndrome is characterized by a direct bilirubin value of >2 mg/dl and elevated liver enzymes. There is evidence that the secretory cell membrane is damaged, perhaps by high sugar infusion, toxic amino acids, or deficits in taurine. Elevated levels of bile acids and alkaline phosphatase usually coexist. This rarely occurs in infants who receive enteral feeds as well as PN and is usually reversible once feeding is resumed and amino acid infusions are reduced. The frequency of occurrence increases with lower gestational ages and longer duration of PN (16).

Ordering TPN

The mechanics of ordering TPN can be fraught with complications. Several approaches have been taken to minimize risks. The first approach has been to formulate standard solutions ordered at standard infusion rates. The weakest solution is given at a low rate, the rate is increased daily for 2 to 3 days, and a stronger solution is begun and then gradually increased. Finally the complete formulation is administered at 50 ml/kg/day. The major problems with this approach have been difficulty in adjusting the electrolyte composition and in dealing with changing fluid requirements. It is not uncommon to find an infant receiving over 4 g/kg/day of amino acids because of increased infusion rates meant to correct dehydration.

A somewhat more tedious but flexible procedure is to construct a specific solution to meet each baby's particular nutritional needs. Figure 3.1 is an example of a worksheet used at Columbia Hospital for Women. Each morning the laboratory results are entered and decisions about nutrient requirements made. The calculations are checked by a physician, a nurse, and the pharmacist. Once the PN solution is running, the rate may be reduced if necessary or may be supplemented with sterile water if increased water intake is necessary.

FIGURE 3.1 **Example of TPN worksheet used at Columbia Hospital for Women.**

Patient Name _____
Na: _____ K: _____ Cl: _____ HCO$_3$: _____ Ca: _____ PO$_4$: _____ Mg: _____ BUN: _____
Caloric intake/kg/day: _____ Clinitest: _____ Weight: _____ (kg) Fluid volume (ml/kg/day): _____
Calculate standard dose correction factor:
_____ kg × _____ ml ÷ _____ ml = . . . (enter on all dotted lines below)
  (wt.)   (to be made)   (to be given)

			Usual maximum amounts (ml) in 200/500/1000 ml of TPN solution
Glucose:	$\begin{bmatrix} \text{\_\_\_ g/kg/day} \times \ldots \times 2 \\ \text{OR} \\ \text{\_\_\_ \% } \times \text{\_\_\_ ml to be made} \div 50 \end{bmatrix}$	= ___ ml D$_{50}$W	80/200/400
Amino acids:	___ g/kg/day × . . . ÷ 0.085	= ___ ml Freamine II (8.5%)	60/150/300
Acetate:	___ mEq/kg/day × . . . ÷ 2.0	= ___ ml NaAc (2 mEq/ml)	2/5/10
PO$_4$:	[(___ mmol/kg/day × . . .) − (.01 × ___ ml)] ÷ 3.0 Freamine	= ___ ml KPO$_4$ (3 mmol/ml)	1.5/3.5/7.0
Na:	[(___ mEq/kg/day × . . .) − (0.1 × ___ ml) − Freamine (2 × ___ ml)] ÷ 2.5 NaAc	= ___ ml NaCl (2.5 mEq/ml)	4/10/20
K:	[(___ mEq/kg/day × . . .) − (4.4 × ___ ml)] ÷ 2.0 KPO$_4$	= ___ ml KCl (2 mEq/ml)	4/10/20
Ca*:	___ mEq/kg/day × . . . ÷ 0.9	= ___ ml Ca gluceptate	4/10/20
Mg:	___ mEq/kg/day × . . . ÷ 0.83	= ___ ml MgSO$_4$ (10%)	2/5/10
MVI:	___ ml/kg/day × . . .	= ___ ml MVI	1.5/3.5/7.0
Folate:	___ mg/kg/day × . . . ÷ 5.0	= ___ ml folate (5 mg/ml)	0.04/0.1/0.2

Trace elements   1 ml
Sufficient quantity of sterile water to reach full volume to be made

* Ca should be added only after most of the sterile water has been added to avoid precipitation.

PROBLEM	The baby is receiving 120 cc/kg/day of PN fluid with 12 g/kg/day of glucose and 2.5 g/kg/day of amino acid. Clinical exam shows that the baby is dehydrated. You wish to administer 144 cc/kg/day of PN fluid (20% increase). What should you do?
SOLUTION	At 144 cc/kg/day the IV rate is 6 cc/kg/hour. An 8-hour volume of fluid would be 48 cc/kg. At the previous rate 40 cc of PN would have been given over 8 hours. By adding 8 cc of sterile water to 40 cc of PN solution and infusing over 8 hours, you have maintained the same PN rate and provided additional free water. To have simply turned up the rate to 6 cc/kg/hour would have increased the intake of all nutrients by 20%, risking hyperglycemia, azotemia, and electrolyte imbalance.

Transition to Enteral Feedings

When making the transition from parenteral to enteral feeding, care should be taken to prevent over- or underdosing of nutrients. Transition is easiest if PN is providing full protein and calories. Simply reducing the intake of PN fluids by 1 cc for each 1 cc of feeding will provide comparable levels of nutrients. Although milks usually have a greater concentration of nutrients than PN, the unabsorbed nutrients in the stool and the calories needed for digestion and absorption will result in comparable net levels of protein and calories. Difficulties may arise if dilute formulas are used or if feedings are introduced before PN has achieved maximal nutrition. In this case it may be necessary to calculate intakes of protein and minerals from both the IV and oral feeds in order to increase the IV strengths without overdosing. Unusual electrolyte needs may require supplementation of formula.

When IV fluid intake is restricted, as in symptomatic PDA, or with concomitant enteral feedings, care must be taken to avoid overly concentrated IV solutions. If an infant is receiving 10 g of glucose, 8 mEq of total salts, and 125 ml of water for each kilogram, reduction of the water to 100 cc/kg/day will increase the osmolality from about 575 to 720. This solution is more than twice normal serum tonicity and very irritating to tissues and veins. It may be necessary to reduce the sugar or electrolyte dose in such instances.

Enteral Feeding

Programs of enteral feedings for premature or sick infants are as varied as are choices in formula. The following discussion is necessarily brief and personalized. Presented first are some basic principles of digestion and absorption and a discussion of breast milk, then some suggestions for instituting feeding with vitamin and mineral supplements. Table 3.7 presents one approach to the enteral feeding of the infant.

Digestion

The enzymes required for digesting disaccharides or polysaccharides develop throughout fetal and neonatal life (17). Sucrase develops first and reaches adult levels by 24–26 weeks gestation. Lactase activity is below adult values until approximately 32 weeks. Full absorption of lactose is not achieved until 2 to 3 weeks of life in preterm infants. Despite this, overt lactose intolerance is rare in neonates of any gestational age. Balance studies show over 98% of the carbohydrate is absorbed. Enzymes for starch digestion develop during the first 6 months of life. Corn syrup solids, partially hydrolyzed or digested, have been added to formulas to increase calories without increasing the osmolality. Current evidence indicates that these oligosaccharides (glucose polymers) are completely processed, although more slowly absorbed than glucose alone.

Protein digestion is dependent on a number of enzymes that also mature late in gestation. The period from 26 to 32 weeks appears to be a critical time. Studies in growing tiny premature infants fed mothers' milk have shown that about 65% of protein nitrogen is retained and 25% is excreted via the kidney, leaving only 10% in the GI tract. The source of protein does not seem to affect digestion, but metabolic efficiency for different proteins is quite variable. For similar amounts of protein,

Table 3.7 Gastric Nutrition: Calorie and Route Recommendations

	Gestational age and birth weight		
	30 weeks (<1251 g)	31–34 weeks (1251–2000 g)	35+ weeks (>20,000 g)
First feed: sterile water	2 cc	3–5 cc	5–10 cc
followed by milk	—	5 cc	5–10 cc
Second feed (milk)	2 cc (½ strength)	5 cc	15–20 cc
Route	gavage	gavage	nipple
Frequency	every 2 hours	every 3 hours	every 3–4 hours
Rate of increase	every 12 hours	every 6–9 hours	every 4 hours
Volume increase	1 cc	2 cc	2–5 cc
Switch to full strength	at ½ desired final volume	—	—
Switch to "hypercaloric"[a] (reduce before discharge)	when growing (if not on breast milk)	when growing	—
Desired calories/kg	110–130	100–120	100
Desired volume (cc)/feed/kg			
0.67 cal/cc	14–16 (every 3 hours)	19–23 (every 3 hours)	25 (every 4 hours)
0.80 cal/cc	12–14 (every 2 hours)	16–19 (every 3 hours)	

[a] Breast milk may be supplemented with formula or medium-chain triglycerides to increase caloric intensity if desired.

breast milk, then whey-predominant cows' milk protein, and finally casein-predominant cows' milk protein seem decreasingly supportive of growth. Vegetable proteins (soy formulas) do not appear to be satisfactory for preterm infants. Casein-predominant formulas are also associated with higher blood urea nitrogen values, lower pH values, and more abnormal plasma amino acid levels in preterm infants when compared to breast milk.

Digestion of lipids depends greatly on the type and source of lipids (18). The longer and more saturated the fatty acid chain, the more lipid is excreted in the stool as FFAs or calcium soaps. Butterfat is poorly absorbed, whereas medium-chain triglycerides (MCT) are the most completely absorbed. Most formulas now contain vegetable oils and MCTs. Breast milk contains long-chain fatty acids with variable saturation, but it also contains lipases activated in the GI tract. These enzymes remain active even when stored in the refrigerator. Lipases allow almost complete (90%) fat absorption. Premature infants also have a preduodenal (lingual) lipase that augments the relatively small amounts of pancreatic lipase. This may explain why nonnutritive sucking during gavage feedings helps weight gain (19).

In the usual intensive care nursery patient, feedings are introduced gradually. The major risks are regurgitation, aspiration, and GI damage. The first is related to the volume introduced into the stomach and the speed of gastric emptying. The ability to coordinate sucking, swallowing, and breathing develops late in gestation; therefore, before about 34 weeks most infants require gavage feeding (see Appendix

3.5 for information). Swallowing and lower esophageal sphincter tone are independent of gestational age; the latter increases as the baby ages. The resting volume of the stomach is about 7 ml/kg (the same as lung tidal volume); therefore, relatively low feeding volumes are indicated when feeding begins. Preterm infants have delayed gastric emptying only during the first 4–12 hours of life, in comparison to term infants. The higher the sugar or fat concentration of the milk, the longer the gastric emptying time. For this reason dilute feedings should be given. Formula dilution also may lower the risk of GI mucosal damage by lowering the osmolality of the milk. The feeding of each baby must be individualized, but Table 3.7 lists suggestions for starting and advancing feedings for different gestational ages and birth weights. The larger the baby, the more quickly feedings can be advanced.

Transpyloric feeding is used infrequently. There are a number of digestive complications reported (20). This type of feeding is best reserved for those infants intolerant of intragastric feedings. (See Appendices 3.6 and 3.7 for information on gastric/jejunal and gastrostromy feeding.) Do not feed infants by any route until at least 24 hours after umbilical catheters have been removed. Expect the abdomen to be soft and bowel sounds to be present; however, stools may not occur until after feeding is started. It may not be desirable to feed infants who are acutely ill (for example, with acute respiratory problems or a symptomatic PDA), but it is acceptable to feed infants who require chronic mechanical ventilation. Specifically, an endotracheal tube does not contraindicate oral feedings.

Breast Milk

Breast milk is the standard against which all formulas fed to term infants have been judged. For preterm infants, controversy rages. Studies about pooled human milk regularly reveal relative deficiencies of protein, calories, and minerals. More recent studies of milk from mothers who deliver prematurely suggest that growth is more than adequate, and overt deficiencies rare. A comparison of mother's milk of 20 cal/oz (67 cal/100 ml) with "premature" formula showed no differences in somatic growth, most serum chemistries, or acid-base balance (21). Serum phosphorus levels were lower and alkaline phosphatase levels higher in the human milk–fed group. No baby developed rickets. A third group fed pooled "mature" milk grew less well and had more abnormal serum chemistries. Balance studies in infants under 1300 g at about 3 weeks of age showed retention rates of fat and protein, as well as weight gain, comparable to fetal accretion rates (22).

Trace elements are found in human milk, and their bioavailabilities are so good that deficiencies while on breast milk feedings are rare. Human milk carnitine levels are higher than formula levels. Because premature infants may be unable to synthesize carnitine, breast milk may be important for maintaining adequate FFA metabolism, which is carnitine dependent. Although formula feeding usually results in plasma amino acid levels consistently higher than human milk feedings, taurine is one notable exception. Taurine levels in breast milk are about 10 times higher than those in formula. Serum taurine levels are 25% higher and urine taurine values three to four times as great on human milk feedings as on formula feedings. The exact significance of relative taurine deficiency is unknown. Taurine alters bile salt metabolism and may lead to high serum cholesterol levels. Animal models of taurine deficiency point to the central nervous system and retina as major sites of taurine incorporation.

In addition to lipases, breast milk also contains an amylase that can process intestinal oligo- and polysaccharides. Much has been written about the anti-infective properties of human milk and the role the mother can play in her infant's care as she provides her milk. Heating breast milk alters several potential beneficial properties, including anti-infective and fat-absorptive properties. Storage of breast milk can also affect its immune properties. Freezing destroys cellular components, and the use of glass bottles reduces the number of white blood cells, which apparently adhere to a glass surface.

Formulas

None of the currently available formulas are ideal for all infants. For term or larger preterm infants almost all modified cow's milk formulas are satisfactory. Even soy-based formulas work; these are occasionally used when there is a strong family history of allergy. There also are lactose-free formulas for infants with lactase deficiency. The small preterm infant (1500–1800 g) has different nutritional requirements. As discussed above, human milk from mothers who deliver prematurely seems acceptable in all but a few ways, because it has higher amounts of protein and electrolytes than "term" milk.

Efforts to modify commercial formulas have been based on the fast growth patterns of preterm infants, higher electrolyte and mineral requirements, and an apparently increased protein requirement. The newer premature formulas seem adequate for the growing low birth weight infant. Current evidence suggests that whey proteins are more easily metabolized than casein proteins. It is important to emphasize that these 24-cal/oz formulas contain larger amounts of minerals and protein nitrogen that, if not utilized for growth, must be excreted by the kidney. Use of these formulas is therefore not recommended for introductory feedings. A reasonable alternative might be to use either standard formula or 20-cal/oz versions of the premature formulas. Lactobezoars have been associated with several hypercaloric formulas. Balance studies in formula-fed premature infants suggest that 115–145 kcal/kg/day are needed for maintenance (50–75 kcal), immature absorption (15 kcal), and to maintain intrauterine rates of growth (50–75 kcal).

Supplementation

Supplementation of formulas to increase caloric density may be indicated when volume restriction is necessary. Both MCT and glucose polymers have been used. MCT should constitute no more than 40% of fats (about 19% of calories). Further substitution of MCT for long-chain triglycerides does not enhance growth despite improved nitrogen and fat absorption. Aspiration pneumonia can occur after MCT oil feedings. Glucose polymers appear well tolerated but might cause hyperglycemia and diarrhea. Another technique is to add powdered formula (concentrate) to liquid formula. This preserves the balance of protein, calories, and minerals but may stress renal concentrating ability. Dosage calculations must be exact.

Even with newer formulas, there is a need for vitamin and perhaps calcium supplementation. Vitamin E is important for its antioxidant property, which influences red cell stability and probably reduces the severity of retinopathy of prematurity. Doses of 10 IU/kg/day by mouth seem necessary for such effects. Intramuscular doses may be necessary for some weeks after birth to maintain the serum levels of 3–7 mg/dl found effective in prevention studies of retinopathy of prematurity. Vitamin E requirements increase when polyunsaturated fats or iron are added to the diet (23).

Since the majority of fetal iron reserves is acquired in the last trimester of pregnancy, preterm infants are at risk for iron deficiency. During acute illnesses, anemia is treated by red blood cell transfusion. Once the infant is feeding, low-iron (1.2–3 mg/L) formulas are used until about 2 months of age, when supplementation with 2 mg/kg of iron as ferrous salts (total dose 4 mg/kg/day at 3 months of age) is begun (24). Larger infants may begin with iron-fortified formula at the time of discharge. Serum iron, total iron binding capacity, transferrin saturation, and serum ferritin remain in the normal range, although hemoglobin levels may not begin to rise until 4 months of age nor rise to "term" levels until 8 months.

Vitamin D, Ca^{2+}, and PO_4^{2-} intimately interact to influence the formation of bone. Intrauterine accretion rates (2.75 mmol/kg/day for PO_4^{2-}) are difficult to achieve, although this has been reported for Ca^{2+} in infants supplemented with calcium lactate (5 mmol/kg) or fed newer premature formulas (25, 26). These contain, per 100 kcal, 178 mg of calcium and 89 mg of phosphorus (Similac Special Care) or 117 mg of calcium and 58.5 mg of phosphorus (Mead Johnson Premature Formula). A little less than half of ingested calcium is absorbed. More than 90% of phosphorus is absorbed (exclusive of soy formulas). Vitamin D levels are also higher in these formulas, but the required dose of vitamin D in the low birth weight infant is unknown.

Several studies suggest that conversion of vitamin D_3 to $25\text{-(OH)-}D_3$ and perhaps of $25\text{-(OH)-}D_3$ to $1,25\text{-(OH)}_2\text{-}D_3$ is impaired in preterm infants. Oral or IV administration of D_3 does not raise serum $25\text{-(OH)-}D_3$ levels until the 36th to 38th postconceptual week. Treatment with 1 μ/kg/day (but not 0.05 μg/kg/day) of $1,25\text{-(OH)}_2\text{-}D_3$ significantly improved calcium homeostasis and absorption in infants $\leq$37 weeks gestation (7). Administration of vitamin D_2 (550–1150 IU/day) beginning at 14 days of life reduced but did not eliminate the incidence of rickets in Japanese infants of 2000–2500 g birth weight, perhaps because of malabsorption and poor conversion to $25\text{-(OH)-}D_3$ (27). Four of 24 supplemented infants who did have rickets had $25\text{-(OH)-}D_3$ levels lower than those without rickets. These values were the same as those in unsupplemented infants, with or without rickets. The use of water-soluble $1\text{-}\alpha\text{-(OH)-}D_3$ (0.1–0.15 mg/kg/day) reduced the incidence of rickets to 0% ($n = 8$) in these infants and to 15% ($n = 13$) in infants of less than 2 kg birth weight. Levels of $1,25\text{-(OH)}_2\text{-}D_3$ were clearly higher in infants supplemented with $1\text{-}\alpha\text{-(OH)-}D_3$ than with vitamin D_2. No infant ($n = 7$) with levels in the normal range or higher (>45 pg/ml) had rickets, whereas all three infants with rickets had low $1,25\text{-(OH)}_2\text{-}D_3$ levels.

Perhaps three recommendations can be made from this confusing literature on vitamin D:

1. Breast milk should be supplemented with vitamin D_3 for term infants if maternal deficiency is likely, skin color is dark, or birth occurred in the spring.
2. Vitamin D_3 is not the formulation of choice in preventing rickets in premature/low birth weight infants. Newer forms of water-soluble, active D_3 metabolites, such as $1\text{-}\alpha\text{-(OH)-}D_3$ or $1,25\text{-(OH)}_2\text{-}D_3$ are preferable.
3. Small infants are at greater risk for rickets, and supplemental minerals are probably more important than vitamin D in its prevention.
4. Phosphorus may yet be shown to be the limiting nutrient in the rapidly growing infant. Early introduction of phosphorus in PN or as enteral feedings is essential. There is little doubt that current feeding regimens will not prevent all cases of rickets.

PROBLEM

A 1000 g infant is now 1 week old and has regained birth weight. The umbilical artery catheter was removed 2 days ago. His ductus arteriosus recently closed. The baby is receiving a PN solution at 135 cc/day that contains 10% dextrose (13.5 g/day) and 2.0 g/day of amino acids. The infant receives 6 mEq/day of NaCl. How do you start feedings?

SOLUTION

Table 3.7 suggests that this infant might be able to tolerate 30 cc [(2 × 6) + (3 × 6)] of water and dilute formula (e.g., 10 cal/oz Similac). This would also provide 0.23 g protein, 1.1 g lactose, and 0.3 mEq sodium. It would be reasonable to rewrite the PN solution to give 2.0 g/day of amino acids, 5.5 mEq/day sodium, and 12.4 g/day glucose in 105 cc/day of water. If PN is given by peripheral vein, the amount of sugar may be reduced to 10 g/day (10% solution) to prevent injury to the vein. The total protein intake rises to 2.2 g/day protein. The next day, at 4 or 5 cc/feed, 20 cal/oz formula is used. This will increase protein to 2.7 g/day. Because the IV rate has been reduced to 75 cc/day to accommodate the 60-cc/day oral feeding, sugar intake is only 11.8 g/day (0.75 dl × 10 g/dl via IV, 0.60 dl × 7.2 g/dl by mouth). The missing calories have been more than replaced by enteral fat. From this time onward, the dose of IV amino acids should be reduced as feedings progress. Each 100 ml of formula contains 1.5 g of protein. At a final volume of 135 cc/day (11 cc every 2 hours achieved at about day 6 or 7), 2.11 g/day of protein is ingested; therefore IV protein should be ≤1g/day. About this time 24 cal/oz formulas may be introduced.

Breastfeeding Premature Infants

Many mothers of preterm infants pump their breasts for months in anticipation of eventually breastfeeding. This pumping experience can be frustrating, but with careful preparation, teaching, and a little luck, many mothers eventually breastfeed their convalescing sick or preterm infants. The following recommendations are based on our own experience, feedback from women who tried to breastfeed their "premies," and routines followed by other institutions.

Pumping Breast Milk

An initial step is to inform the parents that it is very possible to eventually breastfeed their sick or preterm infant. Many women are surprised to learn that they will be able to breastfeed eventually even though there will be delay. The advantage of breast milk must be weighed against the expense of a breast pump and the time commitment required by long-term pumping. Amazingly, many women do opt to pump their breast milk, often reporting later that this was their only tangible tie to their newborn during his acute illness. For some this is painful, because the mother is regularly reminded of the absence of the infant. One mother reported feeling like she had given birth to a machine, another reported that she had intense crying episodes during pumping, but was able to keep calm the rest of the time. Not surprisingly, the latter woman decided to stop pumping her breasts. Nursery personnel need to be aware of such responses so they can give appropriate feedback and support to the woman who is pumping her breasts for milk. For those who can get through this period, however, pumping can eventually lead to the intimacy of breastfeeding mothers long for.

Some concrete information about pumping that needs to be shared includes:

1. Pumping must occur at regular intervals throughout the day (every 2–4 hours) if milk production is to be established and maintained.
2. Each session of pumping should last only as long as milk flows.
3. The volume of breast milk is increased by increasing the frequency of pumping, *not* by pumping the breast after flow has stopped (i.e., increase from pumping every 3 hours to pumping every 2 hours).
4. Decrease milk volume by pumping less often.
5. Showering daily and handwashing prior to pumping is sufficient "prep" of the breasts. Harsh drying soaps or antiseptic agents should not be used on the breasts or nipples.
6. Sterilize the collection bottle on the pump daily.

7. Store milk in sterile plastic containers. The white blood cells in breast milk adhere to glass so the infant will not receive them if the milk is stored in glass containers.
8. Refrigerate milk until delivered to the hospital if it can be used within 24 hours.
9. Freeze milk that cannot be used within 24 hours. Breast milk is nutritionally stable in a home freezer for 2 weeks and bacteriologically stable for 3 months.
10. Label each bottle with the infant's name, the date, and the time that the milk was pumped.

We usually use only fresh breast milk (milk pumped within 24 hours) for sick infants. Fresh breast milk seems advantageous over frozen milk because it contains active immune and enzymatic materials. There are several commercial breast pumps available. In our experience women who use electric pumps have better luck than those who use manual pumps.

As with any kind of patient teaching, repetition and follow-up increase the patient's success. Many women experience a decrease in milk supply at some point during this time. They need to be encouraged to increase the frequency of pumping and to try to rest more. Speaking to another woman who got through this period successfully helps bolster their morale.

Advancing from Gavage to Nipple Feedings

Preterm infants usually will have been tube fed for some period of time before being nipple fed. As a general guideline nipple feedings are not introduced until the infant:

1. Is equal to 34 weeks gestation.
2. Sucks vigorously on a pacifier during gavage feedings. (Interestingly, it has been found that sucking during gavage feeding accelerates the development of an effective suck reflex.)
3. Has no evidence of respiratory distress at rest.

If each of these criteria are met, nipple feedings are gradually introduced. First the infant is fed by nipple once a day, then twice, three times, every other feeding, and so on until the infant is totally nipple fed. One technique is to put a gavage tube in place and taped to the infant's cheek prior to the nipple feeding. Then, if the infant cannot finish feeding by mouth, the tube can be used to complete the feeding. Some infants may have difficulty sucking with a tube in place and need to have the gavage inserted after sucking. Remember, any foreign object in the pharynx can trigger gagging and bradycardia.

We generally do not allow a previously sick infant to suck for longer than 30 minutes. They tend to get exhausted when pushed beyond this time interval. Instead they are nipple fed for 30 minutes, until they finish their feeding, or until they stop suckling, whichever comes first. Parents need to be encouraged during this time to believe that their infant will eventually develop sufficient strength to suck vigorously.

Advancing from Nipple to Breast Feedings

When nipple feeding by bottle begins the parents should be prepared for the introduction of breast feedings. Even after weeks and sometimes months of pumping breast milk, this possibility can seem unreal to parents. Mothers may even find themselves reluctant to attempt breastfeeding when it becomes a reality even though they had dreamed of it for months. This is an understandable reaction considering the extent of anxiety associated with the infant's survival and perceptions about her own capacity to be a successful parent. Warning mothers well before attempting to put the infant to breast will allow them time to overcome some of these feelings. The criteria we use for putting the infant to breast are:

1. The infant is able to finish at least one bottle feeding per day within 30 minutes.
2. The infant has been gaining weight regularly since nipple feedings were introduced.

Both of these criteria are reflections of how well the infant is able to suck and how much work it is for him. We feel that once the infant has met these criteria he can be breastfed. We find the sooner breastfeeding is introduced the more successful mother and baby are at it.

   Preterm infants often take more time to adjust to breastfeeding than term infants. It is important that parents be aware of this so they do not become discouraged when the infant is acting like a "premie." We generally tell parents it can take as long as 2 weeks before their baby is totally breastfed. This allows the infant plenty of time to learn. In fact, parents of babies who learn in less time are pleased that their babies are so "smart." Parents who are not informed of the difference between term and premature infants in this regard may give up after the first or second discouraging try. In otherwords, breastfeeding will become a negative rather than a positive experience unless you anticipate problems the infant might have in learning this task.

   Several hints may help both the mother and baby learn breastfeeding successfully:

1. Make sure the mother has not pumped immediately prior to putting the infant to breast.
2. Have the mother manually express a few drops of milk before offering the breast so the infant will smell the milk, root more successfully, and receive milk with the first suck.
3. If the infant is small, have the mother hold her baby in a "football" grip with the infant's body in the crook of her arm and the infant's head in her hand. In this position the infant's mouth can be directed toward the breast and the baby will be less likely to become frustrated because of random rooting. The infant's nose is also less likely to become covered by the breast in this position.
4. Provide the mother with a quiet area to breastfeed. Ideally a room adjacent to the NICU would be helpful, but if this is not possible a screen can be used to reduce distractions.
5. Supplement after breastfeeding with the mother's own breast milk, but do not force feed. Supplementation can be stopped when the infant is breastfeeding a total of 15 minutes.
6. Weigh infants daily for growth, but avoid weighing the infant before and after feedings to judge the amount of milk taken. Instead, encourage the mother to observe the amount of urine and stool the baby passes as a measure that the baby "got something."
7. Encourage the mother to plan on breastfeeding as often as possible.
8. When possible, put the baby to breast on demand rather than allowing the infant to become exhausted from crying while waiting for the next feeding.

Conclusions

Fluid therapy and nutrition are clinically intertwined. Consideration of both must be made when IV or enteral support is provided. The smaller the patient, the more narrow his tolerance limits. Water and electrolyte balance in such neonates is very important. Many technical difficulties must be overcome before homeostasis is maintained in the smallest infants. Deficiencies of almost all minerals and vitamins are unusual and easily prevented; Ca^{2+} and PO_4^{2-} are exceptions. Parenteral nutrition may be lifesaving, but has complications and an uncertain impact on the developing brain. Breast milk, always the feeding standard for infants over 5 pounds, fell into disfavor when the use of pooled human milk during the 1960s and 1970s to feed very premature infants proved inadequate. Research during the past 5 years has shown that mother's milk is more effective for nourishing premature infants than pooled breast milk. As the use of mother's milk for preterm infants regain favor, it is rewarding to recall old advice:

> The food for the child in this artificial nursing, is the same we have already recommended . . . namely, the cow's milk, water, and sugar. . . . But the nearer we can approach the qualities of the breast milk, the better will be our compound; for nature has declared that to be the best possible pablum for the child. . . . (Dewees, 1825)

Breast milk may yet prove to be best!

References

1. Harkavy KL: Water and electrolyte requirements of the very low birthweight infant. Perinatal Press 6:47–50, 1982.
2. Jones MD Jr., Gresham EL, Battaglia FC: Urinary flow rates and urea excretion rates in newborn infants. Biol Neonate 21:321–329, 1972.
3. Bell EF, Rios GR: A double-walled incubator alters the partition of body heat loss of premature infants. Pediatr Res 17:135–140, 1983.
4. Sulyok E, Varga R, Gyory E, et al.: On the mechanism of renal sodium handling in newborn infants. Biol Neonate 37:75–79, 1978.
5. Arant BS: Developmental patterns of renal functional maturation compared in the human neonate. Pediatrics 93:705–712, 1978.
6. Tsang RC, Steichen JJ, Brown DR: Perinatal calcium homeostasis: Neonatal hypocalcemia and bone demineralization. Clin Perinatol 4:385–409, 1977.
7. Steichen JJ, Gratton TL, Tsang RC: Osteopenia of prematurity: The cause and possible treatment. J Pediatrics 96:528–534, 1980.
8. Dancis J, O'Connel JR, Holt LE Jr.: A grid for recording the weight of premature infants. J Pediatr 33:570–572, 1948.
9. Harkavy KL, Scanlon JW: Hypernatremia in the very low birthweight infant. Int J Pediatr Nephrol 4:75–78, 1983.
10. Heird WC, Anderson TL: Nutritional requirements and methods of feeding low birth weight infants. Curr Probl Pediatr 7:8, 1977.
11. Zlotkin SH, Bryan MH, Anderson GH: Intravenous nitrogen and energy intake required to duplicate in utero nitrogen accretion in prematurely born human infants. Pediatrics 99:115–120, 1981.
12. Raiha NC: Biochemical basis for nutritional management of preterm infants. Pediatrics 53:147–155, 1974.
13. Committee on Nutrition, American Academy of Pediatrics: Use of intravenous fat emulsions in pediatric patients. Pediatrics 68:738–743, 1981.
14. Dhanireddy R, Hamosh M, Sivasubramanian KN, et al.: Postheparin lipolytic activity and intralipid clearance in very low-birth weight infants. Pediatrics 98:617–622, 1981.
15. Vileisis RA, Inwood RJ, Hunt CE: Prospective controlled study of parenteral nutrition associated cholestatic jaundice: Effect of protein intake. J Pediatr 96:893–897, 1980.
16. Black DD, Suttle EA, Whitington PF, et al.: The effect of short-term total parenteral nutrition on hepatic function in the human neonate: A prospective randomized study demonstrating alteration of hepatic canalicular function. Pediatrics 99:445–449, 1981.
17. Lebenthal E, Lee PC, Heitlinger LA: Impact of development of the gastrointestinal tract on infant feeding. Pediatrics 102:1–9, 1983.

18. Hamosh M: Fat digestion in the newborn: Role of lingual lipase and preduodenal digestion (a review). Pediatr Res 13:615–622, 1983.

19. Bernbaum JC, Pereiria CR, Watkins JB, et al.: Non nutritive sucking during gavage feeding enhances growth and maturation in premature infants. Pediatrics 71:41–45, 1983.

20. Whitfield MF: Poor weight gain of the low birthweight infant fed nasojejunally. Arch Dis Child 57:597–601, 1982.

21. Gross SJ: Growth and biochemical response of preterm infants fed human milk or modified infant formula. N Engl J Med 308:237–241, 1983.

22. Atkinson SA, Bryan MH, Anderson GH: Human milk feeding in premature infants: Protein, fat, and carbohydrate balances in the two weeks of life. J Pediatr 99:617–624, 1981.

23. Bell EF, Brown EJ, Milner R, et al.: Vitamin E absorption in small premature infants. Pediatrics 63:830–831, 1979.

24. Siimes MA, Jarvenpaa A: Prevention of anemia and iron deficiency in very low-birth weight infants. J Pediatr 101:277–280, 1982.

25. Atkinson SA, Radde IC, Anderson GH: Macromineral balances in premature infants fed their own mothers' milk or formula. J Pediatr 102:99–106, 1983.

26. Shenai JP, Reynolds JW, Babson SG: Nutritional balance studies in very-low birthweight infants: Enhanced nutrient retention rates by an experimental formula. Pediatrics 66:233–238, 1980.

27. Seino Y, Ishii T, Shimotsuji T, et al.: Plasma active vitamin D concentration in low birthweight infants with rickets and its response to vitamin D treatment. Arch Dis Child 56:628–632, 1981.

Suggested Reading

American Academy of Pediatrics: Pediatric Nutrition Handbook. American Academy of Pediatrics, Evanston, IL, 1979.

Easton LB, Halata MS, Dweck HS: Parenteral nutrition in the newborn: A practical guide. Pediatr Clin North Am 29:1171–1190, 1982.

Fischer JE (ed): Total Parenteral Nutrition. Little, Brown, Boston, 1976.

Fomon SJ (ed): Infant Nutrition, 2nd ed. Saunders, Philadelphia, 1974.

Lebenthal E (ed): Textbook of Gastroenterology and Nutrition in Infancy. Raven Press, New York, 1981.

Measel CP, Anderson GC: Non nutritive sucking during tube feeding: Effect on clinical course in premature infants. JOGN Sept/Oct:265–272, 1979.

Wing JP: Human versus cow's milk in infant nutrition and health. Nutrition and health update. Curr Probl Pediatr 8:3–50, 1977.

Winters RW (ed): The Body Fluids in Pediatrics. Little, Brown, Boston, 1983.

Appendices

The following appendices provide Columbia Hospital for Women nursing care guidelines for specific techniques for fluid and nutritional support. They can be modified as required.

Appendix 3.1
Intravenous Therapy

Purpose

1. To provide fluids and nutrients to an infant unable to tolerate GI intake, or to supplement oral feedings.
2. For the administration of drugs by the parenteral route.

Policy

1. All IVs must be infused with a pump.
2. All infants with an IV must have intake and output measurements: weigh diapers dry, then weigh again after voiding (1 g equals 1 cc of urine).
3. Check urine for specific gravity, Clinitest, glucose, blood, protein, ketones, and pH at least every 8 hours.
4. Dextrostix every 8 hours with IV fluids, every 4 hours with TPN.
5. Any peripheral IV site that appears infiltrated may be removed by a nurse.
6. Change tubing every 24 hours.

Procedure

1. To start IV, assemble the following equipment:
   a. Infusion
   b. Needle
   c. Sterile syringe with flush solution: dextrose (5%) in water (D_5W)
   d. Arm board
   e. Tape cut to appropriate sizes
   f. Sterile 2 × 2, alcohol, and Betadine swabs
   g. Rubber band
   h. Razor blade (for scalp vein site)
   i. IV tubing with 22 mμ filter
   j. 50-cc syringe with ordered solution
   k. Medicine cup cut in half with padded edges
2. To prevent heat loss, place infant under radiant heat source while procedure is in progress.

3. Set up pump with filled tubing in place, set rate, and switch to "on" position. Eliminate all air from tubing. Label the syringe with date, time, initials, type of solution, and amount and type of any additives (i.e., electrolytes).
4. Prepare IV site for placing needle:
   a. Shave head, *or* tape extremity to board
   b. Prep site with alcohol or Betadine
5. Apply pressure above vein with a rubber band tourniquet or finger. Insert the needle. Tape the needle securely to prevent accidental dislocation.
6. Reconfirm patency of IV needle by checking for blood return and/or flushing needle with D_5W.
7. IV orders are to be written in cubic centimeters per hour. Each hour check and record the amount of fluid infused.
8. All IV tubings, stopcocks, and filters are to be changed daily. The tubing changes should be noted in the comment column of the IV sheet.
9. When an IV needle is removed, pressure should be applied to the IV site until the bleeding stops and then a Band-Aid applied.

Appendix 3.2
IV Filter Procedure

Purpose

To filter IV solution being administered to infant to prevent contaminants from entering the circulatory system.

Recommendations

1. A 22-mμ filter is to be used on all parenteral solutions.
2. Intralipid should not be infused through a filter.
3. All filters are changed every 24 hours along with all IV connecting tubes.

Procedure

1. Using aseptic technique, assemble syringe with IV solution and extension tubing.
2. Attach IV tubing to filter.
3. Remove protector from extension set adapter.
4. Hold filter upright, fill set, and expel air bubbles.
5. Attach to umbilical catheter or IV.
6. Put syringe in IV pump and adjust setting.
7. Change filter every 24 hours with tubing.

Appendix 3.3
Parenteral Lipid Administration

Purpose

To provide adequate calories and lipid for growth and repair of cells.

1. Intralipid (Cutter) is a 10% soybean oil fat emulsion that provides 1.1 cal/ml.
2. Liposyn (Abbott) is a 10% safflower oil fat emulsion that provides 1.1 cal/ml.
3. Travamulsion (Tavenol) is a 10% soy base fat emulsion that provides 1.1 cal/ml.

Procedure

General:

1. Order the amount from the pharmacy required for each 24-hour period.
2. Refrigerate when not in use.
3. Check the bottle for lipid/solute separation. Do not give if any separation is noted.

Nursing care:

1. Infuse lipid piggyback in main IV line with 25-gauge needle inserted into rubber stopper using aseptic technique. Do not filter. Keep lipid line elevated above TPN line to keep lipids from floating up and clogging TPN filter.
2. Daily triglyceride levels must be drawn to monitor the infant's ability to metabolize intralipids. Blood triglyceride level should not be drawn sooner than 2 hours after the infusion has ended to prevent an erroneously high level.
3. No blood work should be drawn *while* lipid is infusing, unless it is an emergency situation (i.e., blood gases). Lipids interfere with many lab tests.
4. Medications should not be given while IV lipid is infusing. Clear line if necessary to give medication during fat infusion.
5. Observe for adverse effects of lipid:
   a. Infection or infiltration at IV site.
   b. Misinterpretation of lab values drawn while lipid is infusing.

Appendix 3.4
TPN Guidelines

General

1. Reorder solution every 24 hours.
2. Keep refrigerated when not in use.
3. Discard after 24 hours.

Nursing Care

1. Clinitest, Multistix, and specific gravity on urine every 4 hours.
2. Dextrostix every 4 hours.
3. Examine the infant for signs of adequate fluid intake (see "Observations for Hydration Status," Table 3.3).
4. Check to see that daily and weekly blood work ordered is drawn by laboratory:
   a. Daily: electrolytes, hematocrit, glucose, blood urea nitrogen, calcium.
   b. Weekly: bilirubin, serum glutamic-oxaloacetic transaminase (SGOT), serum glutamic-pyruvic transaminase (SGPT), albumin.
5. Use a 22-mμ terminal filter; change every 24 hours.
6. Change pump syringe, filter, and tubing every 24 hours. Mark with name of solution and date. Draw up solution in laminar flow hood and keep bottle capped when using syringe pump system.
7. Do not interrupt line unless absolutely *necessary* and use strict aseptic technique when doing so.
8. Check to see that infant is receiving weekly vitamin therapy as ordered, including vitamin K and vitamin B_{12} IM.
9. Use caution when giving sodium bicarbonate IV push. If there is calcium in the solution, the sodium bicarbonate will combine with it to form a precipitate. Flush the line before and after giving bicarbonate.
10. Cover hyperalimentation solutions containing multivitamins with aluminum foil to prevent destruction of vitamins by photoxidation.
11. Observe infant for such adverse effects of TPN as:
    a. Electrolyte imbalance
    b. Hyperglycemia
    c. Hypoglycemia—usually associated with IV infiltrates or when the appropriate TPN solution is not available
    d. Fluid overload or dehydration
    e. Liver cholestasis: reflected in rising bilirubin, SGOT, and/or SGPT levels
    f. Metabolic acidosis
    g. Infection—local (at infusion site) or septicemia
    h. Incompatibility with other drugs—TPN solutions are usually acidic and so should not be mixed with drugs with an alkaline pH
    i. Infiltration of IV, and slough of tissue

Appendix 3.5
Feeding by Gavage

Purpose

1. To provide a method of meeting the nutritional needs of infants unable to feed by nipple.
2. To give medications directly into the stomach when desired.

Recommendations

All infants in the following groups should be enterally fed by gavage at least initially:

1. Infants <34 weeks gestational age
2. Infants unable to coordinate suck-swallow actions
3. Infants with respiratory distress
4. Infants on mechanical respiratory support
5. Nipple-fed infants showing signs of nipple intolerance (at the discretion of an R.N.)

Equipment

#5 or #8F feeding catheter
20-cc syringe
5-cc syringe
Container with measured amount of formula
Any *per os* medications ordered at this time
Sterile water
Stethoscope

Procedures	*Rationale*
1. Procedures such as measuring abdominal girth and weights, and Dextrostix testing should be done before feeding.	
2. Before each feeding measure tube for placement: a. Turn head to side and measure from tip of ear lobe to nose, then to xyphoid process. b. Label this length with tape on the tubing.	2. To place tube into stomach and avoid accidental insertion into the duodenum and possible perforation.
3. Insert tube through the mouth after lubricating tip with sterile water to measured length. Observe infant's heart rate while tube is passed. a. If bradycardia occurs persistently with each feeding, the tube may be taped and left in for 8 hours. b. Tube must be labeled with time and date.	3. Lubrication reduces irritation from insertion of foreign object. Bradycardia may occur from vagal stimulation. The oral route of tube feeding should be used because an infant's nares are easily traumatized. Infants who gag continuously when an oral-gastric tube is inserted may require a nasal gavage tube.

Procedures

4. Check for tube placement:
   a. Inject small amount of air while listening with stethoscope for bubbling in stomach area.
   b. Gently aspirate for gastric content with the 5-cc syringe.

5. Aspirate the stomach after the tube is placed and assess the character and quantity of gastric contents.
   a. If blood- or bile-stained mucus or solid milk curds are aspirated, notify M.D. before proceeding with feeding.
   b. Liquid undigested milk should be refed. If the volume of residual is <1 cc, refeed it and give total feeding. If the residual is >1 cc, then refeed it and check with the physician as to whether to subtract the volume of residual from the feeding volume or whether to feed the ordered amount of feeding.

6. Medications should be given first in a small volume of milk. Do not mix them together. *NOTE:* Medium-chain triglyceride oil should be mixed with formula.

7. Remove the 5-cc syringe from the gavage tube. Remove the plunger from the 20-cc syringe and attach the 20-cc barrel to the gavage tube.

8. Elevate the head of the bed; then, with the infant positioned on his right side, fill the syringe barrel with the appropriate amount of formula. Hold the syringe 4–6 inches above the infant's head. Start the feeding by gentle pushing with plunger, but once milk flow starts remove the plunger and feed by gravity.

9. Time allowed for feeding should be the same time as allowed for a nipple feed.
   a. Offer pacifier while milk is going in.
   b. If regurgitation or bradycardia occurs, stop the feeding imme-

Rationale

4. Ensuring proper placement of the tube in the stomach reduces the potential for aspiration.

5. Checking abdominal contents before meals will demonstrate whether character or amount is abnormal.
   a. Blood or bile in residual may indicate a seriously compromised GI tract; feeding orders need to be reevaluated in light of this.
   b. Gastric contents are rich in electrolytes and should *not* be routinely discarded.

6. Since some medications will react when put in solution together, each should be fed separately. *NOTE:* Vitamin E and iron will interfere with the absorption of each other and should be given at different feeding times.

7. Be sure to remove plunger before attaching the feeding tube to prevent tissue damage from excessive negative suction.

8. The feeding may create vagal stimulation or vomiting if given too fast or pushed. Gastric trauma may result from pushing.

9. Avoid expanding the stomach rapidly because this could cause vagal bradycardia, respiratory compromise, and/or emesis. *NOTE:* By offering a pacifier to the infant during tube feedings the infant is encouraged to establish the suck-swallow

Procedures

diately and proceed only if the infant restabilizes promptly.

10. To remove tubing after completion of feeding, pinch off or cap the tube and remove slowly and gently. (It may be left in for as long as 8 hours. This is recommended only if a hypersensitive vagal response is noted when the tube is passed.)
11. Burp the infant after feeding if the infant's condition permits.
12. Place the infant in a prone position, or alternatively, on the right side, with the head elevated and well propped so the infant cannot roll backward.

13. Chart the amount, type, time of feeding, and any medication or additive on flow sheet along with the amount of any residual. Chart character of residual, whether refed, and regurgitation or any other unusual occurrence on the nurses' notes.

Rationale

reflex. Sucking also helps the infant relax, which enhances milk flow.
10. To prevent vagal response as well as reflux, regurgitation, and/or aspiration.

11. To remove air from stomach and simulate oral feeding routine.
12. To reduce potential for spitting up and aspirating and to improve digestion. Digestion occurs maximally in a prone position and more effectively on the right than the left side.
13. Maximize communication so that trends in feeding problems can be identified early or tolerance documented so that nutrition can be advanced.

Appendix 3.6
Continuous Feedings: Gastric or Jejunal

Purpose

1. To instill small amounts of milk into the stomach when larger volumes compromise respirations.
2. To provide feedings to the infant when it is necessary to bypass the stomach.

Procedure

Insertion of oral-gastric tube—follow gavage procedure but use a soft Silastic tube and tape securely.

Insertion of jejunal tube

1. Equipment
   a. Silastic tubing—lumen size as prescribed by infant's age and weight and premeasured to infant's heel-to-nose length
   b. 15- or 18-gauge Intramedic Luer Stub Adapter
   c. Adhesive tape
   d. 5-cc syringe
   e. Saline
2. Tube placement
   a. Cut side holes at jejunal end of tube.
   b. Premeasure and flag the tubing the length of the infant's nose-to-heel measurement.
   c. Insert the tube as with a gastric tube. When the tube is in the stomach, place the infant on the right side and stroke his abdomen from the left side of the abdomen toward the right side to encourage the tube to pass through the pyloric valve. Stop at premarked point.
   d. Position the infant on his right side, as perpendicular to the bed as possible, until the tube is passed into the jejunum.
   e. Advance the tube 1 cm at a time to the tape marker; aspirate after the tube is in. Measure and record the pH of the fluid obtained.
   f. If an alkaline pH (>6) is obtained, the tube is in the jejunum.
   g. If the fluid pH is acidic after 2 hours, remove the tube. It is most likely curled in the stomach.
3. Tape the tube securely to cheek with adhesive tape. Place stockinette mittens on an active infant's hands to keep him from pulling out the tube.
4. Assist with x-rays for the tube placement if ordered. If Gastrografin solution is to be instilled for x-ray, draw up 1 cc of Gastrografin in a 5-cc syringe and add 4 cc of sterile water to the Gastrografin. Mix this solution thoroughly in syringe. Attach the syringe to the adapter of the feeding tube. Inject 1 cc of solution immediately before the x-ray is taken and aspirate the entire amount of radiopaque dye immediately after the film. (*NOTE:* Use of Gastrographin is not routine and is done only with a specific order.)

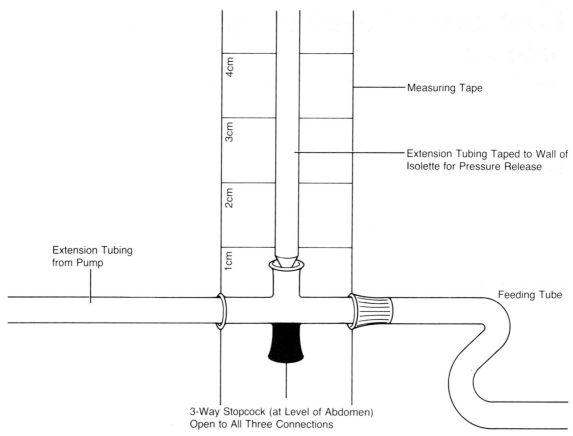

FIGURE 3.2   **Stopcock setup for continuous feeding.**

Continuous Feeding

1. Measuring pressure—Connect 3-way stopcock to the feeding tube adapter, and attach extension tubings as Figure 3.2 indicates. Note that placement of a 3-way stopcock in the line between the feeding tube and extension tube creates a pressure release point.
   a. Change extension tubings and 3-way stopcock once every 24 hours.
   b. Tape a centimeter measuring tape or stick to the side of the isolette with the zero at the level of the infant's midapical line. The third tubing attached to the stopcock should be taped along side the measuring tape. Any resistance to the feeding will be reflected in milk backup in this "pop-off" line (see Figure 3.2).
   c. If milk backs up higher than 10 cm, the infusion pump should be shut off, the line flushed, and the feeding stopped until the backup is less than 10 cm.
2. Maintain continuous feedings as ordered at the hourly rate prescribed with an infusion pump. Keep a running total volume of feedings on the data sheet.
3. Record pertinent nursing observations on nurses' notes. Observe for, record, and report immediately any of the following:
   a. Vomiting
   b. Distention
   c. Backup of more than 10 cm of feeding into pressure release tubing
   d. Blood in gastric aspirate
   e. Frank blood in stools or guaiac-positive stools (guaiac-test all stools)
   f. Loose stools
   g. Apnea or bradycardia

Appendix 3.7
Gastrostomy Feeding

Purpose

To provide GI feeding to an infant through a surgically established gastrostomy.

Equipment

1. 20-cc syringe
2. Feeding solution as prescribed
3. Medications as prescribed

Procedure

Prepare infant:

1. Take vital signs.
2. Prop infant on right side.

Administer feeding:

1. Attach 20-cc syringe.
2. Unclamp gastrostomy tube.
3. Aspirate gastric contents to check for residual or prior feeding. *NOTE:* Check with physician about whether residual should be refed or discarded.
4. Inject any medications directly into the tube ahead of the feeding.
5. Attach barrel of 20-cc syringe to gastrostomy tube.
6. Pour desired volume of feeding into barrel.
7. Allow feeding to flow into stomach by gravity very slowly.
   a. If infant begins to regurgitate fluid at any time, terminate feeding immediately.
   b. After the feeding is in, suspend syringe barrel from side of isolette 10 cm above level of the infant and leave unclamped for 1 hour.
   c. If no reflux has been noted for an hour after feeding, the tube should then be clamped.
   d. Offer a nipple to the infant during the feeding. Infants deprived of sucking may not establish appropriate sucking reflexes. Sucking also enhances peristalsis.

Nursing Care of Gastrostomy Site

1. Cleanse stoma daily with water and a small amount of soap. Peroxide should be used to clean any crustiness from the site.
2. Examine the sutures that secure the tube to determine if they are intact. The surgeon should be informed if the sutures appear to be deteriorating or have become loose.
3. Dress stoma with Betadine ointment while it is healing. Once the stoma is healed postoperatively, no antibacterial ointment will be necessary.
4. After each feeding, wipe the stoma and skin free of formula.
5. The stoma should be checked periodically for leakage of gastric contents around the tube. If this occurs, Vaseline should be used to protect the skin and the stoma, and the surgeon should be notified. (A pH <4 would indicate gastric contents.)

4

Central Nervous System Development and Dysfunction in the Newborn

Kathleen B. Scanlon

In order to understand the nursing needs of infants with central nervous system (CNS) dysfunction, it is important for the nurse to have a working knowledge of fetal growth and development. The first section of this chapter addresses this issue. Then detailed discussions of asphyxia and major problems of the CNS, including intracranial hemorrhage, seizures, and drug withdrawal, are presented. Nursing care of the infant at high risk for neurological problems is discussed next. Finally, an explanation of the Brazelton Neonatal Behavioral Assessment Scale and infant stimulation presented. Three case studies summarize and complete the chapter.

Brain Development

As survival of premature infants of earlier gestational ages increases, the need for the intensive care nurse to understand CNS development is crucial. Development of the CNS is a continuous process beginning 3 weeks after conception and continuing into the second or third decade of life. CNS development can be broken down into six major events:

1. Dorsal induction
2. Ventral induction
3. Neuronal proliferation
4. Migration
5. Organization
6. Myelination

Dorsal Induction

Dorsal induction is the initial formation of the neural tube. It begins on the dorsal aspect of the embryo as a plate of tissue that differentiates in the middle of the ectoderm (outer layer) during the third and fourth weeks after conception. The lateral margins of the neural plate close in to form the neural tube. The fusion begins centrally and proceeds in both cephalic and caudal directions. Fusion of the lumbar area occurs last. Different regions of the brain develop as a series of flexures in the neural tube. The midbrain flexure appears during the third week. Brainstem flexures appear at about 30 days of gestation. Disorders during this period of CNS development include anencephaly, myelomeningocele, and encephalocele. They are often accompanied by alterations in skeletal, meningiovascular, and dermal coverings.

Ventral Induction

Ventral induction is the second major event of CNS development. This takes place during the fifth and sixth weeks of gestation. There are four major developments during this time. The face and forebrain evolve from prechordal mesoderm. The prosencephalon divides into paired optic vessicles and olfactory bulbs and tracts. The telencephalon divides into paired cerebral hemispheres, lateral ventricles, and basal ganglia. The diencephalon divides into the thalamus and hypothalamus at this time.

Disorders of development during this period fall into two major categories, holoprosencephalies and faciotelencephalic formations. Holoprosencephalies are severe and involve malformation of both telencephalon and diencephalon. In 30% of holoprosencephalic infants there is no unusual facial anomaly. Facial anomalies in the most severe cases are a single eye or no nose. Less severe cases may show widely set eyes with a flat, single-nostril nose and cleft lip.

The clinical features of holoprosencephaly are frequent apnea, stimulus-sensitive tonic seizures, almost total absence of neurological development, and death during infancy. Abnormalities in other organ systems occur in three-fourths of these cases. Holoprosencephaly occurs in trisomy and mosaic trisomy 13, deletion 13, trisomy and deletion 18, and ring 18, and may occur sporadically in the general population. Holoprosencephaly also occurs in families as an autosomal recessive disorder.

Faciotelencephalic malformations are diseases characterized by odd facies and abnormal brains. The neuropathology of many of these has yet to be discovered (1). The most severe form, atelencephalic-aprosencephalic microcephaly, is characterized by absence of cerebral hemispheres and thalamus. It is extremely rare. These infants show no neurological development and die during infancy.

Neuronal Proliferation

Neuronal proliferation is the third phase of CNS development. It is divided into two phases. The first begins at about 10 weeks gestation and continues to about 18 weeks. The second phase, which is called glial proliferation, begins at about 30 weeks gestation and continues beyond 1 year of age postnatally. This second phase is discussed under the fifth phase of development: organization.

At about 10 weeks, neuronal cells lying deep in the ventricular area of the developing CNS begin to increase their deoxyribonucleic acid content, migrate toward the surface to the neural tube lumen, and divide into two cells. Then both cells migrate back to the outer edge of the ventricular zone.

Major disorders during this period of development include microencephaly and macroencephaly. The microencephaly of this disorder is caused by disruption in the neuronal proliferation in the fetus and is not the same type of microcephaly associated with maternal viral disease such as rubella or with early neonatal disease in the infant. It may be caused by teratogenic agents such as irradiation. Intellectual development is affected, but motor problems and seizures are not present. The macroencephaly of this phase of development results in an infant who has an abnormally large head at birth. The head continues to grow at an abnormally rapid rate. Neurological deficits may not be present, and motor development and intelligence are in the normal range in 50% of the cases.

Migration

Migration is the fourth event during normal CNS development. Its peak occurrence is between 12 and 24 weeks of gestation. During this phase millions of cells migrate from their sites of origin in the ventricular and subventricular zones to their permanent sites in the CNS. There are two forms of cell migration: radial and tangential. These occur in both the cerebrum and cerebellum. Radial migration in the cerebrum involves migration of cells from the ventricular and subventricular zones to form the cortex and deep nuclear structures. Tangential migration in the cerebrum involves migration from the germinal zones, over the external surface of the cortex and then inward. This layer of cells reaches its maximum width at 22 weeks and gives rise to small cells of the superficial cortex. In the cerebellum, radial migration of cells forms the external granular layer. These cells then migrate inward to form the internal granular layer of the cerebellar cortex.

All disorders at this stage of development lead to mental retardation, seizures, and spasticity. In schizencephaly there is agenesis of part of the cerebral wall with bilateral clefts. In lissencephaly the brain has few or no gyri. In pachygyria the gyri are few and have an abnormally thick cortical plate. In ploymicrogyria the gyri are many times the normal number but extremely small, and infants with this disorder have generalized weakness with absent higher level responses to visual, auditory, or tactile stimuli. Neuronal heterotropias, which are collections of arrested nerve cells in subcortical white matter, are found to accompany the more severe migrational disorders.

Organization

Organization is the fifth phase in normal CNS development. The peak time for its occurrence is from 24 weeks gestation to a year or more after birth. Organization continues to take place for many years in the human cerebrum. During this phase there are four major events: 1) attainment of proper cortical neuronal alignment, orientation, and layering; 2) development of axonal and dendritic spines; 3) establishment of synapses; and 4) proliferation and differentiation of glial cells (or supporting cells). The rapid increase in dendritic and axonal spines resulting in synapse formation during the last part of gestation is associated with increase in the cortical area and an increasing complexity of the convolutional pattern in the cortex. During this period the cerebral ribonucleic acid content multiplies. These maturational changes occur rapidly in the hippocampus, which includes the olfactory lobes. They occur more slowly in limbic and supralimbic lobes where major neuronal association areas are located.

Disorders of the organization phase show as severe defects in dendritic branching and synapses, particularly decreased number and length, and abnormal spatial arrangement. Children with these disorders show severe mental retardation, infantile myoclonic seizures, and hypsarrhythmia on an electroencephalogram. Dendritic and axonal abnormalities have been reported in children with trisomy 21 (2). Organizational defects have also been shown in congenital rubella, phenylketonuria, trisomy 13–15, and Rubinstein-Taybi syndrome (broad toe, broad thumb, beaklike nose, hypotonia, and mental retardation).

Myelination

Myelination is the sixth process of normal CNS development. It continues for the longest period, beginning during the second trimester of pregnancy and continuing into the third decade of adult life. This process begins with the rapid production of oligodendrocytes, which are the cells responsible for myelin formation. After their formation, myelination of nerve cells begins in the peripheral nervous system where motor roots myelinate before sensory roots. Myelination in the CNS begins in the sensory system before major motor systems and occurs well before birth. Myelination in the cerebral hemispheres, especially in the regions of associative functions and sensory discrimination, does not begin until after birth and continues for decades. There is no known developmental disorder of myeline formation in humans. However, there is one disease in which the primary disturbance is in myelination—cerebral white-matter hypoplasia (3). Early in life these infants demonstrate spastic quadriplegia and severe mental impairment that is nonprogressive. Seizures are present from the newborn period onward.

Disturbances in myelination have been reported in other conditions such as phenylketonuria and other amino or organic acidopathies, congenital rubella, and Rubinstein-Taybi syndrome. There are also data demonstrating reduction of myelin lipids in cerebral white matter in premature infants who have been malnourished during the neonatal period. What effects perinatal insults may have on the developing nervous system of the premature infant needs further investigation.

Asphyxia

Brain function is dependent upon a constant input of oxygen and nutrients from the blood. There are two major ways in which oxygen flow may be interrupted. The first is by hypoxemia, a diminished amount of oxygen in the blood. The second is by ischemia, which is diminished blood perfusing the brain. Most of the time during the perinatal period, hypoxemia and ischemia occur as a result of asphyxia. Asphyxia is an impairment in the exchange of oxygen and carbon dioxide, resulting in decreased levels of oxygen and acidosis.

The vascular network in the human cerebrum is composed of paired carotid arteries joining with the basilar artery to form the circle of Willis. Three major branches (anterior, middle, and posterior cerebral arteries) supply the cerebral hemispheres and the diencephalon. Branches of the basilar artery and the paired vertebral arteries supply the brainstem and cerebellum. Although the major cerebral arteries communicate with each other on the surface of the cortex, branches that feed the inner cortex end in the specific areas they serve. There is little or no overlap from neighboring blood vessels in these areas. These isolated "border zones" are particularly sensitive to ischemia. There are also similar border zones in the cerebellum and brainstem.

Venous drainage of the cerebrum is into small surface sinuses that empty into the superior sagittal sinus. Other venous drainage is into interior veins that in turn form the great vein of Galen and empty into the superior saggital sinus.

Cerebral blood flow (CBF) is defined as the amount of blood delivered to brain tissue per unit time. Two factors are involved in regulating cerebral blood flow: 1) blood pressure, both systemic and local; and 2) the resistance to flow in cerebral blood vessels. Under normal conditions cerebral blood flow is maintained at a constant rate despite changes in systemic blood pressure. This is called autoregulation. Autoregulation is presumed to be due to changes in the caliber of blood vessel size, although the exact mechanism is unknown. CBF autoregulation provides an important buffer protecting the brain from variations in the systemic blood pressure.

When hypoxia or asphyxia occurs, CBF autoregulation is lost. This is probably the result of blood vessels becoming maximally dilated in reponse to hypoxia, which overrides attempted changes in vascular resistance in response to increased perfusion pressure. This is also the probable pathogenesis of hypoxic-ischemic brain damage and severe intracranial hemorrhage during the newborn period.

Hypoxemia (arterial $pO_2 \leq 50$ mm Hg) may cause a 200% to 400% increase in CBF through vasodilation. Hyperoxia may cause a 10% to 15% decrease in CBF. Carbon dioxide causes cerebral vasodilation, but unlike hypoxia its effect is linear. There is no critical level required before response begins. Although the relationship is linear, further increases in CBF do not occur with arterial pCO_2 levels above 70 to 80 mm Hg.

There are two proposed pathways for pathogenesis of brain edema and hemorrhage. The first pathway begins with an anoxic insult, which in turn damages arteriolar smooth muscle and causes loss of CBF autoregulation. Intracranial hypertension may ensue from an increase in capillary blood flow, resulting in capillary distension. From this point two things can occur: endothelial cells in brain capillaries open up their normally tight intercellular junctions, or pinocytosis occurs in endothelial cells. Either process leads to interstitial edema.

The second pathway for cerebral edema and hemorrhage begins with anoxic insult, which causes brain cell damage. These damaged cells either become a focus for seizures or release proteases that damage the capillary basement membrane. The effect of this autolysis is rupture of the capillary wall, which produces brain hemorrhage. Cellular hypoxia also allows electrolyte influx (Na^+), which causes intracellular edema.

Neonatal Hypoxic-Ischemic Encephalopathy

Most CNS damage during the intrapartum period occurs as a result of asphyxia. (Trauma has declined as a significant cause of brain damage as obstetric care has improved.) Three separate sites of asphyxial damage have been identified:

1. Cortical and subcortical gray matter
2. Subependymal germinal matrix
3. Periventricular white matter

Incidence of injury to these areas differs between premature and term infants. Damage in term infants occurs mainly in the peripheral and dorsal areas of the cerebral cortex in the gyri at the depths of sulci and in the nuclei of the basal ganglia. Damage of this type is called hypoxic-ischemic encephalopathy (HIE).

In the premature infant, damage occurs at the center of the cerebral cortex in the germinal matrix along the periventricular region. There is relative sparing of the outer cortical mantle. These injuries are hemorrhagic. Damage to the white matter in the periventricular region is called periventricular leucomalacia. It may occur in either term or premature infants. It represents necrosis of white matter around the posterior and anterior ends of the lateral ventricles. With smaller lesions there is a small area of absent glial cells. With moderate-size lesions there will be decreased myelination and ventricular dilation. With large lesions, the cerebral white matter may be filled with cystic cavities.

The decrease in the incidence of cerebral palsy over the last 25 years has been mainly in infants weighing under 2500 grams at birth. Although the rate of cerebral palsy is greater in premature infants who survive perinatal asphyxia, the actual number of affected infants is greater among term infants.

Conditions predisposing a term infant to HIE are shown in Table 4.1. Many infants will have experienced an abnormal delivery, required resuscitation, and had a low Apgar score, a low cord pH, intrapartum asphyxia, and/or the appearance of abnormal neurological signs within a few hours of birth. These abnormal neurological signs also are listed in Table 4.1.

The Apgar score is likely to be the first information the nurse will have about possible HIE in the infant. A 1-minute Apgar score of 0–3 is foreboding. However, the

Table 4.1 Factors Associated with Increased Fetal Risk of HIE and Major Signs

Placental factors
1. Abruptio placentae
2. Placenta previa
3. Prolapsed cord
4. Nuchal cord
5. Postmaturity
6. Intrauterine growth retardation
7. Placental insufficiency
8. Placental infarctions
9. Placental malformation
10. Prematurity

Maternal factors
1. Maternal hypertension
2. Maternal hypotension
3. Maternal hypoxia and hypoventilation
4. Material cardiovascular disease
5. Abnormal uterine contractions

Major signs in HIE
1. Seizures
2. Abnormal state of consciousness
3. Abnormal tone
4. Abnormal posture
5. Abnormal reflexes
6. Bulging anterior fontanelle
7. Abnornal breathing
8. Abnormal oculovestibular response

longer the score is low, the greater its significance. As was discovered in the National Institutes of Health Collaborative Perinatal Project, term infants with Apgar scores of 0–3 at 1 minute have a mortality rate of 5–10%. If the 0–3 Apgar score is maintained for 20 minutes, the mortality rate jumps to 53%. The incidence of cerebral palsy in a term infant with a 1-minute Apgar score of 0–3 is 1%. If the 0–3 Apgar score is maintained for 15 minutes, the incidence is 9%. If the 0–3 Apgar score is maintained for 20 minutes, the incidence jumps to 57%. Note that even with 15 minutes of low Apgar score, 91% of infants will not have cerebral palsy, if they survive.

It is important to remember that a low Apgar score may be due to causes other than asphyxia. Drug depression, trauma, infection, and/or congenital anomalies may also cause low scores. Thus it is important to be looking for an antecedent asphyxial incident while ruling out other causes of a low Apgar score.

There are three clinical patterns of HIE that have been described (1): severe, moderate, and mild.

Severe HIE

In severe HIE the infant has a low 5-minute Apgar score and may appear to be moderately well on admission to the intensive care nursery. However, upon closer examination, the infant has mild hypotonia, shows poor sucking, and is lethargic. Hypotonia may increase and in 3 to 4 hours eye-blinking and/or lip-smacking episodes may be evident. Tonic-clonic seizures may not appear until 12–18 hours of age. The anterior fontanelle may be tight and seizures may continue. The infant's state of consciousness goes from mild lethargy to stupor. The anterior fontanelle bulges over the next 48 hours. Abnormal breathing with periods of apnea and bradycardia develops. Pupils become fixed and dilated, with no oculovestibular response. Seizures are uncommon at this point except for decerebrate posturing. Death usually follows.

Moderate HIE

The infant with moderate HIE has low 1- and 5-minute Apgar scores, scores of 5 and 6 at 10 and 15 minutes, and 9 by 20 minutes. He is floppy with decreased reflexes, shows "frog" posturing with extended arms and legs, and is lethargic. Seizures develop within 6 hours of age, and apnea may or may not develop. Seizure activity increases in intensity over the next 24 hours but can be controlled by medication. The hypotonia persists over the next couple of weeks, but the seizures gradually diminish. The infant must be gavage fed because of a poor suck. At the time of discharge, these infants may remain hypotonic and still require tube feedings. However, seizure activity is decreased. These infants are at increased risk for cerebral palsy and must be followed up.

Mild HIE

In mild HIE the infant has poor 1- and 5-minute Apgar scores, 5 and 6 Apgar scores at 10 and 15 minutes, and a 20-minute Apgar score of 9, similar to the moderate HIE. However, the infant has increased tone and reflex activity and good flexion, but some decreased spontaneous activity. The infant may have one or two clonic seizures over the next 24 hours, but that is all. Tone and reflex activity gradually return to normal after 24 hours. The infant is able to nipple feed by 48 hours. Follow-up is necessary, but long-term sequelae are unusual.

Care of an Asphyxiated Infant

The first and most obvious step is to establish adequate oxygenation. [For a detailed explanation of resuscitation practice refer to Dazé and Scanlon (4).] The second step is to evaluate systemic perfusion by monitoring heart rate, capillary filling time, blood pressure, and urine output. It is important to remember that vasoconstriction initially may result in near-normal blood pressures. As the peripheral vascular bed opens up, blood pressures may fall. At this point, volume expansion becomes necessary. If no cross-matched blood is available, uncross-matched O-negative blood or placental blood can be used. If no blood is available, fresh frozen plasma may be used as a temporary measure.

Because autoregulation of CBF may be impaired by severe asphyxia, it is important to keep the infant's blood pressure in the normal range for his birth weight. Table 2.6 shows normal values for blood pressure by birth weight. The hematocrit should also be closely monitored and kept in the normal range. It is important to realize that blood loss may be initially compensated for by vasoconstriction. After 6–12 hours the infant may appear anemic and may need blood at that time; recheck the hemotocrit.

Once oxygenation has been established, a persistent metabolic acidosis may remain. Sodium bicarbonate may be infused gradually (1–2 mEg/kg as a dilute solution) over 15 to 20 minutes to help correct this.

Fluid balance should be carefully monitored to prevent overload. Both volume and content should be adjusted according to serum electrolyte levels, serum osmolality, urine output, and body weight. These values may need to be obtained as often as every 6 hours (see Chapter 3 for specific details).

Intracranial Hemorrhage

There are four types of CNS hemorrhage in term and preterm infants: subdural, subarachnoid, intraventricular, and intracerebellar. All four may occur in term infants secondary either to trauma or asphyxia. Preterm infants most commonly suffer from two varieties, intraventricular and intracerebellar hemorrhage.

Subdural Hemorrhage

Subdural hemorrhage is the result of:

1. A tear in the tentorium with bleeding into the straight or lateral sinuses or into the vein of Galen.
2. A tear of one of the superficial veins in the cerebral hemispheres.
3. A laceration of the falx with rupture of the inferior sagittal sinus.

Subdural hemorrhage in the neonatal period is the result of a traumatic delivery: when the pelvis is rigid (as in an older primiparous or elderly multiparous mother); when the baby is large and the mother's pelvis small; or when the duration of labor is prolonged, causing increased compression and molding of the head. It may also be seen after a precipitous delivery or in breech presentation when cervical dilatation is incomplete. Subdural hemorrhage may also occur when the head is subjected to unusual pressure such as face or brow presentations. Or it may occur when a difficult forceps extraction or rotational maneuver is used during delivery. Excessive anterior-posterior pressure on the firm skull of the term infant is more likely to cause a tear in the dura than is the same pressure on the soft, pliable skull of the premature infant. Bleeding into the posterior fossa from a tear in the tentorium is usually a catastrophic event leading to death of the infant from brainstem herniation. Subdural hemorrhage resulting from the rupture of superficial cerebral veins may not cause any clinical signs at first, or these infants may present with seizures and focal signs.

Subarachnoid Hemorrhage

Primary subarachnoid hemorrhage, caused by bleeding into the subarachnoid space resulting from damage to small veins from trauma or hypoxia, was once the most common variety of neonatal intracranial hemorrhage in term infants. It is now seen more often in premature infants following hypoxic events. A second, rare type of massive subarachnoid hemorrhage leads to rapid death. This is usually seen in infants who have received massive trauma or experienced severe hypoxia at birth.

Sequelae of subarachnoid hemorrhage are related to hydrocephalus secondary to obstruction of cerebrospinal fluid by adhesions around the outflow of the fourth ventricle. Precise diagnosis of this type of bleeding is difficult because it occurs along with other types of intracranial hemorrhage. However, term infants who develop seizures around the second day of life or a seemingly well baby with seizures often have this condition.

The prognosis for infants with primary subarachnoid hemorrhage without serious traumatic or hypoxic injuries is good. Those with minimal signs in the neonatal period also do well. Often up to 90% of those with seizures go on to be neurologically normal.

Periventricular Hemorrhage

Periventricular (or more commonly, intraventricular) intracerebral hemorrhage is characterized by hemorrhage into the cerebral white matter at the floor of the fourth ventricle. It is most often seen in premature infants in the area of the developing brain called the subependymal germinal matrix. This is a gelatinous area of primitive cells located near the head of the caudate nucleus. Supporting tissues in this area are weak. Arterial blood supply to this part of the developing brain between 24 and 32 weeks is greater relative to cortical areas. After 32 weeks, the arterial bed in the cerebral cortex dramatically increases in complexity, and blood supply to that area becomes relatively greater. Until 32 weeks, any factor causing an increase in cerebral blood flow will send increased blood flow to the subependymal germinal matrix. This includes the initial stages of asphyxia, where a rise in blood pressure is one homeostatic response, and loss of CBF autoregulation is another.

Other factors contributing to intraventricular hemorrhage include the immature capillary network in the germinal matrix and the impaired vascular autoregulation of premature infants; both are vulnerable to rapid changes in systemic or cerebral blood flow and pressure. Elevations of arterial blood pressure and cerebral blood flow have been identified in routine handling and movement of premies. Another factor is excessive blood or colloid administration. Hypoxia is a strong precipitating factor for intraventricular hemorrhage in infants with severe respiratory distress, hyaline membrane disease, and apnea. Hypercapnia has also been demonstrated to increase cerebral blood flow and contribute to increased incidence of intraventricular hemorrhage. The extent of bleeding, its pattern, and its rate of spread are variable in the subependymal germinal matrix bleeds of premature infants. Often bleeding does not break through to the ventricles.

There are two syndromes associated with intraventricular hemorrhage. One presents as a rapidly evolving deterioration in which the infant becomes suddenly comatose, hypotensive, and bradycardic, has metabolic acidosis, and suffers respiratory arrest and generalized seizures. Finally, the infant exhibits decerebrate posturing, fixed pupils, flaccid muscle tone, and a bulging anterior fontanelle. This deterioration process may last from 24 to 48 hours and is usually fatal. In the second syndrome, the infant may exhibit partial deterioration with alteration in level of consciousness, changes in spontaneous or elicited movements, and hypotonia, plus deviation of eye movements, especially downward. Brief, vacillating periods of deterioration or improvement may follow.

Management of progressive ventricular dilation may include serial lumbar punctures to lower cerebrospinal fluid (CSF) pressure, or compressive head wrapping to increase CSF absorption and force open the blocked aqueduct of Sylvius. Drugs may be given to decrease CSF production, such as acetazolamide, furosemide, digoxin, glycerol, or isosorbide. Ventricular tapping and a ventriculoperitoneal shunt may eventually be needed. Many of these therapies have not been clearly shown to improve outcome, however.

The long-term outcome of infants with intraventricular hemorrhage appears to be improving as neonatal intensive care improves. The immediate outcome relates to the severity of the bleed. Fifty to sixty-five percent of infants with severe intraventricular hemorrhage died in a study of 173 cases documented by computed tomography (CT) scan (1); 65–100% to of survivors in this group had progressive ventricular dilation. Only 5–15% of infants with moderate intraventricular hemorrhage died; 15–25% of such survivors had progressive ventricular dilation. There were no deaths of infants with mild intraventricular hemorrhage; up to 10% of them showed progressive dilation on follow-up.

Intracerebellar Hemorrhage

Intracerebellar hemorrhage now appears more frequently because it is seen in small premature infants below 1500 g birth weight and under 32 weeks' gestation. Location of the bleed does not appear to be consistent. Destruction of both cerebellar cortex and underlying white matter have been reported. Pathogenesis is similar to intraventricular hemorrhage: vascular fragility, a compliant skull, impaired vascular autoregulation, and the presence of subependymal and subpial germinal matrices. It is often seen along with intraventricular hemorrhage.

Diagnosis of this problem is mostly at autopsy in premature infants. Most cases showed catastrophic deterioration with apnea, bradycardia, falling hematocrit, and bloody CSF. Onset varies from 1 to 21 days, and death occurs within 12 to 36 hours.

Intracerebellar bleeds are also seen in term infants. Of those who survive, many are treated by surgical removal of the hematoma using a posterior fossa craniotomy. Many survivors develop hydrocephalus and require shunting. Spontaneous recovery has been reported also.

Diagnosis of Intracranial Hemorrhage

The CT scan has facilitated diagnosis of intracranial hemorrhage as a noninvasive x-ray procedure. It has become an invaluable tool for early diagnosis and treatment. It effectively shows sites and extent of bleeds, patterns of ventricular dilitation, and the presence of white-matter and other intracranial lesions. However, the infant must be transported to the machine, posing logistical and management problems.

Ultrasonography can be done in the intensive care nursery using a portable sector scanner unit. A transducer is placed over the anterior fontanelle, where it can detect intraventricular blood and ventricular size. The infant does not have to be disturbed and serial studies are easily obtained. It offers no radiation exposure to the baby or personnel.

Neonatal Seizures

Table 4.2 lists the various causes for neonatal seizures and is discussed in detail later. It is important to realize that seizures themselves may lead to brain injury. A seizure is the result of excessive synchronous electrical discharge or depolarization of neurons in the CNS. This may cause cell damage. Hypoxemia, ischemia, and hypoglycemia precipitate dramatic decreases in energy production and may be associated with seizure activity. Seizures in premature infants are different from those in term infants. These differences exist because premature infants exhibit incomplete cortical organization and lack of synaptic development, whereas term infants exhibit incomplete cortical organization and myelination.

Types of Seizures

Five types of seizures have been described by Volpe (5): subtle, tonic, multifocal clonic, focal clonic, and myoclonic. Each has its own presentation, with different observations for assessing each.

Subtle Seizures

These commonly consist of one or more of the following movements:

1. Tonic horizontal deviation of the eyes with or without their jerking
2. Repetitive fluttering or blinking of eyelids
3. Drooling, sucking, or other movements of the mouth
4. Pedaling movements of legs

Less common subtle seizure activity includes:

1. Apnea: in premature infants apnea is less likely to be the result of seizure activity than to be related to other mechanisms
2. forced vertical deviation of the eyes (more commonly down) with or without jerking movements

Table 4.2 Some Causes of Seizures in the Newborn

Perinatal asphyxia (HIE)
Intracranial hemorrhage
Hypoglycemia
Hypocalcemia
Hypomagnesemia
Intracranial infection: meningitis, encephalitis
CNS developmental disorders
Drug withdrawal and intoxication
Inborn metabolic errors
Fifth-day fits, benign familial seizures, and other esoterica

3. rapid breathing
4. vasomotor activity or tonic posturing in the limbs

Tonic Seizures

Commonly tonic seizures consist of generalized activity involving tonic extension of all limbs, are found in premature infants, and are associated with severe intraventricular hemorrhage. They sometimes include:

1. Flexion of upper limbs and extension of lower limbs that mimic decorticate posturing
2. Associated eye movements
3. Apnea or stertorous (snoring-like) breathing
4. A few clonic movements

Multifocal Clonic Seizures

Multifocal clonic seizures are found most often in term infants. They commonly consist of:

1. Clonic movements of one limb that migrate to other body parts or may involve another body part simultaneously
2. Irregular migration of movements unlike the ordered movements seen in Jacksonian seizures; may include one or both sides

Focal Clonic Seizures

Focal clonic seizures commonly consist of localized clonic movements and occur in infants in a conscious state. They indicate focal trumatic injury, such as cerbral contusion, in term infants. Focal clonic seizures are relatively uncommon but accompany other types of seizures; such as those resulting from generalized cerebral dysfunction and metabolic encephalopathies.

Myoclonic Seizures

Myoclonic seizures are rarely seen during the newborn period. They commonly consist of single or multiple jerks of arms and/or legs, and are indicative of later development of hypsarrhythmia on the infant's electroencephalogram. More massive myoclonic seizures occur at several weeks or months of age.

Jitteriness versus Seizure Activity

Jitteriness is often confused with seizure activity. A clear distinction between the two must be made to prevent 1) delay in treating seizures and 2) undue treatment of jitteriness as seizures. With jitteriness there is:

1. Tremulous movements with occasional clonus
2. Normal eye movement
3. Activity triggered by a stimulus
4. Rhythmic movements that are usually inhibited by flexion of the affected limb

Conversely, seizure activity may be identified by:

1. Deviation of the eyes or other types of rhythmic eye movements
2. Absence of a specific triggering stimulus

3. Common seizure movement of clonic jerking with fast and slow rhythm that cannot be inhibited by gentle passive flexion

Most commonly, jitteriness occurs as an aftereffect of HIE, or as a result of hypocalcemia, hypoglycemia, or drug withdrawal.

Common Etiologies of Seizures

Perinatal asphyxia with resultant HIE is the most common cause of neonatal seizures in both premature and term infants. Seizures occur most commonly in these infants within the first 24 hours and rapidly become very severe. Infants with seizures from HIE usually have subtle seizures. Prematures also often have tonic seizures. Term infants frequently have multifocal clonic seizures.

Intracranial hemorrhage is difficult to distinguish as a separate cause of seizures because it usually accompanies hypoxia or trauma. However, it has been found as a separate cause in primary subarachnoid hemorrhage, which is the most common form of intracranial hemorrhage. It is also observed much more often in premature than in term infants. Seizures from subarachnoid hemorrhage occur later than those caused by hypoxia, usually on the second day of life. While the bleed is occurring, the infant appears well, leading him to be referred to as "well baby with seizures."

Intraventricular hemorrhage of the subependymal veins in the germinal matrix is a lesion of premature infants. Onset of seizures is 1½ days. The predominant seizure type is the generalized tonic variety and usually accompanies a rapid deterioration of the infant to coma and respiratory arrest within minutes to hours.

Subdural hemorrhage secondary to a traumatic tear of the falx or tentorium occurs in large infants. It occurs less frequently than the other types of hemorrhage. Seizures occur with subdural hemorrhage in about half the cases and appear within the first 2 days of life if they are going to occur. These seizures are focal because they are secondary to cerebral contusions.

Various metabolic disturbances may also lead to seizure activity. Hypoglycemia, hypocalcemia, and hyperbilirubinemia are discussed this chapter. *Hypoglycemia* is defined in term infants as a blood glucose level below 30 mg/100 ml and in preterm infants as below 20 mg/100 ml. It is seen frequently in infants who are small for gestational age and in large infants of diabetic or prediabetic mothers. Duration of the hypoglycemia is the critical factor in determining neurological consequences. The amount of time elapsed before treatment begins is also important. Symptoms of hypoglycemia are jitteriness, stupor, hypotonia, apnea, and seizures. It is difficult to establish hypoglycemia as a single etiological agent for seizures in small infants because perinatal asphyxia, intracranial hemorrhage, hypocalcemia, and infection are often found concomitantly. However, infants of diabetic mothers often escape without any neurological sequelae, probably because the duration of their hypoglycemia is much shorter since their blood sugar is observed closely from birth.

Hypocalcemia is defined as a serum calcium level below 7 mg/100 ml. Its incidence has two major peaks. The first occurs during the first few days of life and is found in low birth weight infants, or those who have suffered a traumatic delivery or HIE. In such seizures hypocalcemia is never the only etiology. Hypocalcemia that appears later appears most commonly in large term infants at about the sixth day of life who are on cow's milk formula. Cow's milk has a suboptimal ratio of phosphorus to calcium and to magnesium for human infants. Infants with this problem exhibit hyperreactive deep tendon reflexes; knee, ankle, and jaw clonus; and jitteriness plus seizures. They do not demonstrate the hypotonia and stupor seen in infants with hypocalcemia of early onset.

Hyperbilirubinemia is rarely a cause of seizures because of improved recognition, the use of phototherapy, and prevention of erythroblastosis fetalis. However, among those infants who do sustain kernicterus (yellow staining of the basal ganglia and other brain cells), 50% have seizures. Subtle early symptoms of hypotonia, lethargy, and depressed suck reflex are difficult to recognize. Once bilirubin deposition in the brain has occurred, opisthotonos, spasticity, seizures, and elevated body temperature are seen.

Drug withdrawal from the more commonly abused substances is an unusual cause of neonatal seizures. These substances include heroin, methadone, phenobarbital, and alcohol. Infants may also be toxically affected by the local anesthesia administered to the mother. These infants usually present with bradycardia, hypotonia, apnea, and seizures.

Drug Therapy for Seizures

Because of the increased need for glucose by the brain during seizure activity, a Dextrostix determination of blood glucose should be done when seizures are observed. If the infant is hypoglycemic, dextrose should be given IV immediately. A bolus dose of 250 mg/kg is followed by a maintainance dose of 0.5 g/kg/hour. A 10% glucose solution, at most, is adequate for such therapy.

To terminate the seizure activity, a loading dose of phenobarbital is given at 20 mg/kg divided in two 10-mg/kg doses administered over 5 to 10 minutes IV. The respiratory rate needs to be carefully monitored. Respiratory arrest may occur secondary to phenobarbital use. The potential need for intubation and mechanical ventilation should be anticipated whenever phenobarbital is given. Phenobarbital is the drug of choice for infants with HIE. Measuring drug levels is useful for efficient therapy.

Phenytoin is given in a loading dose of 15–20 mg/kg. It is often used when the loading dose of phenobarbital has not stopped seizure activity after 20 minutes. Heart rate and rhythm need to be carefully monitored during IV administration. Slow IV administration is recommended because phenytoin can cause severe phlebitis and sloughing of tissue. Maintainance dosage is 3–4 mg/kg/day. Paraldehyde, magnesium sulfate, calcium gluconate, and diazepam may be used in selected cases.

Drug Withdrawal

Drug withdrawal may also be called the abstinence syndrome. It is a generalized disorder involving CNS excitation and respiratory and gastrointestinal malfunction, which begins during the newborn period. It is associated with a maternal history of continuing addictive drug use during pregnancy. Withdrawal occurs when the CNS tissue level of the substance become critically low compared with previous exposure. Recovery is gradual and occurs when the infant's CNS adjusts to absence of the drug (6).

Infants of mothers addicted to narcotics may show fetal distress and be meconium stained. The 1-minute Apgar may be low. Intrauterine growth retardation is reported in approximately one-third of such infants. Hypertonicity, irritability, tremors, vomiting, and respiratory distress are the most common signs of withdrawal. Not all infants have involvement; some may have only one or two signs, whereas some have five or six. Zelson (7) compared infants of heroin- and methadone-addicted mothers and found that methadone-addicted babies have more withdrawal signs

Table 4.3 Symptoms of Drug Withdrawal

CNS
1. Frantic restlessness: overactivity in supine or prone position
2. Crying: continuous, high pitched, may cry out
3. Tremors: may have myoclonic jerking
4. Hypertonia: may be difficult to hold
5. Hyperreflexive: spontaneous mouthing, rooting, hand-to-mouth activity, startles, Moro reflex
6. Fever: associated with increased activity
7. Sneezing, hiccoughs, yawning
8. Increased sensitivity to sound, change of position

Respiratory
1. Irregular breathing: may be rapid, may hyperventilate
2. Excessive secretions

Gastrointestinal
1. Suck may be weak and disorganized, depressed, poor suction
2. Hunger: appears hungry between feedings
3. Vomiting: sensitive gag reflex
4. Diarrhea or loose stools
5. Hyperphagia with constant sucking: appears day 2 to 5, may last 2–3 months

Skin
1. Flushes with crying
2. Cirumoral pallor with cessation of crying
3. Scratches and abrasions from increased activity
4. Excessive sweating: may last for months
5. Mottling: may last for months

than heroin-addicted babies. Hypertonicity, irritability, vomiting, and fewer were found often in infants of mothers addicted to methadone.

In general, the signs of drug withdrawal are nonspecific with a wide range in severity. Table 4.3 lists common groups of withdrawal symptoms. Gastrointestinal symptoms may occur alone, but CNS excitability is usually present. It is important to remember that signs of withdrawal may be modified by prematurity or disease.

There are several signs that may persist after these infants are discharged from the hospital: a continuous desire to suck, sweating, diarrhea, irregular sleep patterns and increased sensitivity to sounds. These characteristics make them difficult and unsatisfying infants to raise or to place in foster care. Coupled with the mother's drug dependency and aberrant life style, such characteristics set the stage for abuse and neglect.

There are seven complications that may occur in infants of drug-addicted mothers:

1. Jaundice or hyperbilirubinemia, often seen in infants of methadone-addicted mothers, less frequently in infants of heroin- or barbiturate-addicted mothers.
2. Infection, including herpes, syphillis, and hepatitis, as a result of maternal infection.
3. Respiratory problems, including aspiration pneumonia and nasal congestion due to increased secretions.
4. Electrolyte disturbances, including hypoglycemia, hypocalcemia, and dehydration; this last problem may result from hyperventilation, feeding disturbances, or diarrhea.
5. Seizures from hypoglycemia, anoxia, hypocalcemia, or severe withdrawal.
6. Temperature instability and fever in severe withdrawal.
7. Cardiovascular collapse may also be seen in cases of severe withdrawal.

In recent years, the fetal alcohol syndrome has received attention. Although the actual number of infants with this problem is small, the findings are severe enough to deserve mention. Decreased fetal weight and prematurity in surviving infants have been described. In addition, epicanthic folds, maxillary hypoplasia, cleft palate, micrognathia, altered palmar crease pattern, anomalous external genitalia, and capillary hemangiomas have been reported.

Nursing care of infants of drug- or alcohol-addicted mothers requires careful observation in an intensive care nursery during the first 48 hours for development of withdrawal signs and symptoms. Severe withdrawal can occur as late as 10 days of age in infants of methadone-addicted mothers. The infant, wearing only a diaper, should be observed in an isolette until withdrawal signs become evident; then he should be observed with greater frequency, as needed. Some physicians advocate collecting urine samples to be examined for morphine, quinine, methadone, barbiturates, and other suspected drugs when an accurate drug history is not available. However, since withdrawal occurs at low tissue drug levels, such testing is not often helpful and should not be routine.

Once withdrawal begins, supportive care needs to be given to the infant based on those symptoms that are present. Swaddling is particularly effective for quieting the mild to moderately affected infant. Placing sheepskin under the infant helps prevent severe breakdown of the skin over the knees and elbows, which results from constant movement. The diaper area should be protected with an ointment (A & D or Vaseline) since loose stools can irritate skin. The baby's hands may also need to be covered to prevent scratching of skin by fingernails. Temperature instability can occur when the infant cools with diaphoresis after warming during increased activity. A pacifier is often useful with hyperphagia, and picking up and carrying around an irritable infant helps stop the crying during long periods of wakefulness.

Often drug therapy is begun once withdrawal symptoms become moderately severe. Opium drops, paregoric, methadone, barbiturates, or chlorpromazine have been used. A loading dose may be given at first, and the daily doses can be adjusted according to the infant's response. Drug therapy may continue for a few days or a few weeks. It should be individualized to maintain the infant midway between the two extremes of agitation and drug-induced sleep.

Nursing Care of the Newborn with Acute CNS Dysfunction

Nursing care of the newborn infant at risk for acute neurological problems should begin with a careful assessment. The first part is an examination of the head, which may help to identify the infant with a neurological disorder. The second part is testing specific neurological functions.

Examination of the Head

1. Look for signs of trauma: bruises, depressions, abrasions, cuts, cephalohematomata.
2. Measure and record the head circumference (measure at widest diameter when molding is present).
3. Palpate the anterior fontanelle for evidence of increased or decreased intracranial pressure (bulging fontanelle, widely separated sutures).
4. Carefully look for dysmorphic physical features:
    a. Anencephaly: absence of the cerebrum and skull.
    b. Encephalocele: saclike structure containing meninges and portions of the cortex or cerebellum.

     c. Cranial meningocele: saclike structure containing only meninges, no nervous tissue.

     d. Abnormal facies: includes facial clefts, low-set ears, hypertelorism.

     e. Nevus flammeus: reddening along the trigeminal nerve distribution may signify the presence of an intracranial vascular lesion.

5. Auscultate the head: listen for murmurs over the skull; when present, these may signify the presence of an arteriovenous malformation.

Evaluation of Neurological Function

A thorough neurological examination by the nurse caring for the infant at risk for neurological problems consists of evaluating seven separate areas: state of alertness, posture, muscle tone, spontaneous movement, primitive reflex activity, autonomic nervous system, and cranial nerves.

State of Alertness

Specific states of alertness should be noted throughout the neurological exam. An infant who is constantly asleep or awake and crying is abnormal. The state affects how the infant responds during the neurological exam. Sleeping infants are usually flaccid and hyporeflexive. Crying infants are usually rigid and may be either hyporeflexive or hyperreflexive. State of alertness may be a good prognostic indicator for infants who have suffered HIE. Asphyxiated newborns who do not reach a stuporous state and are lethargic for less than 5 days usually appear normal in later follow-up. Newborns who become stuporous or remain lethargic for more than 7 days either die or show significant neurological problems on follow-up. A more detailed discussion of states of consciousness may be found under the section "Brazelton Neonatal Behavioral Assessment Scale."

Posture

Posture is the position assumed by the undisturbed infant. It shows the balance between flexor and extensor tone when the infant is at rest. Since newborn posture is influenced by gestational age, it is important to be aware of the different amount of flexor tone to expect at each gestational age. The posture item on the Dubowitz scale of gestational age assessment (8) is an excellent reference. Opisthotonus, obligatory thumb flexion, and extension of the legs are abnormal postures in term newborns.

Muscle Tone

Muscle tone is related to both gestational age and state. The optimal state for assessing muscle tone is either quiet alert or awake and moving. When the infant is in sleeping or crying states, his tone cannot be adequately assessed. In the term infant, muscle tone can be tested by suspending the infant in a prone position with hands under his chest. He should be able to hold his head in line with his trunk for 2–3 seconds with straight back and slightly extended hips.

If the infant is preterm, being ventilated, and cannot be suspended in a prone position, passive extension and recoil of arms and legs may be done to assess muscle tone. In a term infant little resistance to extension and little or no recoil of arms and legs is abnormal. Tight flexion with inability to extend arms and legs without dragging the infant across the mattress is abnormal hypertonus. In premature infants the smoothness of resistance and recoil should be assessed rather than the angle of flexion. In infants who have been asphyxiated, the length of time for tone to return is a good indicator of the severity of the episode. A delay in return of muscle tone of greater than 2 hours is associated with increased risk of long-term neurological problems (9).

Spontaneous Movement

Spontaneous movements of arm and legs by the infant are important to note. Their symmetry, fullness of range, and smoothness are the qualities to observe. Movement can be observed in all states but is easiest in alert states. Characteristic types of movement differ according to gestational age. The very immature infant of 24–28 weeks' gestation has few periods of spontaneous activity; these consist of rapid large arcs of the whole limb, slow twisting of arms and legs, and overall jerky movement. Facial grimaces are also part of his repertoire. The premature infant of 32 weeks is beginning to demonstrate symmetrical flexor movements in his knees and hips. He also demonstrates improving head control by being able to turn it to the side. His arms show less flexion than his legs. By 36 weeks the premature infant shows much more flexor movement in the legs and arms, and his leg movement is no longer symmetrical. The term infant exhibits much activity when awake and alternates movement in all limbs.

Primitive Reflexes

Primitive reflex activity is routinely assessed by the physician. However, there are three primitive reflexes with long-term significance that the nurse can monitor on a daily basis to look for recovery from CNS insult (10): 1) asymmetric tonic neck reflex, 2) placing response, and 3) Moro reflexes.

Asymmetric Tonic Neck Reflex The asymmetric tonic neck reflex (ATNR) is often referred to as the fencer's position. When the infant is supine and his head is passively turned from side to side through the midline, he assumes a position in which the arm and leg on the side toward the face are extended and the arm and leg toward the occiput are flexed. Although there is some controversy as to whether or not the ATNR is present at all in normal premature or term newborn infants, there is general agreement that it is abnormal if the infant exhibits it in an obligatory manner. In other words, a normal infant can move out of the fencer's posture unassisted.

Placing Response The placing response is elicited by holding the infant under both arms and stroking the dorsum of one foot by passing it under a protruding edge—either a table top or crib edge. The unstimulated leg may be held flexed, out of the way, depending upon the examiner's preference. The stimulated leg should flex, then extend, and the foot should be placed on the table or mattress. Prechtl and Beintema (11) found the placing response full and strong at 6 days of age in 50% of normal term infants. Other authors (12) have found it present in most infants, even premature ones. They found the placing reaction to be absent in all four limbs of children with mental ages of less than 4 months or with IQs less than 28. This is one primitive reflex that seems dependent upon the presence of a moderate amount of cerebral cortex.

Moro Reflex The Moro reflex is routinely used during the newborn period to screen for problems. Asymmetry between arms suggests a fractured clavicle, brachial palsy, or hemiplegia. Absence of the Moro reflex during the newborn period suggests severe CNS depression or damage. Persistence of the Moro reflex with maximal intensity past 4 months of age correlates with mental retardation and cerebral palsy. The techniques for eliciting the Moro reflex are varied. Moro's original method was to hold the infant supine on one arm, dropping the head suddenly. On dropping the head, there is rapid symmetrical abduction of the arms, followed by their upward movement. The hands open and the arms gradually adduct and flex in a clasping position. The legs may also abduct and extend.

Autonomic Nervous System

Evaluation of the autonomic nervous system is an integral part of the nursing role. Heart rate, blood pressure, respiratory rate and effort, temperature, sweating, skin color, and pupillary response to light are assessed continuously. In the absence of other systemic or peirpheral causes, instability in the above signs may be manifestations of brainstem dysfunction.

Cranial Nerves

Cranial nerves I through XII may be tested during care of the neurologically suspect newborn infant. Careful observation of the infant can take the place of a specific neurological exam. Blinking eyes in response to bright lights tests the optic nerve. Equal constriction of the pupils to light tests the optic and oculomotor nerves plus the retina. Ptosis of eyelids involves the oculomotor nerve. The rooting reflex measures trigeminal nerve function. Facial nerve function is best observed when the infant is crying. The auditory nerve can be tested by noticing how the infant responds to sounds in his environment. Accessory nerve function can be observed by watching the infant right his head when supine. Glossopharyngeal nerve function is reflected in the gag reflex. Hypoglossal nerve function affects the strength of the infant's suck. Absence of any of these reflexes indicates damage to cranial nerves either in their central origin or peripherally.

Obtaining Cerebral Spinal Fluid

Work-up of the infant at risk for neurological problems often includes a lumbar puncture (LP), subdural tap, or intraventricular tap. The basic preparation for all three is similar.

Equipment

The following equipment should be assembled:

> Sterile towels
> Sterile gloves
> Skin prep solution
> Sterile CSF collection containers
> Needles
>> 22–24-gauge needle with stylet for LP
>> 21–22-gauge needle with stylet for subdural tap

In some cases a sterile pressure manometer might be needed to measure intracranial pressures. Prepackaged LP trays are available (Pharmaseal) and are convenient but relatively expensive. For infants receiving taps every day or every other day, it may be more economical to assemble the above equipment from standard supplies.

Infant Preparation

Once all the equipment is assembled, the infant must be prepared for the procedure. The bed should be flat throughout the procedure. A heat source must be provided during the procedure to prevent cold stress. Usually a radiant heat source provides maximal access to the infant. When a subdural tap is to be done, the head must be shaved beyond the level of the back of the anterior fontanelle.

When an LP is done, the infant must be held on his side or in a sitting position with the back flexed. In order to maximally flex the back without obstructing the airway, grasp the infant at the hips and shoulders and round the infant into a "C" shape. It is usually *not* necessary to position the infant's head so the chin is on the chest to achieve optimal CSF flow. Because respirations can be compromised while the infant is in this flexed position, any infant having an LP should be monitored both with an electrocardiogram and apnea alarm system. Additionally, infants with a compromised respiratory status should be monitored throughout the procedure with a transcutaneous pO_2 unit.

Procedure

The site of the procedure must be thoroughly scrubbed with an iodine-based solution and then draped with sterile towels to create a sterile field. Strict aseptic technique must be observed at all times to prevent the introduction of contaminants into the CSF. The site for an LP is between the fourth to fifth lumbar spinous process. Subdural taps, usually performed by a neurosurgeon, are performed through the coronal suture at the midpupillary line (13).

Specimen Collection and Site Care

Once the needle is in place, CSF can be collected and sent for the desired laboratory work. After the needle is removed, apply pressure to the site for approximately 5 minutes to encourage clot formation. Subdural taps may be sealed with collodion and sterile cotton.

Brazelton Neonatal Behavioral Assessment Scale

The Brazelton Neonatal Behavioral Assessment Scale (BNBAS) combines three types of neurological testing. It is intended to score interactive behavior between the infant, his environment, and his caretakers. Brazelton (14) and others feel that the reactions the infant creates in his parents in early weeks after birth may be the best predictors of outcome in the mother-father-infant interaction.

The BNBAS contains three major techniques of neurological assessment: evaluation of reflex activity, habituation, and orientation:

> *Evaluation of Reflex Activity* involves testing the primitive reflexes present in the infant at birth. These reflexes are involuntary motor responses elicited by appropriate peripheral stimuli. They disappear during the first 6 months of life as myelination takes place in the maturing nervous system.
>
> *Habituation* is the ability of the infant to diminish his strongest reflexive response to repetitive applications of the same stimulus. It is a conserving and adaptive behavior. Infants with absent or severely damaged cerebral cortex do not habituate. Most infants habituate to environmental noise, light, and clothing by rousing but remaining in sleep state.
>
> *Orientation* measures the infant's response to visual and auditory stimulation, both human and environmental. Most babies respond by decreasing random activity, focusing on the stimulus, changing facial expression, and changing respiration pattern. Orientation items are designed to test the infant's re-

sponsiveness to social and nonsocial cues and his ability to interact with his family and to learn by observation during the first year.

There are four uses of the BNBAS:

1. Long-term prognosis of high-risk or recovering neurologically impaired infants.
2. Documentation of normal functioning in healthy infants.
3. Research, as an outcome measurement for comparing the difference between control and experimental groups in such areas as drug addiction, maternal medication, cultural differences, maternal intervention, and infant stimulation.
4. Teaching newborn behavior to parents and nursing and medical students.

The main goal of the BNBAS is to score the infant's available responses ot his environment. The score sheet includes 27 behavioral items, each of which is scored on a 9-point scale. There are 20 elicited-response (neurological) items, each of which is scored on a 3-point scale. Most scales are set so that the midpoint is the norm. The norm is related to the expected behavior of a 3-day-old, 3-kg, term Caucasian infant whose normal mother had 100 mg or less of barbiturates and 50 mg or less of other sedatives prior to delivery. The norm had Apgar scores of 7 or greater at 1 minute and 8 or greater at 5 minutes, and required no special care after delivery.

The BNBAS differs from most neurological tests in that all but a few items are scored on the infants' *best* performances, not his average. Therefore during testing, the examiner may use holding, rocking, or cooing to help the infant achieve an optimal score.

States of Consciousness

Assessing the infant's states of consciousness is perhaps the single most important element in the exam. His reactions to all stimulation are dependent upon his ongoing state of consciousness. The infant's use of state to maintain control of his reactions reflects his ability to organize. Thus, control of consciousness state sets a dynamic pattern that affects the infant's full range of behavior.

State of consciousness depends upon physiological variables such as hunger, nutrition, hydration, and time within the infant's sleep-wake cycle. Both the pattern of states and the number of state changes are related to the infant's mental ability on the Bayley Scales of Mental Development at 3 months of age (15).

There are six states of consciousness used in the BNBAS: two are sleep states and four are awake states.

> *State 1: Deep Sleep*   Eyes closed, no eye movements; breathing regular; little or no spontaneous activity except startles at regular intervals; state change is less likely than from other states.
> *State 2: Light Sleep*   Eyes closed, rapid eye movements; low-level, random activity; movements are smoother than in state 1; external stimuli may produce change of state.
> *State 3: Drowsy*   Eyes may be opened or closed, eyelids may flutter; activity level variable; reactive to sensory stimuli but response often delayed; state change after stimulation often occurs; movements are smooth; fussing may be present.
> *State 4: Alert*   Bright look; attention focused on source of stimulation; stimuli may break through with some possible delay in response; motor activity is minimal.

State 5: Active Eyes open; motor activity with thrusting movements of limbs; few startles; stimuli cause increased activity; discrete reactions difficult to see because of activity level; fussing may be present.

State 6: Crying Intense and difficult to interrupt; must last for at least 15 seconds.

The BNBAS Assessment

The BNBAS should be done in a quiet, dimly lighted room. When this is impossible, the interfering variables item should be scored accordingly. The exam usually takes 30 minutes and should be done midway between feedings. Although it is recommended that the items be administered in order, it is important for the examiner to take cues from the infant and to present the items in a manner that makes best use of the infant's state and level of organization.

Habituation Items
The examiner is looking for change from initial response.

1. Flashlight (3 to 10 times) through closed eyelids
2. Rattle (3 to 10 times)
3. Bell (3 to 10 times)
4. Pinprick softly on heel (5 times)

Reflexive Items
The examiner is looking for strength and completeness of each reflex. Uncover infant and gently turn onto back.

1. Ankle clonus: absent or present beats.
2. Plantar grasp: toe grasp.
3. Babinski reflex: movement of big toe up or down, fanning of other toes.
4. Undress: look for skin color change and waking passive movements and general tone—moderate is normal.
5. Resistance and recoil.
6. Palmar grasp: hand grasp.
7. Pull to sit: head control.
8. Standing (positive support reflex): elicit with tactile stimulation.
9. Walking: alternating steps; elicit by tactile stimulation, placing, flexion at knee, extension, toe fanning.
10. Incurvation (Galant reflex): paravertebral stroking of infant's, back noting lateral truncal movement; holding infant in prone suspension, check truncal tone against gravity.
11. Cuddling: pick up and hold to see how well infant molds when held.
12. Glabella-brow tap: single blink of eyes.
13. Rooting and sucking: strength and completeness.
14. Spin: tonic deviation and nystagmus, eighth nerve response, turns in direction of spin, controlled nystagmus.

Orientation Items
The most sophisticated response is circular following of visual stimuli and repeated turning to sounds with eyes and head, searching.

1. Inanimate auditory: rattle.
2. Inanimate visual: red ball.
3. Animate auditory: examiner's voice.

4. Animate visual: examiner's face.
5. Animate auditory and visual: both voice and face.

Adversive Reflex

1. Defensive reaction: cloth on face, infant swipes at cloth to free face.
2. Asymmetric tonic neck reflex: fencer's position.
3. Moro reflex: startle with arm and leg movement; observe symmetry.

General Behavior

1. Smiles.
2. Hand to mouth spontaneously.
3. Tremors.
4. Motor activity.
5. General tone.
6. Motor maturity (arcs and smoothness of movement).
7. Lability of states (number of changes), highest state reached, irritability, and rapidity of build-up to crying state.

Although this chapter cannot train the reader to be a qualified Brazelton examiner, it provides information to guide infant assessment. The BNBAS also helps identify five signs of neurodevelopmental disorders during the newborn period. These are:

1. Poor or absent alert state by 24 hours of age.
2. Abnormal movements such as absence of spontaneous activity in awake states, presence of excessive brisk and rapid or slow and wide movements of the extremities, tremors, sustained clonus, or asymmetries.
3. Pathological ocular signs such as fixed or deviated eyes, or abnormal eye movements.
4. Defective tone of the head and trunk extensor muscles, either hypotonic with complete head lag or hypertonic with opisthotonus.
5. Lack of reaction to visual and auditory sensory stimuli described in the orientation items.

A modified form of the BNBAS, called the MABI, was used by Widmeyer and Field (16) to teach high-risk mothers infant behavior. It contained all the behavioral items, using a 5-point scoring scale. The neurological items were the only ones excluded. The MABI was successful when demonstrated by any examiner and repeated weekly by mothers for 4 weeks. Mothers taught this examination method were more responsive to their infants than were control mothers on follow-up.

Early Infant Stimulation

The normal newborn infant is totally dependent upon his caregivers. Generalized motor activity and crying attract attention to needs when he is distressed. His caregivers must come to him; he cannot go to them. Therefore a major nursing goal is to help the parents become sensitive to their newborn infant's cues.

Once the infant leaves the hospital, the parents' responsiveness to the infant's cues become vital. Both timing and appropriateness of response provide feedback to the infant and reinforce his behavior. This behavior in turn reinforces the parents' feeling of self-confidence and enjoyment of the infant. The greater the sensitivity shown to the infants' signals, the higher is the rate of development of object and person permanence. Such children also demonstrate more socially mature behavior by age 10 (18). Infants of parents who are intrusive, punishing, critical, or who direct their behavior show lower scores on intelligence testing. A crowded household with the TV on most of the time and without a quiet place for the infant to escape the noise and activity may lead to delayed language acquisition and delayed sensorimotor development. Most developmental psychologists agree that parents and nurses should respond promptly when the infant cries by coming to the cribside and attempting to solve the problem. This response to crying teaches the infant that his needs will be met, helping instill confidence in his environment.

Visual and auditory stimuli can best be responded to by an alert infant. It is important to remember that newborn infants respond best to human faces. The parent's or caregiver's face will be enjoyed by the newborn. If we consider what is known about habituation, the infant appropriately should tune out visual, auditory, and tactile stimulation when asleep. It is important to consider that appropriateness and timing provide feedback to the infant to reinforce behavior.

One of the infant's main sources of learning during the first year of life is observation. Therefore, one goal of infant stimulation should be to help the infant increase his periods of quiet alert time and to help him lengthen the amount of time he can visually focus. One of the easiest ways to accomplish this task is to establish eye contact with the infant and encourage him to follow your face from side to side. By 2 months of age he should be able to follow objects horizontally, vertically, and in a circle. By 3 months he should be able to follow a rolling ball across a table and glance from one object to another (15).

Vestibular stimulation is helpful in alerting the infant. Intuitively mothers pick up an infant and place him at the shoulder to quiet. Gentle vertical rocking also helps the infant to alert and to quiet. Non-nutritive sucking is a very effective aid in helping a fussy infant to quiet. Many infants will either return to sleep state or to quiet and alert if allowed to suck on a pacifier. Infants given a pacifier at a regular interval in a premature nursery gained weight more quickly than the control group. Many parents are concerned that it will be difficult to stop their infant from using a pacifier. However, this is usually no more of a problem than weaning from the bottle.

The family and the infant are active participants in language acqusition. It is important to reinforce the infant's earliest sounds by imitating them, smiling, and praising his efforts. Parents should speak words to the infant, not baby talk, because their speech has a positive influence on the infant's learning. The rhythm, sound, and structure is specific for the parent's own language. There is a positive correlation between the parents' use of words that identify and describe the infant's environment and the acqusition of language. However, attempts to control and direct the child are negatively correlated with language acquisition (18). The baby's cry varies according to whether he is hungry, tired, wet, or fussy. The parents' response helps the infant to understand what different sounds mean to his parents. It is important that the infant learn that his happy sound are important also.

Physical stimulation is not obligatory for parents to do with their infant, but may be enjoyable for all. Encouraging an infant to relax by placing him supine on a soft mattress and stroking him gently until his flexion tone decreases is one "exercise" (19). This may best be done after bath time, but should not be done during a fussy or irritable period. Another "exercise" for the newborn infant is to place him in a prone position and encourage him to look up. This will strengthen shoulder and neck muscles.

Passive range-of-motion exercises are often recommended for infants who have spent extensive time in an intensive care nursery. The purpose of these is to maintain mobility in all joints of the arms and legs. It is important that these be done only while the infant is *relaxed.* If they are done against resistance, they can be harmful. It is important to stress this point with parents. In passive range-of-motion exercises the shoulders should be moved in a circular motion. The fists should gently be opened and fingers extended and closed. Passive movement of the hips should be done by flexing the knees and moving each hip in a circular, bicycling motion. The knees should be flexed and extended and the ankles moved in a circular motion. It is important to make certain that the ankles flex at least to a 90° angle so that the heel cord does not become shortened.

How the infant is carried can also help develop head control and trunk strength and maintain hip flexibility. He should be lifted some of the time by placing hands under his shoulders with the thumbs in front and the fingertips behind to "catch" the head if it should fall. This way of holding enables the infant to support his own head. He should be carried on both sides of the parent's body. This encourages him to look, listen, turn, and reach evenly to both sides. Placing the infant in a supported sitting position builds trunk strength, encourages head control, and maintains hip flexibility.

Premature infants are born before their nervous system are mature. Even at 40 weeks most premature infants are neurologically different from term infants. Many primitive reflexes are weak or incomplete. Abnormalities of tone (increased, decreased, and variable from one to the other) are common. Many premature infants cannot complete the hand-to-mouth maneuver, focus their eyes to make eye-to-eye contact with parents, regulate their states of consciousness effectively, or control motor activity well. Many are either slow feeders or seem hungry constantly.

It is important for the nurse to evaluate each infant for strengths and weaknesses using the BNBAS as a guideline. Each infant-parent dyad needs to be treated individually, adjusting for parental experience, knowledge, and observations.

Vestibular stimulation or non-nutritive sucking may be needed to facilitate state of consciousness control. Passive range-of-motion exercises, head control exercises, and careful positioning may be needed for help with transient dystonia of prematurity. Encouragement of eye-to-eye contact may be needed to work on focusing and attentional deficits. Many infants need to be awakened and played with prior to feeding, or need a pacifier after feeding to satisfy their need to suck. Feedings need to be planned consistently through the day, every 3 to 4 hours, whether the infant is sleepy or constantly hungry.

In general, premature infants need increased environmental structuring and assistance in order to achieve developmental milestones during the first year of life. It is important that nurses and parents pay particular attention to the special needs of the premature infant.

Case Studies

These case studies of newborns with special needs illustrate follow-up and techniques for instructing parents in the care of their infants.[1]

Case 1: The Irritable Premature Infant

Baby G. was an 1180-gram male infant born at 27 weeks to a gravida III para 0, 26-year-old mother. The parents were married, and until the unexpected delivery both were employed. Baby G. had Apgar scores of 2 at 1 minute and 7 at 5 minutes. He had group B streptococcal sepsis, respiratory distress with pulmonary insufficiency

[1] Refer to Appendices 4.1 to 4.3 at the end of the chapter for outlines describing the nursing care plans for each of the case studies.

requiring ventilation, a pneumothorax, and pulmonary interstitial emphysema. He developed bronchopulmonary dysplasia and was treated with steroids. He had periods of apnea and bradycardia, and was also found to have grade I retrolental fibroplasia, which did not progress. The infant was on a ventilator for 20 days. He remained in the intensive care nursery for 99 days.

During the entire hospitalization his parents visited him daily. His mother pumped her breasts to provide fresh breast milk. She returned to work but visited him during her lunch break and in the evenings. Close to the time of baby G.'s discharge, his mother took a leave of absence from her job and spent each day caring for her son in the hospital. Breastfeeding was well established before discharge.

However, Baby G. slept very little between feedings while in the nursery. He would wake up and cry, and was difficult to console. The nurses reassured Mrs. G. that the love and attention that she was giving her son was important. She was encouraged to carry her son around and to rock him in the rocker. The vestibular stimulation sometimes helped to quiet him. Although the infant tired easily while nursing, he did seem to enjoy breastfeeding, and Mrs. G. was encouraged to persist. At first she expressed feelings that her son seemed not to like her; the nursing staff helped her to see that her son was less fussy when she was there than when she was not. Baby G. was discovered to sleep for longer periods and to cry less frequently once he was moved to a transition room in the nursery where the lights could be dimmed and there was less noise. When this was explained to Mrs. G., she also developed a method of quieting her son by putting her face next to him and cooing to him without picking him up. It was pointed out to her that he was a child who quieted more easily by having less environmental noise and less stimulation. He seemed to respond better to soft voices, dim lights, and being left untouched when out of control.

Baby G. was seen in the developmental evaluation follow-up clinic for 2 years. At 25 months of age he tested in the normal range on the Bayley Scales of Motor and Mental Development. However, at the time he still did not like to be touched or lifted and showed intolerance for sitting quietly during the testing period.

Case 2: The Infant of a Drug-Addicted Mother

Baby C. was born at term weighing 2870 grams. She had Apgar scores of 7 at 1 minute and 9 at 5 minutes. Her mother was in a methadone program at the time of delivery and had taken heroin sporadically during the pregnancy. The infant became increasingly irritable and difficult to quiet during the first 36 hours of life. She developed a temperature of 100°F, was diaphoretic, and had three loose stools at that time. Her neurological exam showed jitteriness, brisk movements, strong sucking, high-pitched crying, and long periods of alertness.

It was decided to place the infant on opium, 3 drops/kg body weight/day, administered in divided dose every 4 hours for 3 days. The opium drops were gradually tapered and discontinued over 20 more days. The infant continued to be awake and irritable throughout her hospital stay but for decreasing amounts of time.

Some of the nursing problems this infant presented were erractic sucking behavior, spitting up feedings, jitteriness, irritability to environmental stimuli, erratic sleep patterns, and irritable crying. The infant required slow, patient feeding with frequent burping. Her jitteriness and irritability were handled by tightly swaddling the infant, placing her in a quiet corner of the nursery, and covering her crib with a blanket. She was picked up and carried around by nursing personnel whenever possible between feedings.

Fortunately, both her mother and a drug counselor visited the infant daily. The nurses encouraged the mother to hold and feed her infant during each visit. At the time of discharge the drug program counselor reported the mother to have been free of any drugs for the month since the infant's birth.

Generally, drug-addicted parents do not keep developmental follow-up clinic appointments. Therefore this infant was not enrolled. However Baby C's mother brought her back to visit the intensive care nursery at 5 months of age. At that time the mother appeared drug free, and the infant was gaining weight appropriately and was very sociable.

Case 3: The Low-Apgar Infant with Asphyxia and Seizures

Baby L. was born at term weighing 3330 grams to a 21-year-old, gravida II, para 0 mother. Meconium was noticed when membranes ruptured. Before the emergency cesarean section could be performed, there was an episode of severe fetal bradycardia. By the time the infant was born, he had suffered complete cardiopulmonary arrest. His Apgar scores were 0 at 1 minute, 4 at 5 minutes, and 8 at 10 minutes. AT 11 hours of age he developed subtle seizures lasting 2 minutes. He required oxygen at 6 hours of age and ventilatory support from 10 to 24 hours of age. He tolerated room air at 25 hours of age.

Baby L. developed asphyxial cardiomyopathy, demonstrated by a heart rate of 190 beats/minute, and pulmonary edema and bilateral rales. His first seizure began with clenched fists, legs jerking towards his face, and eyes rolled back. Throughout the seizure periods at 11 hours, 24 hours, and 48 hours, his fontanelle was firm but not bulging. He was treated with a loading dose of phenobarbital and then was placed on daily maintenance. Because he had more seizures at 24 hours, his phenobarbital was increased, after which no more seizures were noted. Baby L. also had hyperbilirubinemia, which was treated with high-intensity phototherapy.

Additional nursing problems presented by this infant included facilitating maternal-infant interaction (because of his precarious neurological and cardiac status), encouraging breastfeeding, and discharge instructions, including cardiopulmonary resuscitation (CPR) and administration of phenobarbital and diogoxin. Follow-up of the neurological and cardiac problems needed to be arranged.

Baby L.'s mother visited him daily along with his grandparents. Breastfeeding was begun at 6 days of age and was well established by his discharge at 11 days of age. His mother was taught CPR and how to administer both medications successfully. Appointments were scheduled with the cardiologist and neurologist following discharge.

The infant was followed in the developmental evaluation follow-up clinic for 2 years. From his first visit at 3 months of age to his last visit at 24 months of age, his scores on the Bayley Scales of Mental and Motor Development were above average. His neurological exam was normal, and he remained seizure free after being taken off phenobarbital at 2 months of age.

References

1. Volpe JJ: Neurology of the Newborn. Saunders, Philadelphia, 1981.
2. Purpura DP: Normal and aberrant neuronal development in the cerebral cortex of human fetus and young infant. In NA Berchwall, MA Brazier (eds), Brain Mechanisms in Mental Retardation, pp 141–170. Academic Press, New York, 1975.
3. Chattha AS, Richardson EP: Cerebral white-matter hypoplasia. Arch Neurol 34:137, 1977.

4. Dazé AM, Scanlon JW: Code Pink. University Park Press, Baltimore, 1981.

5. Volpe JJ: Neonatal seizures. Clin Perinatol 4:43–67, 1977.

6. Desmond MM, Wilson GS: Neonatal abstinence syndrome: Recognition and diagnosis. In RD Harbison (ed), Perinatal Addiction, pp 113–122. Spectrum Publications, New York, 1975.

7. Zelson C: Acute management of neonatal addiction. In RD Harbison (ed), Perinatal Addiction, pp 159–168. Spectrum Publications, New York, 1975.

8. Dubowitz LMS, Dubowitz V, Goldberg C: Clinical assessment of the gestational age in the newborn infant. J Pediatr 77:1, 1970.

9. Brann AW: Neonatal ischemic encephalopathy. In: Mead Johnson Symposium on Perinatal and Developmental Medicine, No. 17 Perinatal Brain Insult, pp 49–64. Mead Johnson & Co, Evansville, IN, 1981.

10. Capute AJ, Aceardo PJ, Vining PG, et al.: Primitive Reflex Profile. University Park Press, Baltimore, 1978.

11. Prechtl H, Beintema D: The Neurological Examination of the Full-Term Newborn Infant. Spastics Society, London, 1964.

12. Paine RS, Zapella M: Postural reactions in 100 children with cerebral palsy and mental handicap. Dev Med Child Neurol 6:475–484, 1964.

13. Cloherty JP, Stark AR: Manual of Neonatal Care. Little Brown Company, Boston, 1980.

14. Brazelton TB: Neonatal Behavioral Assessment Scale. Spastics Society, London, 1967.

15. Bayley N: Manual for the Bayley Scales of Infant Development. The Psychological Corporation, New York, 1969.

16. Widmayer SM, Field TM: Effects of Brazelton demonstrations on early interactions of preterm infants and their teenage mothers. Infant Behav Dev 3:79–89, 1980.

17. Beckwith L: Caregiver-infant interaction and the development of the high risk infant. In TD Tjossem (ed), Intervention Strategies for High Risk Infants and Young Children, pp 119–139. University Park Press, Baltimore, 1976.

18. Cromer RF: Reconceptualizing language acquisition and cognitive development. In RL Schiefelbush, DD Bricker (eds), Early Language: Acquisition and Intervention, pp 51–138. University Park Press, Baltimore, 1981.

19. Levy J: The Baby Exercise Book. Pantheon Books, New York, 1975.

Appendices

Appendix 4.1
Nursing Care Plan for Case 1: Irritable Infant

Observation/Task	Nursing Action	Rationale
1. Irritability	a. Organize care to minimize handling	a. Decreases tactile stimulation
	b. Place in crib in quiet area; speak in whispers to infant	b. Decreases auditory stimulation
	c. Keep lights as dim as possible	c. Decreases visual stimulation
	d. Swaddle when held	d. Decreases tactile stimulation, restrains motor activity
2. Inability to sleep	a. Reduce noise level and lights when infant asleep	a. Decreases CNS stimulation
	b. Note sleep-wake patterns and organize care accordingly	b. Facilitates infant organization in sleep-wake cycles
3. Facilitation of breastfeeding	a. Swaddle infant	a. Decreases tactile stimulation and increased motor activity
	b. Provide private, quiet, dimly lighted area for mother and infant	b. Decreases infant distractibility
4. Low maternal confidence	a. Reinforce appropriate maternal observation and behaviors	a. Sharpen mother's observational skills and increases her caregiving skills
	b. Teach environmental control and special needs of her infants	b. Increases confidence by better meeting the special needs of her infant

Appendix 4.2
Nursing Care Plan for Case 2: Infant of Drug-Addicted Mother

Observation	Nursing Action	Rationale
1. Irritability, hyperactivity, high pitched cry	a. Tightly swaddle infant	a. Aides in controlling motor activity secondary to CNS irritability
	b. Place crib or isolette in quiet area	b. Reduces auditory stimuli
	c. Organize care to decrease stimulation	c. Reduces stimuli
	d. Observe and record number and severity of withdrawal symptoms	d. Drug therapy dependent upon documentation of changes in sleep-wake cycles
	e. Administer medications as ordered; observe for absent activity or depressed respirations	e. Avoidance or detection of drug overdose
2. Unstable temperature	a. Monitor temperature and weight as needed	a–c. Hypo- or hyperthermia increases O_2 consumption. Hyperthermia caused by hyperactivity can cause excessive water loss by evaporation through the skin
	b. Observe mottling, flushing, tachycardia, bradycardia	
	c. If body temperature ≥99°F, decrease environmental heat; bathe in tepid bath if above unsuccessful	
	d. Increase frequency of skin care; keep clothes and bedding dry; observe for dehydration	d. Perspiration from hyperthermia may cause a rebound hypothermia; perspiration may cause skin breakdown. Clean and dry skin to decrease this effect
3. Frantic sucking: observe for blisters, skin breakdown	a. Dress infant in mits or shirt with sleeve mits	a. Decreases skin trauma

Observation/Task	Nursing Action	Rationale
	b. Keep skin clean and dry; use aseptic techniques for broken-down areas, using Betadine solution	b. Decreases chance for infection
	c. Use sheepskin under infant	c. Prevents decubitus ulcers and friction burns
	d. Change position often when infant awake	d. Decreases skin breakdown from pressure or rubbing
4. Regurgitation, vomiting, loose stools	a. Observe and document precipitating factors such as medication handling, position	a. Minimizes effects of gastrointestinal irritation from the drug
	b. Position upright after feeds and prone with elevated head of bed (crib)	b. Decreases motion and reflex after feeding
	c. Keep accurate intake and output records	c. Detection of electrolyte imbalance or dehydration
	d. Culture loose stools if persistent	d. Rules out bacterial cause of diarrhea
	e. Evaluate type of feeding	e. Rules out other causes of vomiting
5. Jitteriness, tremors, seizures	a. Document time, movements, precipitating factors, state after seizure	a. Determining type of therapy needed
	b. Maintain patent airway	b. Prevents hypoxia
	c. Stimulate infant if apneic during seizure	c & d. Terminates apneic episode and provides O_2 to the brain during seizures
	d. Hope bag and mask should be at bedside and used if stimulation does not terminate apnea. Infant must be ventilated until seizure stops	
6. Poor feeding	a. Feed small amounts more often; gavage as needed	a. Promotes digestion and prevents reflux; maintains fluid and calorie intake
	b. Check Dextrostix	b. Observation for hypoglycemia

Observation/Task	*Nursing Action*	*Rationale*
	c. Observe for poor skin turgor depressed fontanelle, sunken eyes, increased urine specific gravity, weight loss	c. Detection of dehydration
7. Inability to sleep	a. Minimize noise and light; cover crib	a. Decreases irritability from sensory stimulation
	b. Record sleep-wake cycles and plan care accordingly	

Appendix 4.3
Nursing Care Plan for Case 3: Asphyxiated Infant with Seizures

Observation/Task	Nursing Action	Rationale
1. Respiratory distress	a. Observe and record heart and respiratory rate and Silverman score frequently	a. Evaluates need for oxygen and ventilatory support
	b. Obtain and record blood gases frequently	b & c. Promotes adequate respiratory status
	c. Once on ventilator, provide optimal ventilator care (see Chapter 5)	
2. Seizures	a. Observe and record onset, activity, duration, frequency	a. Helps evaluate need for medication and type required
	b. Communicate any seizure activity immediately to physician in charge	b. Facilitates rapid administration of medication to minimize brain injury
3. Asphyxial cardiomyopathy	a. Observe and record heart rate	a & b. Evaluates cardiac damage and the presence of congestive heart failure
	b. Listen for rales, murmurs	
	c. Administer digoxin	c. Slows heart rate and increases cardiac efficiency
4. Facilitation of maternal bonding	a. Encourage early and frequent visitation	a. Minimizes adverse effects of separation and intensive care nursery on bonding
	b. Encourage touching and stroking whenever possible	b–d. Encourages early involvement
	c. Encourage naming of infant	
	d. Position infant so parents can see infant's face	
	e. Emphasize infant recognition of parental voice, touch, scent	e. Decreases parental feelings of helplessness
	f. Careful explanation of equipment and machinery	f. Educates parents and decreases anxiety

Observation/Task	*Nursing Action*	*Rationale*
5. Breastfeeding	a. Encourage mother to begin pumping breasts immediately	a. Stimulates milk production; builds mother's confidence by giving her task that can be done by no other
	b. Put infant to breast as soon as possible	b. The earlier breast feeding begins, the earlier it becomes established and the easier the transition to home will be
6. Hyperbilirubinemia	a. Check serum bilirubin level if infant appears jaundiced	a. Detects significant icterus early
	b. Remove clothing and diaper	b. Exposes as much skin surface as possible to phototherapy lights
	c. Cover eyes with sterile eye pads and secure them in place	c. Protects retinas from the effects of phototherapy lights
7. Discharge instruction	a. Demonstrate cardiopulmonary resuscitation and have parents practice on mannequin	a. Provides parents with skills necessary to resuscitate high-risk infant at home
	b. Teach techniques for administration of digoxin and phenobarbital; emphasize that exact times and amounts must be adhered to	b. Helps ensure accurate administration of medications at home
	c. See that all necessary follow-up appointments with medical specialists (neurologist, cardiologist), pediatrician, and developmental evaluation clinic are made so that the parents have names, phone numbers, and addresses in hand at discharge; arrange visiting nurse follow-up for at least first 2 weeks after discharge	c. Makes compliance with outpatient therapy as easy as possible for parents

5

Respiratory Development and Disease in the Newborn

Anne Marie Dazé

An understanding of the pathophysiology of newborn respiratory diseases is essential in order to respond appropriately to an infant's physical needs and to keep his family appropriately informed about the infant's status. This chapter provides basic information required by a nurse who cares for an infant with respiratory disease. It also describes a variety of ways to assess and respond to the infant's needs.

Development of the Lung

The most common cause of respiratory difficulties in the neonatal period is an immature lung. As those who have worked with preterm infants know, the infant born at 27 weeks' gestation does not necessarily follow the same course as an infant born several gestational weeks later. There is a spectrum of problems that can be best explained by fetal lung development and the variable rates at which individual infants mature.

Table 5.1 reviews pulmonary embryology in some detail. Through the first 4 months the lung is a solid glandular mass. It is during this phase that canalization of the lung occurs. By the end of the canalicular phase, terminal air spaces appear as outpouchings from bronchioles. These terminal air spaces are not true alveoli, but through several generations of division eventually give rise to clusters of true alveoli. During this phase the lung becomes highly vascularized. Between the 17th and 21st weeks, the mesenchyme thins so that capillaries, which were embedded in the mesenchyme, begin to fuse with alveoli.

With the appearance of terminal air spaces (at about 24 weeks), the final or alveolar phase of lung development begins. During this period several critical events occur that allow the lung to function as an organ for gas exchange. The surface area for gas exchange increases by the proliferation of capillary loops, and the original sacular terminal air spaces mature into true alveolar clusters. The appearance of true

Table 5.1 Fetal Lung Development

Phase	Age	Characteristics
Glandular phase	24 days	Outpouching from foregut appears
	26–28 days (4 weeks)	Two primary bronchial branches appear[a]
	10 weeks	Cartilage deposition begins; branching of bronchi continuing
	12 weeks	Lobes of lung demarcated; cartilage rings reach the lobular and segmental bronchi
	16 weeks	Formation of new bronchi nearly complete
Canalicular phase	18–20 weeks	Mesenchyme begins to thin and the distance between capillaries and airways begins to decrease; septa appear between lobes
	20 weeks	Canalization of airways; appearance of cuboidal cells lining airways
	24 weeks	Terminal air sacs appear as outpouching of the bronchioles; cartilage deposition complete
Alveolar phase	24–26 weeks	Beginning differentiation of type I and type II epithelial cells lining alveolus
	26 weeks	Capillary network proliferating close to the developing airway and thinning of capillary lumen
	28 weeks	Alveoli increase in number to form multiple pouches of a common chamber: "alveolar ducts"
	37 weeks	Production of surfactant sufficient to prevent atelectasis

Adapted from Avery ME, Fletcher BD: The Lung and Its Disorders, 3rd ed. WB Saunders, Philadelphia, 1974; and Hamilton WJ, Mossman HW: Human Embryology. Williams & Wilkins, Baltimore, 1972.

[a] Parallel development of pulmonary vasculature.

alveoli is not consistent but usually occurs at around 27 weeks. Capillary proliferation keeps pace with increasing alveolar numbers. The numbers of capillary loops increase proportionately with alveolar divisions. In addition, capillary lumens increase in diameter as the endothelial cells of the capillary wall begin to thin with maturity. There is increased pulmonary vascular perfusion as gestation increases. Postnatally, alveolar divisions continue through the first months of life, giving rise to six or seven additional generations of alveolar units (1). This ability to produce new alveoli postnatally may account for the remarkable ability of neonates to repair damaged lung tissue, as demonstrated in the capacity of some infants to resolve bronchopulmonary dysplasia (BPD).

Besides increasing the surface area for gas exchange, the alveolar phase of development is characterized by maturation of alveolar structures. During the third trimester the early cuboidal cells differentiate into two types of alveolar cells. Type I cells make up the thin walls of the alveolus, its structural unit. Type II cells, fewer in number but metabolically more active than type I, produce surfactant. The commencement of surfactant production in sufficient quantities varies, but usually occurs at around 36 weeks. External agents such as steroids or heroin can cause precocious development of surfactant, whereas maternal factors such as diabetes or phenobarbital use may delay its production. With the dominance of mature forms of thin-walled alveoli, adequate surfactant production, and matched perfusion, the neonate is ready for independent respiration. Infants born before this sequence of events require ventilatory help.

Surfactant

As the lung matures anatomically, it is also maturing biochemically. The critical biochemical process for normal lung function is the lung's ability to synthesize and secrete the major surfactant dipalmitoyl lecithin. Without sufficient lung surfactant the newborn will develop respiratory distress syndrome (RDS). The effect of surfactant on alveolar function is to diminish the surface-attractive forces of the alveolar wall. Surfactant overcomes the tendency of alveolar walls to collapse or to overexpand.

Dipalmitoyl lecithin is a phospholipid that aligns itself on the alveolar surface. During expiration, when no force for expansion is being applied, the lecithin molecules are tightly packed, creating a uniform surface on the cells lining the alveoli. In this configuration surface-attractive forces are eliminated and the alveoli remain open. While the alveoli remain partially distended at expiration, a small volume of gas, known as the functional residual capacity (FRC), remains in the lung. If the alveoli collapse at expiration (eliminating FRC), the pressure required to open the adherent alveolar walls at the next inspiration is greatly increased. Surfactant thus acts to prevent collapse at expiration and ensures that relatively low opening pressures are required at inspiration.

The surface-active properties of surfactant on the alveolar wall are reversible. During inspiration surfactant has the reverse effect on alveolar function: as alveoli expand, the lecithin molecules are spread out, thereby diminishing their surface-active force. In other words, when the alveoli distend, surface-attractive forces rise. These surface forces will increase at a fairly constant rate in lungs with adequate surfactant production. This means that surface tensions will aid elastic recoil during expiration by enhancing passive emptying of the lung. Surfactant also ensures uniformity of alveolar distension during inspiration. Finally, as the alveoli empty, lecithin molecules become more tightly packed and emptying slows. This allows additional time for gas exchange that would not be available without surfactant (2). In essence, the pulmonary surfactant stabilizes or "buffers" the alveoli from emptying too much or overdistending through an accordionlike action with inspiratory/expiratory cycling.

Prediction of Lung Maturity

Mature lung function depends on the presence of sufficient lung surfactant. Fetal lung cells produce a liquid that fills the alveoli. This liquid constantly flows outward, eventually making its way into the amniotic fluid. Knowledge that fetal lung fluid contributes to amniotic fluid has led to testing samples of amniotic fluid for surfactant. The measure most widely used is the lecithin-sphingomyelin (L:S) ratio. This test compares two phospholipids found in the amniotic fluid: sphingomyelin (a nonsurface-active material that remains constant in amniotic fluid) and lecithin. An L:S ratio greater than 2 is generally accepted as a measure of lung maturity.

Two other measures have recently been used to improve the predictive value of lung maturity tests. These additional measures of lung maturity are the phosphatidylinositol (PI) and phosphatidylglycerol (PG) concentrations. These have been helpful because phospholipids from sources other than the fetal lung can be found in amniotic fluid, creating the possibility of false-positive and false-negative results. At 26–30 weeks PI concentrations begin to rise slowly, parallel with lecithin production. PI peaks at about 36 weeks gestation, then levels and declines (3). PG does not appear until 35–36 weeks gestation and rises as PI falls. Table 5.2 shows interpretations of these tests.

Table 5.2 Testing for Lung Maturity

Interpretation	L : S ratio	PI	PG
Immature	<1.0	Absent	Absent
Intermediate maturity	<1.5–2.0	Small amount	Absent
Mature with some susceptibility	≥2.0	Large amount	Absent
Completely mature	≥2.0	Small amount	Large amount

The L : S ratio requires nearly 12 hours before results are reported. This does not decrease its practicality as a tool for predicting the risk of RDS in unborn fetuses, but does render it impractical for an infant who has already been born, since a newborn infant will be sick from RDS by 12 hours of age if he has inadequate surfactant. A test that has the advantage of speed and simplicity is the foam stability test or "shake test." This test can be done on amniotic fluid or gastric aspirate. Appendix 5.1 describes the procedure for collecting a gastric specimen, and Appendix 5.2 describes the procedure for conducting and interpreting this test. We routinely obtain a shake test on all infants of less than 35 weeks gestation to help determine the amount of monitoring indicated in the first hours of life. Blood and meconium contamination may alter the measured amount of surfactant in a mature specimen. This may cause a false-negative result and lead to delayed delivery of a mature, but endangered fetus if used prenatally. On the other hand, blood or meconium may tend to lead to more falsely mature results in specimens from immature fetuses. Care must be taken when interpreting bloody or meconium-stained specimens.

Respiratory Distress Syndrome

The role of alveoli surfactant in preventing atelectasis is well documented. The infant who lacks adequate surfactant becomes symptomatic within minutes or a few hours and shows progressive respiratory distress.

At birth the lung is fluid filled and with each breath air is introduced. Some of the fluid is expelled outward and swallowed but most is absorbed via pulmonary lymphatics. Alveoli will remain partially distended by fluid so that atelectasis does not occur immediately. Instead, the infant with RDS may appear to breath normally at birth but develops increasing respiratory distress as more fluid is eliminated and alveoli collapse. Symptoms commonly exhibited in RDS are grunting, tachypnea, xyphoid and intercostal retractions, nasal flaring, and seesaw breathing (abdominal asynchrony). All are symptoms of the increasing work of breathing caused by progressive atelectasis. The Silverman score describes a system useful in standardizing the observations of respiratory effort (see Table 2.4 for details). It is not uncommon for a healthy newborn to display mild nasal flaring or retractions after birth. These may disappear spontaneously or after suctioning. Progressive deterioration indicates a pathological process; Silverman's scoring system helps differentiate normal from pathological breathing patterns by rating respiratory effort. Besides progressive evidence of increased breathing work, hypoxia and acidosis will develop early in RDS. This compounds the disease, since asphyxia increases the incidence and severity of RDS.

The incidence of RDS is highest among infants whose birth weights are less than 1500 grams and who are of less than 36 weeks gestation. The chest x-ray of an infant with RDS shows a typical "ground glass" appearance that, in the most severe cases, progresses to complete opacification or "white out." White out indicates that atelectasis is so severe that the border of the heart cannot be distinguished from the lung. For those with a special interest in x-ray patterns in newborn lung disease, Miller et al. (4) presented a succinct review. RDS infants typically show progressive respiratory deterioration that peaks at about 72 hours. In uncomplicated cases the disease will run its course in 7–10 days.

Initial nursing care of all preterm infants includes identifying infants at risk for RDS. This can be done by routinely sending gastric contents at birth for a shake test and observing the infant closely for symptoms of increasing respiratory effort. (See Table 5.3 for steps of respiratory assessment.) Once an infant has exhibited symptoms of RDS, a capillary blood gas sample should be obtained (see Appendix 5.3). Early identification of RDS is essential so that constant positive airway pressure (CPAP) or other appropriate ventilatory support may be used to alleviate atelectasis, and so that oxygen may be used to prevent hypoxia. Procedures for basic nursing care of an infant with lung disease are summarized in Appendix 5.4. (Nursing care for infants treated with nasal CPAP or intubation is discussed in detail under "Interventions for Infants with Respiratory Disease.")

Infants of less than 30 weeks gestation will often have a more protracted respiratory illness than "older" premies. Their disease is complicated by severely immature pulmonary anatomy. In this group, surfactant deficiency plus decreased alveolar size, shape, and number significantly contribute to inadequate respiratory function. Severely preterm infants are compromised to varying degrees by each of the following:

1. Inadequate numbers of true alveoli: dominance of cuboidal end-airway saccules
2. Decreased gas exchange surface
3. Increased alveolar capillary distance, causing a diffusion barrier
4. Diminished respiratory muscle mass, reducing endurance for the work of breathing
5. Minimal calcium bone deposition: soft, collapsible chest wall
6. Immature central respiratory control
7. Inadequate nutritional reserves

Severely preterm infants with RDS might follow the initial acute course described earlier, but they often will require prolonged mechanical ventilation. This

Table 5.3 Infants at Risk for Acid-Base Imbalance

Premature fetal malnutrition (small for gestational age)
Hypoxia: acute, chronic, or intermittent
Asphyxia (low Apgar, low cord pH)
Hypotension: hypovolemia/dehydration; cardiogenic, hemorrhagic, and neurogenic shock
Anemia
Cold stress
Septicemia
Disseminated intravascular coagulation
Tissue necrosis
Renal failure
Liver failure
Inborn metabolic errors
Congenital cardiac disease
CNS injury
Bowel disease (necrotizing enterocolitis)

increases the risk for BPD, since they may require mechanical ventilation and supplemental O_2 for many weeks. In addition, small infants (<1800 grams) undergoing prolonged O_2 administration are at risk for retrolental fibroplasia (see Appendix 5.5 for preventative protocols). Chronic ventilation will compound the potential complications and nursing care. Growth is essential for these infants before they can breath independently. The problems of adequate nutrition then are added to those of standard pulmonary care (see Chapter 3).

Ventilation

Ventilation refers to the movement of volumes of gas, resulting in elimination of CO_2. Perfusion refers to the ability of the lung to saturate hemoglobin with oxygen for delivery. These two seem, at first glance, to be inseparable. However, specific properties of the two gases and the mechanism of gas exchange allow separation. Understanding mechanisms that affect both CO_2 and O_2 exchange clarifies disease pathophysiology and nursing management.

The removal of CO_2 from the alveoli is achieved by the exchange of a volume of CO_2-rich alveolar air for a volume of atmospheric air, which is an essentially CO_2-free gas. Atmospheric air contains 21% oxygen and 0.3% CO_2; alveolar air contains 13% oxygen and 5% CO_2. (See definitions of respiratory terms in Appendix 5.6.) When arterial partial pressure of CO_2 (pCO_2) increases, the minute volume must also increase to prevent accumulation of CO_2. Minute volume can be increased either by increasing the rate *or* depth of breathing. The body normally responds to increased partial pressure of CO_2 (pCO_2) in this manner, but this requires a mature central nervous system (CNS).

Total lung capacity is finite and ventilation occurs within its limitations. Figure 5.1 illustrates theoretical volumes for the lung, so-called "pulmonary function." The

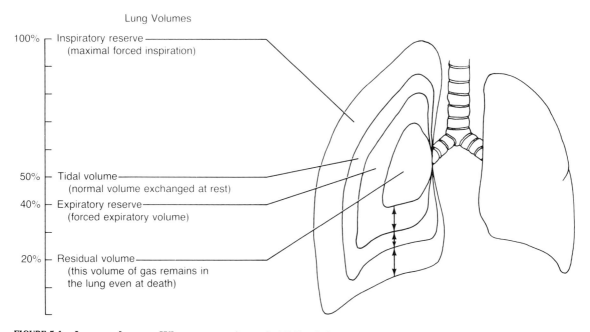

Lung Volumes

100% — Inspiratory reserve
       (maximal forced inspiration)

50% — Tidal volume
       (normal volume exchanged at rest)
40% — Expiratory reserve
       (forced expiratory volume)

20% — Residual volume
       (this volume of gas remains in
       the lung even at death)

FIGURE 5.1   Lung volumes. When approximately 70% of the total lung capacity is exhaled, the closing volume is reached and a small airway collapse begins to occur.

depth of inspiration is limited to the volume of the inspiratory reserve; the depth of forced expiration is limited to the expiratory reserve. The FRC is composed of the expiratory reserve and the residual volume. The FRC prevents collapse (atelectasis) at the end of expiration. In neonates the lung capacity can be estimated by body size. Since there is a very small inspiratory reserve volume in neonates, this estimation is considered the tidal volume (TV):

$$TV = 10 \text{ cc} \times \text{body weight (kg)}$$

Another concept to consider when describing lung volumes is dead space. Dead space is that portion of the tidal volume that is functionless because it is not in contact with an air exchange surface. In a normal breath a portion of the tidal volume is contained in the nose, pharynx, trachea, and conduction bronchioles. This is considered physiological dead space. Any process that increases dead space will increase the work of breathing. An example is an endotracheal tube that extends outside the mouth: the volume of gas that the tube occupies beyond the normal airway increases dead space. This increases the tidal volume requirements proportionate to the length of the tube. In BPD, emphysematous blebs form functionless air sacs that do not contribute to gas exchange. Dead space is increased and larger volumes of gas must be moved to eliminate CO_2. Increased work of breathing is exhibited by the infant with advanced BPD and eventually CO_2 retention occurs.

To some degree the lung resists distension by tidal volume. Compliance describes the lung's rigidity, or the amount of pressure needed to introduce a given volume of gas. Any process that alters lung compliance will affect ventilation. Clearly, as compliance decreases less gas can be introduced, unless greater pressure is exerted. Decreased compliance increases the work of breathing and eventually leads to CO_2 retention. This process is demonstrable in the infant with acute RDS: lung compliance decreases as aveoli collapse. The symptoms induced by this process of decreased compliance are tachypnea and retractions as the infant struggles against an increased opening pressure. Infants with early RDS will have clinical signs of increased work before their blood gases reflect rising pCO_2. This increased effort takes its toll, even though an infant may temporarily compensate for the decreasing compliance by increasing effort.

Mechanical Ventilation

Presently there are two general categories of neonatal ventilators: volume ventilators and pressure/flow ventilators. (For a discussion of hand ventilation, see Appendix 5.7.) Both are capable of delivering a set rate of ventilation, CPAP or positive-end expiratory pressure (PEEP), and a preset oxygen concentration (FiO_2). They differ in a significant way, however. Volume ventilators will deliver a fixed volume by increasing or decreasing the inspiratory peak to compensate for changes in total compliance; they allow for a precise volume to be delivered with each breath. Pressure ventilators deliver an exact peak pressure, but the volume delivered at each breath changes with compliance. As compliance decreases, the pressure ventilator will deliver less volume, and as compliance increases, more volume will be delivered even though the peak pressure remains the same. The actual volume delivered by a pressure ventilator is unknown.

Arterial pCO_2 provides a guide to the adequacy of ventilation. If the minute volume is inadequate, there will be CO_2 retention. If the delivered volume is excessive, it will be reflected by hypocarbia. Other indicators of excessive tidal volume delivery are a flat diaphragm and overdistended lungs on x-ray, and the presence of an air leak. Besides being able to precisely regulate peak inspiratory pressures, most pressure/flow ventilators have accurate timing mechanisms that allow precise regulation of inspiratory times. This allows precise regulation of the mean airway pressure, as discussed on page 122. Manipulation of inspiratory times has been found to be a significant way to minimize exposure to high peak pressures and the resultant barotrauma (5).

The effectiveness of ventilation is measured by the pCO_2. Transcutaneous pCO_2 monitors are becoming more widely available, but arterial or capillary sampling is still the major means of determining the pCO_2. Abnormalities in the arterial pCO_2 can be treated with changes in the rate and/or the depth of ventilation. The depth or volume of ventilation is changed by altering either the peak pressure in the pressure/flow ventilator or the volume setting on a volume ventilator. There is increased use of neuromuscular paralytic agents such as pancuronium bromide (Pavulon) to improve the effectiveness of the mechanical ventilation delivered by decreasing muscle resistance. (See Appendix 5.8 for drugs used in neonatal respiratory disease.) When paralyzation is indicated, the paralytic agent should be administered as soon as slight movement is observed. Because pancuronium bromide has the potential to accumulate at the myoneural junction, the interval of time between doses may increase with successive doses. Side effects include increased salivation, tachycardia, hypertension (occasionally), and a transient rash (6).

The indications for mechanical ventilation include CO_2 retention, apnea, and severe hypoxia. The amount of support required depends on the individual infant and must be adjusted according to the pCO_2 obtained with any particular pressure, volume, or breaths-per-minute setting.

Air Leak Syndrome

Air leaks are common in the neonatal period. Just as a 20-cc balloon ruptures when 25 cc of air are forced into it, alveoli that receive a volume of air greater than their capacity break. Air escapes into the interstitial tissue and from there dissects into the thoracic or the mediastinal space. When air leak results in a pneumomediastinum, it may follow one of four courses:

1. It may remain in the mediastinal space. This rarely causes problems.
2. It may travel from the mediastinum into subcutaneous tissue around the neck or chest, resulting in subcutaneous emphysema.
3. The mediastinal air can enter the pericardial space (pneumopericardium), resulting in cardiac tamponade.
4. If the air leak enters the thoracic space, a pneumothorax results. Pneumothorax may or may not have a significant effect on the infant; the amount of difficulty depends upon the amount of air entering the chest and its pressure.

Each of these conditions—pneumomediastinum, pneumopericardium, pneumothorax, and subcutaneous emphysema—results from the same problem, and they are grouped as the air leak syndrome.

Air leaks occur from overdistention of alveoli. The overdistention and rupture may occur spontaneously, or they can occur secondary to mechanical ventilation if excess volume is delivered. The chance of delivering an excess volume is greater when a ventilator that does not measure or control the delivered volume is used. The chance of delivering an excessively large volume can be reduced by limiting the peak pressure during inspiration. However, there are no guarantees that an excessive volume will not be delivered with any system, since the volume of gas delivered also depends upon the compliance of the lung and airway resistance. Hand ventilators and pressure/flow ventilators are commonly needed for neonatal care, so the nurse must be aware of the potential hazard and monitor infants carefully for air leak signs. Particular attention must be paid when peak measures are being steadily increased during the acute phase of disease. An equally risky period is during resolution of lung disease: compliance may improve more rapidly than the pressures are reduced. Under these circumstances excess tidal volumes may be delivered despite reduction in the peak pressures.

Sometimes air leaks result from hyperdistention of a lung segment. This occurs when a plug partially blocks a bronchiole. With each breath the alveoli distend without completely emptying until rupture occurs. This "ball valve" mechanism occurs most commonly with meconium, but any "sticky" material (blood, vernix) can do it. Keeping the airways free of such materials prevents this sort of air leak syndrome. Chest physiotherapy and suctioning are indicated for the infant with meconium or other material aspiration to help reduce the risk of pneumothorax.

Identifying and locating air in the chest are essential before treatment can occur. The following are findings identified by examination:

Pneumothorax
1. Loss of breath sounds
2. Shift of apical pulse *away* from loss of breath sounds
3. Abrupt tachycardia or bradycardia
4. Cyanosis
5. Hypotension or hypertension of abrupt onset
6. Subcutaneous air (crepitus)
7. Change in peak pressure in mechanical ventilator

Pneumopericardium
1. Narrowing pulse pressures
2. Distant heart sounds on auscultation
3. Weak peripheral pulses

Once an air leak is suspected, transillumination can be used for rapid bedside diagnosis and to assess the removal of air. An x-ray is the definitive means of diagnosing the extent and location of the air leak. Besides the usual anteroposterior view of the chest, a cross-table lateral or decubitus view can help determine the location of air in the chest.

If an air leak is compromising the infant's vital signs, it must be drained immediately. One quick way to remove air is needle thoracentesis. To perform this procedure prep the chest with Betadine and insert a 23-gauge butterfly needle attached to a three-way stopcock into the chest in the third intercostal space on the affected side in the anterior axillary line. Aspirate air using a 20-cc syringe. By putting a stopcock between the needle and the tubing, the syringe can be emptied without disconnecting it from the line. (See Appendix 5.9 for emergency thoracentesis procedure). Once air has been removed by this method, chest tube insertion and water seal drainage can be performed under nonemergency conditions.

After the chest tube has been placed, the infant must continue to be monitored for reaccumulation of air or a second air leak in the other side. In addition, there are special nursing considerations when caring for an infant who has a chest tube in place; these are outlined in Appendix 5.10.

Perfusion and Oxygenation

Any time significant amounts of unoxygenated blood enter the systemic circulation, hypoxemia can occur. This mixing of unoxygenated with oxygenated blood in the systemic circulation is known as "shunting." Shunting can either be pulmonary or cardiac in origin. The causes of cardiac shunts include the cyanotic heart lesions and persistant fetal circulation. The cardiac lesions are discussed in Chapter 8. Pulmonary shunts occur when segments of the lung are perfused without oxygenation occurring or when perfusion-ventilation mismatch occurs. An example is an atelectatic lung segment. Blood will flow past the collapsed alveoli but oxygenation will not occur. When unoxygenated blood mixes with oxygenated blood in the pulmonary vein, the result is a lowered average pO_2 in the left atrium.

Another example of pulmonary shunting is the formation of a diffusion barrier. Because oxygen is not as soluble as CO_2, thickening of the alveolar-capillary surface will be reflected in a lowered pO_2. Thus a ventilation-perfusion mismatch will occur, and blood returning to the left atrium will have a low pO_2 wherever the diffusion barrier exists. Diffusion barriers can result from:

1. Aspiration: inflammation and interstitial edema
2. Infection: inflammation
3. Heart failure: pulmonary interstitial edema
4. Severe prematurity: wide alveolar-capillary space

Treatment of Hypoxemia

The movement of O_2 from the alveoli into the blood depends on a number of variables, including:

1. Percentage of oxygen inhaled (FiO_2)
2. The driving force of inspired gases: mean airway pressure (MAP)
3. Separation of the pulmonary and systemic circulation
4. Blood flow through the pulmonary capillary bed
5. Adequate hemoglobin

The presence of inadequate perfusion is measured by the arterial pO_2. When the arterial pO_2 is low relative to the amount of inspired O_2 (increased alveolar-arterial gradient), oxygenation is impaired and this must be treated. Symptomatic treatment of hypoxemia includes:

1. Increasing the FiO_2 (a crucial initial step)
2. CPAP or PEEP
3. Increasing MAPs (if mechanically ventilated)
   a. Increasing inspiratory times
   b. Increasing peak pressure

Conversely, when an infant is hyperoxic (arterial pO_2 >100 mm Hg), decreasing each of the above elements will decrease the arterial pO_2.

Increasing FiO_2

Room air is 21% oxygen. At sea level, with an atmospheric pressure of 760 mm Hg, the pO_2 of inhaled oxygen is approximately 150 mm Hg.[1] At the alveoli the pO_2 is approximately 100–120 mm Hg. This creates an average arterial pO_2 of 80–100 torr in the healthy mature lung. The driving force (alveolar-arterial gradient) is therefore 20–40 mm Hg. The severity of a shunt is determined by measuring how much oxygen is required to normalize the pO_2. Good nursing management dictates promptly increasing FiO_2 when transcutaneous monitoring or clinical evaluation suggests that hypox-

---

[1] $760 - 60$ (water vapor) $\times 0.21$ (% O_2) = 140 to 150 mm Hg.

emia is present. (See "Transcutaneous pO_2 Monitors.") Increasing the FiO_2 is the first step in correcting hypoxemia.

Increasing MAP

When increasing the FiO_2 is insufficient for supporting the paO_2, positive pressure ventilation is indicated. Increasing MAP values to treat hypoxemia is the next available means of improving oxygenation.

The driving force of oxygen into the airway and into the blood is calculated as the MAP. When various airway forces are calculated, MAP can be derived. This calculation considers centimeters of water pressure delivered by PEEP/CPAP or intermittent mandatory ventilation (IMV), the number of breaths per minute delivered, and the inspiratory times of mechanical breath:

$$MAP = \frac{(R \times IT \times Pip) + [(60 - R) \times IT \times PEEP]}{60}$$

where R is the respiratory rate, IT is the inspiratory time, and PIP is the peak inspiratory pressure.[2]

Theoretically, increasing or decreasing any one of the variables in the MAP equation will cause a change in the pO_2 in the same direction. Controversy exists over which variables are most efficient for improving oxygenation, but the importance of MAP is accepted as a basis for treating hypoxemia with positive pressures.

Manipulation of all the variables of the MAP as a means of improving oxygenation has helped eliminate the need for excessively high peak pressure. This has led to a reduction in the incidence of BPD, reported in several studies where peak pressures were limited (7, 8). However, there do remain risks with increasing the MAP, including air leak, mechanical lung injury, interstitial emphysema, and obstruction of pulmonary blood flow. Because of these potential risks, increases in MAP should be made judiciously and with the above potential problems in mind. In particular, the nurse caring for an infant who has had an increase in MAP must observe not only for improvements in oxygenation but also for acute deterioration from a pneumothorax or redistribution of circulation.

CPAP and PEEP

The application of PEEP or CPAP during spontaneous breathing will have several effects on oxygenation. Both prevent the collapse of alveoli during expiration; this maintains the FRC when there is deficient surfactant or any other process predisposing to alveolar collapse. Early application of CPAP or PEEP may be desirable when there is evidence of an atelectatic process, since these are more efficient at preventing rather than reopening collapsed alveoli. There are some potentially negative effects of CPAP and PEEP on ventilation even though it improves oxygenation. If distending pressure is excessive, either PEEP or CPAP will retard expiration. CPAP increases the work of breathing, and, because it facilitates inspiratory volume, this increased work can lead to air leak. CPAP and PEEP have four postulated effects that improve oxygenation in neonates:

1. Prevention of atelectasis
2. Improvement of MAP

[2] This MAP formula is very cumbersome for clinical use. Recently, constant pressure monitors have been produced that provide automatic readings of MAP; thus minute-to-minute variations in MAP may be observed.

3. Improvement of cardiac output and decrease in right-to-left shunting through the foramen ovale
4. Sparing surfactant production in RDS

Appropriate CPAP settings range from 3 to 10 cm H_2O, with a usual beginning setting of 5 cm H_2O. There are three routes of administration: nasal prongs, endotracheal (ET) tube,[3] and pharyngeal tube.

Inspiratory-Expiratory (I : E) Ratios

The spontaneous normal I : E ratio is usually about 1 : 2; in other words, the expiratory phase of respiration is twice as long as the inspiratory phase. Increasing the I : E ratio by lengthening inspiratory time has been found effective in improving oxygenation during mechanical ventilation for some babies with RDS (9). The ratio generally starts at 1 : 1, then changes as clinical circumstance dictates.

The concept of I : E ratios is applicable only to relatively rapid intermittent positive pressure ventilation rates. When low IMV is used, an inspiratory time should be set at a constant interval, irrespective of the expiratory time of the ventilator, to achieve similar results. Remember, expiration is passive. Expiratory time is determined by the inspiratory time set on the ventilator subtracted from total ventilator time per cycle. With too much time in inspiration (high I : E), expiration may be compromised and CO_2 retention occurs. Also, remember basic arithmetic when contemplating I : E ratios: If the IMV is 60 breaths/minute, there is only 1 second for both inspiration and expiration. Thus, when the IMV is 60 and the I : E ratio is 1 : 1 the inspiratory time is 0.5 second and the expiratory time is 0.5 second.

Transcutaneous pO_2 Monitors

Transcutaneous pO_2 ($TcpO_2$) monitors provide continuous information about the oxygenation status of the infant. This is different than random blood samples, which may or may not reflect the infant's steady state. Premature infants characteristically have labile oxygenation status; episodes of procedure-induced hypoxia have been reported (10). A $TcpO_2$ monitor will detect these episodes. In turn, caregivers can adjust their interventions to prevent or terminate the hypoxic episode. Additionally, the incidence of prolonged hyperoxemia can be decreased with pO_2 monitors.

These monitors have an oxygen-sensitive skin probe that is attached with adhesive. A heating element in the probe warms the skin to a selected temperature (44.0°C), arterializes the tissue under the probe, and measures diffused oxygen. A digital readout displays the measured $TcpO_2$. $TcpO_2$ is generally lower than direct arterial pO_2 but higher than capillary pO_2. The thickness of the skin and adequacy of blood flow to the probe site will affect how closely the $TcpO_2$ reading approaches the arterial pO_2. The use of $TcpO_2$ monitors does not totally replace blood gas studies, but it can cut down on the number of specimens needed.

Any infant who is on a ventilator, on CPAP, receiving oxygen supplementation, and/or experiencing frequent apnea is a candidate for $TcpO_2$ monitoring. All infants of this category are routinely $TcpO_2$ monitored at Columbia Hospital for Women. The following are recommendations for the use of $TcpO_2$ monitors:

1. Ensure monitor accuracy:
    a. Observe a strict schedule of recalibration of the unit according to manufacturer's recommendations.

---

[3] When the infant's respiratory disease can be adequately treated with CPAP and enriched FD_2 alone then nasal CPAP rather than endotracheal CPAP can be used to avoid complications associated with E.T. tubes.

b. Record the $TcpO_2$ reading at the exact time of blood gas sampling to compare the two readings.

c. Keep the probe heat point at a precise standard temperature. The recommended probe temperature is 44.0°C. Variations as small as 0.1°C can affect monitor accuracy and replicability.

2. Prevent local burns or skin breakdown from the heat probe:

a. Change the probe site no less than every 4 hours.

b. Infants of less than 29 weeks gestation generally require probe site changes every 1–2 hours for the first 2 weeks of life to prevent burning.

c. Use adhesive solvent (Detachol, Ferndale Laboratories, Inc., Ferndale, MI) or saturate the tape with water before removing the probe so that skin is not removed when the site is changed.

3. Document oxygenation status:

a. Routinely record $TcpO_2$ reading every 15–30 minutes.

b. If a hypoxic episode occurs, document time, precipitating events (if any), and your intervention.

c. Record the high and low point of the $TcpO_2$ during the time blood is drawn for a gas sampling.

4. Interventions for hypoxemia:

a. If the $TcpO_2$ is less than 40 torr, give additional oxygen, increasing FiO_2 5% every 30 seconds until hypoxemia is terminated.

b. Suction the infant, stimulate respirations, stop other treatment, and/or calm the infant as necessary to alleviate the problem.

c. Reduce the FiO_2 to the previous setting when the hypoxemic episode is terminated. If the infant is unable to maintain a $TcpO_2$ within normal limits, draw a blood gas on the new FiO_2 setting.

5. Interventions for hyperoxemia:

a. If the probe is loose, air will get under it and the monitor will record atmospheric pO_2 (140–160 mm Hg). Ensure that the probe is secured to the skin if $TcpO_2$ values greater than 100 torr are recorded.

b. If the probe is secure and the $TcpO_2$ is still greater than 100 torr, reduce the FiO_2 2–3%. If the $TcpO_2$ remains above 100 torr, reduce the FiO_2 again and draw a blood gas. Once a blood gas has confirmed the accuracy of the $TcpO_2$ monitor, use the monitor to slowly reduce the FiO_2 until the $TcpO_2$ is 70–80 torr. Repeat blood gas sampling to document the arterial pO_2.

General guidelines for O_2 administration are listed in Appendix 5.11.

Anemia

Anemia is defined as too few circulating red cells to adequately oxygenate tissues. The packed cell volume [hematocrit (Hct)] or hemoglobin (Hgb) concentration is used as a measure. If a booster transfusion is needed, the blood replacement calculation is:

$$\frac{\text{Weight in kg} \times \text{blood volume/kg} \times (\text{Hgb desired} - \text{Hgb observed})}{\text{Hgb of transfusion blood}} = \text{transfusion volume in cc}$$

The blood volume estimate for term infants is 80 cc/kg, and for preterm infants, 90 cc/kg. If an infant does not require oxygen supplementation, has a normal acid-base balance, is gaining weight appropriately, and is otherwise asymptomatic, blood replacement may not be indicated despite a Hct or Hgb level below some arbitrary accepted limits. In an asymptomatic infant, the potential complications from transfusion outweigh the benefits. Symptoms of neonatal anemia include:

1. Pallor of lips and nail beds
2. Poor weight gain
3. Tachypnea or tachycardia
4. Lethargy
5. Apnea
6. Heart failure
7. Increased oxygen requirement
8. Unexplained metabolic acidosis

Each infant with a low Hct should be frequently assessed for the presence of any of these signs. The nurse must be an objective observer of the infant in order to identify those infants who do require transfusion.

Acid-Base Balance

The internal environment of neonates must be precisely regulated. One component requiring regulation is the pH. The pH measures the concentration of hydrogen ions. Normally the serum pH is maintained within a narrow range by pulmonary and renal mechanisms. There are two major categories of serum acids: respiratory (carbon dioxide) and metabolic. The list of metabolic acids is long. The body produces many under both normal and abnormal conditions (such as hypoxemia or inborn metabolic errors). There are serum buffers that compensate for production. Included among these are the CO_2/bicarbonate mechanism, Hgb, serum proteins, and large anion complexes. Buffers accept hydrogen ions to prevent lowering the pH. This reaction is simply depicted by:

$$H^+ + buffer \rightarrow H\text{---}buffer$$

Carbon dioxide dissolved in a solution contributes H^+ by the following sequences:

$$CO_2 + H_2O \leftrightarrow H_2CO_3 \leftrightarrow H^+ + HCO_3^-$$

This is a reversible reaction; CO_2 is removed by ventilation, leaving only water. Normally there is no net gain of H^+ during the process of CO_2 production by cellular respiration because of the ability of the Hgb molecule to be a hydrogen ion acceptor (buffer) (11). Since most of the H^+ molecules released by carbonic acid are bound to Hgb globin, physiological CO_2 production normally contributes to the total amount of bicarbonate in the system. Excess CO_2 production or inadequate ventilation will cause a respiratory acidosis.

Hydrogen ions are also added by a metabolic acid load. Their excretion is through the lung if bicarbonate combines with their free H^+ to form carbonic acid. Carbonic acid produces CO_2 and is excreted through the lung. In addition, the kidney directly excretes H^+ in several ways. The interaction of serum buffers (acute phase), ventilation (subacute), and the renal mechanism (slow) constantly maintain normal acid-base homeostasis.

Compensatory Mechanisms

Change in arterial pH stimulates the CNS respiratory center to regulate the amount of CO_2 eliminated by altering ventilation. CO_2 dissolves freely into the cerebral spinal fluid (CSF), causing rapid shifts in the CSF pH. When CSF pH falls, chemoreceptors in the medullary respiratory center increase the rate and depth of respirations. Conversely, there is a decrease in respirations when the pH becomes alkalotic. Change in respirations is the immediate compensatory response to deviations in pH. If the pH remains abnormal for a prolonged period, the kidney begins to compensate. The mature kidney alters tubular function to regulate hydrogen ion excretion. If the kidney is appropriately responding to acidosis, the urine pH becomes increasingly acidotic. However, the neonatal kidney is relatively limited in its ability to excrete H^+ or conserve bicarbonate, so this compensating mechanism rarely totally corrects the pH. Some of the acidosis encountered will be mixed and will require varying therapies plus a diligent search for the underlying problem.

Buffer Replacement

When respiratory acidosis occurs, ventilation is the treatment. When a metabolic acidosis occurs, then buffer replacement and treatment of the underlying cause are indicated. Sodium bicarbonate is commonly used for metabolic acidoses, but its use is limited in neonates largely because of the inefficiency of neonatal sodium excretion. Remember that with every milliequivalent of bicarbonate given, a milliequivalent of Na^+ is also administered. (See Chapter 3 for limitation of Na^+). Bicarbonate must also be given with caution because of its hyperosmolar properties. To decrease the osmolarity, dilute bicarbonate with equal amounts of water to a 0.5 mEq/cc solution. Then give the dose slowly, over 10 minutes. Once the pH is temporarily corrected, the underlying metabolic cause must be identified and eliminated. An example is the neonate who is suffering cold stress and as a result has metabolic acidosis. The infant will continue to produce excess acids until the cold-stressing environment is corrected.

As mentioned above, Hgb is part of the buffer system, acting as a hydrogen ion acceptor. If anemia is significant, reduction in Hgb carrying capacity may contribute to a metabolic acidosis. Reduction in tissue oxygen delivery may also contribute to a metabolic acidosis through increased lactic acid production. Lactic acidosis from anemia will not be fully treated until sufficient oxygen delivery to the tissues has been established. Blood replacement is the treatment of choice. At all times, blood loss through lab sampling must be accurately recorded so that iatrogenic causes of this problem will be detected early.

Table 5.4 Parameters of Normal Neonatal Respiratory Function

Parameter	Normal values
Clinical	
Respiratory rate	30–60 b.p.m.
Respiratory regularity	Periodic pause <15 sec in length
Respiratory effort	Silverman score <3
Breath sounds	Air entry and audible depth of breath sounds are equal throughout chest
	Clarity: no grunting, rales, rhonchi, or squeaks
Laboratory: Blood gases	
pH	7.35–7.42
pCO_2	35–42 mm Hg
Arterial pO_2	60–90 mm Hg
$TcpO_2$	50–70 mm Hg
Capillary pO_2	40–50 mm Hg
HCO_3^-	18–20 mmol/L
Base excess	0 ± 4 mmol/L
X-ray	Clear lung field

Consequences of acidosis on cellular metabolism are legion. All are potentially life threatening. Early identification and treatment will prevent the most severe consequences of acidosis. Since blood gas analysis is the only means of identifying acid-base imbalance, routine sampling must be done when caring for at-risk infants. Table 5.4 indicates clinical situations that indicate close monitoring of acid-base balance. The frequency of blood gas sampling is determined by the severity of the disorder. It cannot be emphasized too strongly that a blood gas analysis should be obtained any time acid-base imbalance is suspected or is yet uncorrected in any neonate.

In summary, acid-base imbalance can be respiratory or metabolic in origin, and may be due to an excess of serum acids or bases, to *insufficient* serum acids or buffers, or to overzealous therapy. The consequences involve many organ systems. The only real tool for determining the acid-base status of any infant is blood gas sampling.

Transitional Physiology

In utero the placenta is the organ of gas exchange and the lungs are essentially functionless. The fetal lungs receive about 20% of the total output of the right ventricle rather than 100% of the output as in later life. This small amount of blood is sufficient for the fetal lung's growth needs. Specific mechanisms that maintain minimal perfusion of the lungs are:

1. Anatomic shunts: ductus venosus, foramen ovale, ductus arteriosus
2. Normal fetal arterial pH (7.25–7.35) in low range
3. Low systemic blood pressure
4. High pulmonary vascular resistance
5. Low arterial pO_2 (40–50 mm Hg)
6. Low vascular resistance at the placenta (high flow)

Once an infant is born, his cardiopulmonary system must make a dramatic change from its fetal state to one that can sustain extrauterine function. These changes are called neonatal transitional physiology.

What sustains fetal blood flow patterns? In fetal life the pulmonary vascular bed is constricted, creating a higher resistance to blood flow. Because of high resistance in the pulmonary circuit, blood is directed from the right to the left side of the heart via fetal shunts. In addition, the placenta is a low-resistance organ. The low systemic pressure, combined with the high pulmonary vascular resistance, shunts right ventricular blood away from the lungs toward the systemic (aortic) circulation. The relationship between pulmonary and systemic resistence becomes critical when caring for an infant with persistant fetal circulation.

At birth the pattern of blood flow changes acutely. The cord is clamped, removing placental circulation. This increases systemic vascular resistance and blood pressure. With the first few breaths the infant develops large negative pressures in his chest. This pulls air with 21% O_2 into the conducting airways and the pO_2 rises. Blood flow increases in the pulmonary capillaries. The arterial pO_2 goes up with each new breath and the pulmonary circuit further dilates.

Closure of the ductus arteriosus is dependent on elevations in the serum pO_2, the amount of available muscle mass, and circulating levels of prostaglandins. Final ductal closure normally may not occur until 2–3 days of age but functionally closes within 1 hour of birth.

Once the ductus arteriosus is closed, the circulating pattern is the adult variety. The remaining major difference from adult function is that the neonate has, for some time, a potential to revert to a fetal circulatory pattern. Any neonate whose systemic pressures falls and pulmonary resistance rises may do so. Without a placenta to oxygenate blood, this is devastating. The some factors that sustain fetal circulation in utero can cause reversion to fetal circulation in the neonatal period, that is, hypoxia, acidosis, and immaturity. Furthermore, diseases that lower systemic blood pressure below pulmonary artery pressure (shock) can trigger a return to intrauterine-like circulation if the fetal shunts open.

Persistant Fetal Circulation

A profound complication in the neonatal period occurs when an infant fails to convert from, or reverts to, a fetal circulatory pattern. This phenomena is known as persistant fetal circulation (PFC) or more properly, persistent pulmonary hypertension. A review of physiological events that occur in cardiopulmonary transition will help explain the causes and effects of this syndrome. The classic picture of PFC is an infant with severe hypoxemia but who has normal or low pCO_2 readings.

Infants at greatest risk of PFC are those who have been severely asphyxiated in the perinatal period. The pulmonary vasculature constricts in response to acidosis and hypoxemia. Thus perinatal asphyxia is directly related to pulmonary vasoconstriction and resultant PFC. Sometimes PFC is the result of pulmonary arteriolar muscular hypertrophy. This variant is very refractory to treatment.

Before a positive diagnosis of PFC can be made, cyanotic congenital heart defects must be ruled out (see Chapter 8). An adequate work-up includes x-ray, M-mode or 2-D echocardiogram, electrocardiogram, and, if the infant is stable enough, cardiac catheterization. Echocardiogram, particularly, is very helpful not only to rule out structural defects by measuring right and left ventricular ejection intervals, but to "rule in" PFC also.

A test that is helpful in PFC is the comparison of simultaneous blood gases, one from below and one above the ductus arteriosus. Potential "postductal" sites include the umbilical or femoral arteries. Preductal sites include the right brachial, radial, or temporal arteries. Since the aortic origin of the right brachial and common carotid arteries is before the ductus arteriosus, the paO_2 obtained from preductal sites will be greater than the postductal pO_2 if right-to-left shunting through the ductus is present. Also, placement of two $TcpO_2$ monitors on the infant—one one the upper right chest to evaluate preductal pO_2 and the other on the abdomen to evaluate postductal pO_2—will provide similar information.

Once PFC is established as the cause of hypoxemia, treatment is directed toward lowering the elevated pulmonary vascular resistance. The critical event in fetal-neonatal transition is dilation of pulmonary blood vessels. One way to stimulate pulmonary dilation is to force the arterial pH into an alkalotic range. This is done most effectively and safely by hyperventilation. The goal of this therapy is to keep the serum pH at 7.45 or greater. One risk of hyperventilation is massive urinary potassium loss, resulting in hypokalemia.

Pharmacological agents used in PFC include pancuronium and Priscoline (see Appendix 5.8). Many infants with PFC will require paralysis with pancuronium to ventilate them effectively. Priscoline (tolazoline HCl), a nonspecific vasodilator, can be administered to enhance pulmonary dilation. The administration of tozalozine should be through a vein that drains into the superior vena cava because, theoretically, more of the drug will go into the pulmonary artery and pulmonary vasculature. An arm or scalp vein can be used for the administration of tozaloline since both veins drain into the superior vena cava (12). No umbilical or lower extremity vessel is suitable for this purpose. The use of tolazoline HCl carries risks. It is a nonspecific vasodilator and may cause systemic hypotension. When the systemic (left-sided) pressure drops below the pulmonary pressure, right-to-left shunting worsens. We routinely have a dopamine drip ready for administration whenever Priscoline is used to treat systemic hypotension, should it develop.

Nursing care of the infant with PFC is complex. Systemic blood pressure *must* be maintained within a normal range. This may require careful titration with dopamine. The infant may suddenly convert to extrauterine circulatory patterns, resulting in hyperoxia. A continuous $TcpO_2$ monitor is very helpful here, as well as for assessing the severity of hypoxia. Since in PFC the infant tends to hypoxemia, nursing care must minimize increases in oxygen demands by external sources, such as temperature fluxes. Fluid overload can occur when multiple drugs and fluids are being administered continuously by several different parenteral routes. Evaluation of fluid status should be done as described in Chapter 3. The kidneys may have sustained hypoxic injury, complicating maintenance of fluid balance. Careful measurement of urine output and all fluid administered (including flushes) is critical.

Two or more daily weighings are helpful, but using a standard infant balance scale requires interruption of ventilation. This could be devastating for the infant with PFC. For this reason we use scales that fit under the mattress (Scaletronix, Inc., Wheaton, IL) so that the infant can be weighed without being moved. Assessments to detect a developing pneumothorax must be continuous in an infant with PFC being mechanically hyperventilated (see "Air Leak Syndrome").

When the infant converts to normal circulation, paO_2 rises dramatically, but weaning from ventilatory and drug support must be done slowly or reversion to PFC can occur. Again, the use of two $TcpO_2$ monitors can be invaluable. If postductal pO_2 drops, support must be increased until shunting decreases.

PFC carries a significant mortality. Parents must be aware that this is a potentially fatal disease. Although specific therapy is available, the disease or complications of therapy produce a 20% mortality.

Apnea

The normal neonatal respiratory pattern is irregular, with periodic pauses and varying rates and depths of breaths. These periodic pauses are not pathological if vital signs remain stable. However, if the pause is longer than 15 second or is associated with bradycardia, it is called apnea. There are two goals when caring for an infant with apnea of any cause. The first is to protect the infant from hypoxemic damage during the apneic episode. The second goal is to determine the cause of the apnea.

Apnea may result from depression of the CNS centers for respiration. One common type is "apnea of prematurity." The more preterm an infant is, the more immature are his medullary respiratory regulatory centers (13). As a consequence, the neonatal respiratory pattern with periodic pauses is exaggerated and apnea is more likely to occur.

Apnea can be so severe that bag and mask resuscitation is needed. Mechanical ventilation may also be necessary. Rocking water beds and mechanical rocking have been tried and sometimes work, but are not reliable. Studies by Aranda et al. (14) have shown that aminophylline and caffein are effective in treating apnea of prematurity. CPAP is also an effective therapy in some cases. Maturation of the CNS will most usually result in a regular respiratory pattern. Controversy exists about home monitoring programs for these babies to prevent sudden infant death syndrome. This decision must be individualized.

Apnea may also result from specific pathological processes, which requires diagnosis and treatment of the underlying cause. The following are particularly important to exclude:

1. Pumonary insufficiency of any cause (hypercapnia)
2. Seizures
3. IVH
4. Hypoglycemia
5. Sepsis

To detect the presence of apnea and determine its underlying cause, careful observation of at-risk newborns is required. Routinely, an electronic heart rate monitor should be used for all infants who weigh less than 1500 grams. Any larger infant with lung disease, hypoglycemia, or an infection should also be monitored. When observations or an electronic monitor detect an apneic episode the following steps should be taken:

Observation Time the pause between breaths and observe heart rate, color changes, and TcpO$_2$.

1. If the pause is less than 15 seconds and all vital signs are normal, it is a periodic pause without any clinical significance.
2. If the pause is longer than 15 seconds or the vital signs deteriorate, stimulate the infant.
3. Sometimes an infant will become bradycardic and hypoxic even though he is moving his chest. Auscultate the chest to determine if breath sounds are present when the infant breathes. Some infants move their chest but do not move any air and are essentially apneic despite respiratory effort. This phenomenon can be due to opposing abdominal muscle movements that impede the movement of the diaphragm, or it can be due to airway obstruction from mucus in the trachea or pharynx, or from a head position that obliterates the airway.

Stimulation The amount of stimulation it takes to reestablish respirations may be helpful in establishing the cause of apnea. Apnea of prematurity is characterized by apneic episodes easily terminated by stimulation. On the other hand, seizures expressed as apnea may be totally unresponsive to stimulation. Stimulate with increasing vigor by 1) rubbing toes gently, 2) rubbing back or sternum gently, and 3) flicking sternum briskly.

Clearing the Airway Suction the nose, mouth, and throat; reposition the head so the neck is appropriately extended to ensure that the infant's airway is not being obstructed.

1. If the infant is now breathing spontaneously, document the episode after suctioning.
2. If the infant is still apneic, proceed to ventilation.

Ventilation Since this is an observed respiratory arrest, ventilate the infant at an FiO$_2$ approximately what the infant was breathing prior to the apnea. For example, if an infant was breathing 35% O$_2$ before the apneic spell, bag the infant at the 40% adjustment of the resuscitator bag. Do not bag with less oxygen than the infant needed prior to being apneic. The FiO$_2$ can be increased if the infant's color fails to improve at the initial setting.

Documentation The following information about the infant's apnea should be included when describing the episode:

1. The number of apneic episodes
2. Events that preceded the apnea (i.e., feeding, suctioning, emesis, stooling, hy-

poxia, change in ventilator setting, rapid-eye-movement sleep, or state of activity, each of which may precipitate apnea)
3. Length of apnea and changes in vital signs
4. Amount of stimulation required to terminate apnea (or whether self-stimulated)
5. Results of suctioning
6. Amount of additional ventilatory support required to bring the infant back to a stable state

Using this scheme of observations and interventions, consistent information will be obtained and safe care ensured. These observations also must be reported promptly since further medical work-up may be required.

Interventions for Infants with Respiratory Disease

Chest Physiotherapy

Chest physiotherapy (PT) is a widely used technique for removing pulmonary secretions. The elements of chest PT (drainage, vibration, percussion, thinning secretions, and suction) are aimed at removing obstructive debris and reexpanding collapsed alveoli.

Not many studies have been done documenting the benefits of chest PT in neonates, but a few conclusions can be drawn concerning this technique. In general, active chest PT has been found more effective in removing mucus than turning an infant into drainage positions followed by ET suction. Chest PT does significantly increase oxygen requirements during the procedure, but is generally followed by improvement in oxygenation. These observations suggest indications and contraindications for chest PT. Indications for PT include:

1. Meconium aspiration
2. Gastric contents aspirations
3. ET intubation (the ET tube irritates as a foreign body)
4. BPD or other chronic pulmonary inflammation (i.e., cystic fibrosis)
5. Pneumonia
6. Atelectasis
7. R.D.S (after 48 hours)

The most obvious contraindication to chest PT is the severely hypoxemic infant with little apparent mucus. Infants hypoxic from a cyanotic heart lesion or persistent fetal circulation are examples. Recent evidence also suggests that chest PT may significantly increase intracranial pressures of premature infants. Thus, the risk of intracranial hemorrhage may be increased when chest PT is done in the first 72 hours of life, when hemorrhage is is most likely to occur.

Clinically, how does one evaluate the need for chest PT? First, a diagnosis of the above mucus-producing diseases or the presence of an ET tube would indicate a need for chest PT. It is our practice that the frequency of chest PT is individualized to maximize the benefits from treatment but minimize potential risks and stress to the infant. To individualize therapy each infant must be thoroughly assessed. Clarity and equality of breath sounds, volume and tenacity of secretions obtained from suctioning, the appearance of the chest x-ray, trends of blood gases, the presence of a mucus-producing pathophysiology, and the effect of chest PT during and after therapy (as indicated by the transcutaneous and cardiorespiratory monitors) are ways to determine an infant's needs for PT.

Taking each element of assessment individually, the presence of mucus and/or the collapse of a lobe can often be auscultated by a careful exam. Both mechanical and spontaneous sounds should be evaluated, since the loss of spontaneous breath sounds may occur much earlier than the loss of mechanical sounds. Mechanical ventilator sounds can also be misleading. They can be audible over a collapsed segment since the small neonatal chest transmits sounds easily. Expertise in evaluating neonatal breath sounds comes only after frequent auscultation and comparison of the volume of secretions suctioned and the infant's clinical status with the sounds you hear. If breath sounds are diminished or absent over a segment (and the ET tube is properly positioned), or rales and rhonchi are audible, chest PT is indicated. An x-ray often reveals collapse or consolidation not noticeable by auscultation. This also is an indication for vigorous and frequent PT.

The volume of secretions obtained after vigorous chest PT may suggest the need for further chest PT. Remember, the volume of secretions will only be affected by vigorous percussion and/or vibration. If a large amount of mucus is obtained, chest PT should be repeated and the interval between sessions of chest PT shortened. Chest PT should be sufficiently frequent to keep the airways clear. For instance, if large amounts of secretions are obtained when chest PT is done at 3-hour intervals, the frequency could be increased to every 2 hours. Inversely, if little or no secretions are obtained, the frequency can be decreased. Thus, the benefit of keeping the airway clear can be balanced against the adverse effects of hypoxia or exhaustion.

Blood gases can be used as a criterion for frequency of PT. Improvement of blood gases (either pCO_2 or pO_2) following chest PT argues a need for PT. If an individual infant's pO_2 or pCO_2 levels remain normal at the chosen routine for chest PT but deteriorate if chest PT is done less frequently, then chest PT should be done at the chosen routine. This can be an important observation in unintubated infants who swallow secretions and mask the volume mobilized by PT.

To prevent hypoxemia during PT, routinely increase the infant's FiO_2 until the $TcpO_2$ is at least 60 torr. The infant is then placed in one of the drainage positions discussed in Appendix 5.12. Note that there are 11 drainage positions, and each one drains a particular segment of the lung. If a particular collapsed lobe is found by x-ray or auscultation, the infant should be positioned to drain that segment. Once positioned, 1 minute of vigorous percussion and/or vibration should be applied over the elevated segment. Several methods of percussion have been described for neonates; the palm of the hand, a padded cup, and a face mask (15). We could find no comparison study that determined the most effective method. However, that it must be done vigorously to be effective is consistently reported. For percussion, we use a commercially available cup that is easy to hold and is well padded (DHD Medical Products, Div. of Diemolding Corp., Canastota, NY).

Vibration during the expiratory phase is also done over the elevated segment. The techniques for delivering vibration include manual vibration and the use of a cordless electric toothbrush handle padded with a rubber cork. When using an electric toothbrush, the head of the cork should be on the chest and enough pressure applied so that vibration can be felt at a rib distal to the cork head. We have found the toothbrush method effective when done in this fashion, but it is useless if the side of the cork is used and/or only the skin is vibrated rather than transmitting the vibration to the ribs.

Many very small, preterm infants cannot tolerate more than a few minutes of percussion or vibration. In such infants either vibration *or* percussion might be done, rather than both. Vibration is less effective than percussion for moving thick plugs and large airway obstruction. Vibration seems to enhance clearing small airways. Percussion then might be the best method for the infant with mucous or meconium plugs, whereas vibration could be chosen when thin secretions are present. Once one segment has been actively percussed and/or vibrated, the infant's position should be changed to give PT to another segment. Many neonates tolerate active PT to only a portion of their chest at any one time. For such infants, PT done over different segments of the chest should be scheduled so that every segment is actively treated in any 8-hour period. If the $TcpO_2$ reading falls significantly or the arterial blood pressure rises during percussion or vibration then the PT should be stopped until the infant recovers.

Suction and thinning of secretions are important elements of chest PT. Suction should follow chest PT. It should be done between vibration and percussion of different lung segments if the volume of secretions warrants it. ET suction is a sterile procedure, and standard sterile technique should be used. A suction kit containing a glove, catheter, and water container are convenient to ensure that correct technique is followed. The catheter should be chosen so that it enters the ET tube freely. When the catheter completely occludes the ET tube, the infant cannot move air (i.e., cannot breathe). *Minimize this time!* Care should be taken not to suction the wall of the trachea or bronchus. The length of the tube to be passed should be estimated from the ET tube connector to the ear, and from the ear to the mid-sternal level. As a general rule, the distance from lip to tip of the carina by birth weight is 7 cm for <1 kg, 8 cm for 1–2 kg, and 9 cm for >2 kg. Suction catheters with centimeter markings can be used to standardize the length of catheter to be passed. Limiting the amount of negative suction pressure used to 100 cm H_2O may decrease traumatic tissue injury during suction.

Saline should be instilled into the trachea prior to suction, and blown down the ET tube with the ventilator or a bag. Saline thins the secretions to maximize their removal by catheter; however, it must be blown down the ET tube to actually thin secretions, not just left rattling around at the mouthpiece. The saline used should be free of bacteriostatic agents since these may cause pulmonary irritation. A volume of 0.2–0.5 cc can be used. Secretions should then be suctioned after the saline has been blown down the ET tube. Additional mechanical breaths should follow the suctioning. By preceding and following the suctioning with mechanical ventilation, hypoxia can be minimized. $TcpO_2$ monitoring throughout the procedure is recommended. Stop suctioning if hypoxia occurs.

The suction should be repeated until only clear saline is obtained. The mouth and nose can then be cleared. Finally, the infant should be turned to a new position, and the FiO_2 should be decreased to the level needed prior to the treatment. (See Appendix 5.13 for a step-by-step method.) From our experience, we recommend that chest PT and suctioning should be done based on infant requirement, not on an arbitrary routine. When used judiciously it is an essential part of the care of the infant with respiratory disease.

Nasal CPAP

The nasal, pharyngeal, or ET routes can be used to deliver CPAP. Nasal or pharyngeal CPAP is used most often for infants who have mild to moderate RDS or who have just been extubated. Their advantage is that constant positive pressure and oxygen can be delivered without the complications of an ET tube. The major disadvantage of nasal CPAP is the ease with which almost any neonate can terminate it. Whenever the infant cries or dislodges the prongs, the treatment is interrupted. For this reason infants with nasal CPAP are routinely nursed in isolettes and the isolette environment is kept at the same FiO_2 as that being delivered through the prongs. If the infant succeeds in bypassing the CPAP or the prongs must be removed, the infant continues to breath the appropriate amount of oxygen.

Nursing Care of the Infant with Nasal CPAP

Prevention of Complications

1. Assessment of effectiveness:
   a. Improvement in blood gases should occur.
   b. Presence of CPAP flow sounds at auscultation.
   c. Nasal suction every 8 hours and as needed to maintain patency of route.
2. Prevention of local irritation:
   a. Examine nares every 8 hours.
   b. Change size of prongs in presence of bleeding or breakdown sores.
   c. Apply small amount of water-soluble lubricant to prongs to decrease friction.
   d. Position tubing so that prongs are in nares but not pushing them.
3. Examination for potential route of infection:
   a. Observe color and type of secretions obtained from nares.
   b. Culture and gram-stain yellow or purulent nasal secretions.
   c. Clean nasal prongs every 8 hours with sterile water to remove mucus.
   d. Change prongs as needed.
4. Ensuring pressure and oxygen delivery:
   a. Choose prong size that will insert easily into infant's nose: a comfortable fit will decrease infant irritability.
   b. Secure prongs to head with a strap with wide headpiece; a paper surgical face mask fits an infant's head well, and the ties of the mask can be used to secure the prongs. The mask should be spread across the back of the head so there is no single pressure point.
   c. Restraints: sand bags on either side of infant's head can minimize head movement.
5. Preventing abdominal distention—because CPAP flow is entering the stomach as well as the lungs, the stomach may become inflated with air and distention of the abdomen can occur.
   a. Check abdominal girths every 8 hours.
   b. Use a no. 8 French catheter feeding tube to straight drainage.
   c. Change tube every 24 hours.
   d. Do not feed by mouth; can give transpyloric feedings.

Insertion of prongs

1. Suction each nostril to ensure patency of nasal airway (see Appendix 5.14).
2. Lubricate prongs with a small amount of Lubrifax. Do not obstruct CPAP flow with Lubrifax.
3. Insert prongs so that they are at a 90° angle to the infant's face.
4. Set CPAP flow and FiO_2 to ordered amounts.
5. Restrain infant as necessary and stabilize tubing so that there are no pressure points on the upper lip or sides of the nostrils.
7. Using O_2 controller,[4] deliver oxygen into the isolette at an FiO_2 equal to the amount ordered for the CPAP. In this way the infant will receive the prescribed FiO_2 when mouth breathing or crying, or when the prongs are out for nasal suctioning.

Ongoing care

1. Every 8 hours remove prongs, suction each nostril, and clean prongs with sterile gauze and water. Reapply Lubrifax as above and reinsert prongs. Check nose and upper lip for signs of pressure and adjust prong position as necessary.

---

[4] The oxygen controller (IMI Oxygen Controller or Biomarine, Inc.) senses the FiO_2, then increases or decreases O_2 flow so that the desired percent is achieved.

2. Check that the FiO_2 and CPAP settings are as ordered and readjust if needed after repositioning prongs.
3. Prongs should be removed only for very short intervals and while the infant remains in an isolette with the prescribed FiO_2 so that pO_2 will not drop excessively.
4. If excess or purulent mucus is suctioned from the nose, culture the secretions.
5. The infant should be turned every 2 hours and as needed while on nasal CPAP. Chest PT should be done as needed, followed by suctioning.
6. The indwelling feeding tube should be changed daily. Patency should be checked as needed. Do not advance a feeding tube once it has been placed, since the plastic may become rigid and increase the risk of gastric perforation. Mark the tube with the date and change it every 24 hours or more frequently, as needed.
7. Check blood gases and monitor with $TcpO_2$ monitor as condition warrants.

Intubation

If an infant requires mechanical ventilation, an ET tube is placed between the vocal cords into the trachea, and positive pressures are used. Mechanical ventilation via intubation has been associated with the following problems:

1. Vocal cord edema, fibrosis, and/or paralysis
2. Perforation of the trachea
3. Chronic upper lobe atelectasis
4. Infection
5. Tube "accidents": plugged or dislodged ET tubes
6. BPD
7. Pneumothorax

Prevention of complications is the major thrust of nursing these infants. Sterile, atraumatic insertion of the ET tube is the first step to this goal. Table 5.5 lists appropriate ET tube sizes based on birth weight. As a general rule, an ET tube should have a slight leak around it so that the vocal cords are not constantly subjected to pressure, and so that inadvertent gas volume excesses can be "blown off." Stabilization of the inserted tube will decrease the possibility of vocal cord or bronchial trauma. Good fixation also decreases the risk of extubation. Ongoing evaluation of the patency and position of the tube is required. Finally, when the ET tube is removed, particular observations and interventions are required to ensure the infant's safety.

Nursing Care of the Intubated Infant

Assessment of Placement
1. Auscultation: if the ET tube is in the trachea, breath sounds will be clearly audible when a mechanical breath is given.

Table 5.5 Appropriate ET Tube Sizes Based on Infant Weight

Infant's weight (g)	Tube size (cm)	Tube depth (cm)
700	2.5	6
1000	3.0	7
1500	3.0	7
2000	3.5	8
2500	3.5	8
3000	4.0	9

2. Equality of sounds: if the ET tube is placed into the right mainstream bronchus, breath sounds will be muffled or inaudible on the left side.
3. X-ray: the tip of the ET tube should be visible between T_1 and T_3. An ET tube placed below T_3 may slip into the right mainstem bronchus and/or traumatize a bronchus. An ET higher than T_1 may flip out of the cords and into the esophagus, leading to accidental extubation. Loose ET fixation will increase the risk of both problems.

Assessment of Patency
1. Breath sounds present with mechanical ventilations: spontaneous breath sounds can be present even if the tube is blocked if the infant is able to breath around the ET tube; thus spontaneous sounds are poor indicators of tube patency.
2. Development of a mucous plug in the ET tube will prevent a suction catheter from being passed the length of the ET tube. Never push a plug back down into the trachea in an attempt to clear the airway.
3. Unexplained deterioration in the blood gases: partially obstructed ET tubes may allow partial but inadequate ventilation, resulting in deterioration in the blood gases.

Intervention
1. Obstruction or displacement of the ET tube requires that it be removed immediately. The infant should be bagged by mask until reintubated.
2. All ET tubes must be secured to the face in a way that immobilizes it far enough from the mouth to prevent saliva from loosening it. A Logan bar (Storz Instrument Co., St. Louis, MO) fastened to the sides of the head with Betadine and moleskin tape, approximately 1 cm from the mouth, is a method the author uses sucessfully (see Figure 5.2).

Observation for Complications
1. Infection: obtain routine cultures of the ET tube (every 2 to 3 days) while the infant is intubated (see Appendices 5.13 and 5.15).
2. Hemorrhage: large amounts of bright red blood suctioned from the ET tube indicate pulmonary hemorrhage; this may be spontaneous or secondary to trauma.
3. BPD: perform weekly pulmonary lavage for pathology staging (see Appendix 5.16).
4. Pneumothorax: loss of breath sounds on one side with a mediastinal shift away from the loss of sounds is indicative of a tension pneumothorax with a mediastinal shift. Compare equality of breath sounds and location of apical pulse to evaluate. This is an emergency! Prompt action is necessary.
5. Vocal cord trauma: secondary to irritation of vocal cords by the ET tube, this does not become symptomatic until the infant is extubated. Once the infant is extubated, loud, high-pitched inspiratory stridor indicates significant narrowing of the airway. Racemic epinephrine inhalent may relieve symptoms if due to edema. Hypoxia and/or CO_2 retention may develop if the vocal cords are significantly swollen either by edema (transient) or fibrosis (chronic). Chronic intubation may cause loss of laryngeal protection and airway patulousness. If the baby cries, you know he can close his vocal cords. This is a good clue that he can safely guard against aspiration and can be fed orally.
6. Skin breakdown: the mouth or nares may develop pressure-point irritation if the ET tube is positioned incorrectly. These can be relieved only by preventing or removing any pressure by the tube on the mouth or nose. $TcpO_2$ monitors may cause skin breakdown from the heat.

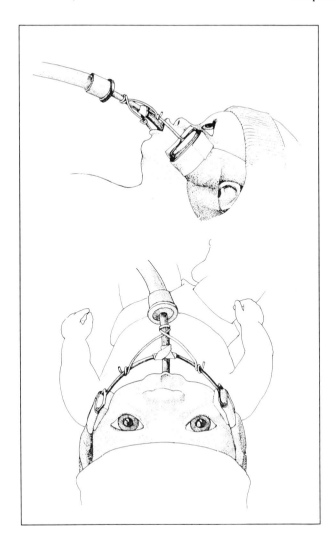

FIGURE 5.2 View of Logan bar method of stabilizing an ET tube. The Logan bar is held in place on the infant's head with moleskin tape. The ET tube is then taped to the bar with ¼-inch adhesive tape. Foam rubber pads the bar where it touches the infant's cheeks.

Environment

1. Radiant heated table: offers maximal access; infants with multiple lines (i.e., umbilical artery catheters, chest tubes, central lines) require a heated table for safe manipulation. The disadvantage is increased fluid loss from the skin by evaporation.
2. Isolette: smaller area in which to nurse infant, but it offers a more controlled environment. The environment can remain at a constant temperature and the air entering the isolette is filtered, offering protection against airborne infection. We routinely nurse intubated infants in isolettes once the umbilical artery catheter is removed.
3. Equipment: every intubated infant should have the following resuscitation equipment at the bedside: bag and mask with oxygen flow; ET tube of the approximate size (see Table 5.5); laryngoscope and blade; emergency thoracentesis setup.

Umbilical Catheters

Umbilical venous (UVC) or arterial (UAC) catheters are commonly placed in sick infants for the administration of fluids, blood sampling, exchange transfusion, and/

or continuous pressure monitoring. Central venous pressures can be obtained from a UVC. It also provides an excellent route for exchange transfusions. Arterial blood pressures can be obtained from a UAC, and when an infant has respiratory disease a UAC is placed both to monitor arterial pressures and to facilitate routine arterial blood gas measurement (see Appendix 5.17 for procedure).

To place a UAC requires sterile technique and experience. A cord tie is put in place and the cord is transected. An artery is probed, dilated, and then catheterized with a no. 3.5 (if birth weight is <1.5 kg) or a no. 5 French catheter. We prefer the "high" supradiaphragmatic position. We do not routinely put heparin in the lines, although some clinicians do so.

Once the umbilical catheter is in place, the nurse caring for the infant must direct her care toward observing for and preventing complications that arise from the presence of an umbilical catheter. The following is an outline of the basic interventions required.

Nursing Care of the Infant with an Umbilical Catheter

Prevention of Excess Blood Loss
1. Keep a padded clamp at bedside in case of an accidental break in the line.
2. Keep an accurate record of the volume of blood removed from the line for lab sampling.
3. Notify the physician if blood loss exceeds 5% of the infant's blood volume (approximately 5 cc/kg).
4. Return volume of blood removed to clear the line of IV fluid prior to lab sampling.
5. Tape the catheter, using a bridge method, and restrain the infant if active to prevent accidental separation or removal of catheter. Mittens may prevent an active infant from grasping a catheter.

Maintenance of a Patent Line
1. A minimal fluid flow of 2 cc/hour is required to prevent clotting of an umbilical catheter.
2. Flush the line with 0.5–1.0 cc dextrose (5%) in water after blood has been withdrawn for lab sampling.
3. If the line becomes difficult to flush or the blood pressure wave form becomes dampened, an order for heparin (1 U/cc fluid) may be needed to prevent total clotting of the line.
4. Do not flush a clotted line since this will introduce a large embolus into the aorta. The line should be changed if it becomes clotted.

Prevention of Sepsis
1. Use aseptic technique when catheter is inserted.
2. Change all tubing and fluid every 24 hours.
3. Apply bacteriostatic solution to umbilical area when catheter is inserted.
4. Every 8 hours and as needed clean umbilical area with alcohol.
5. Observe infant for symptoms of local cellulitis and/or generalized septicemia.

Identification of Vascular Complications
1. Extremities
   a. Observe the color and capillary filling time of both feet and toes.
   b. Notify the physician if the capillary filling time is longer than 5 seconds, or if blue toes or pallor in either extremity develops.
   c. Record normal as well as abnormal observations.

2. Gastrointestinal
    a. Measure abdominal girth every 8 hours.
    b. Guaiac test all stools for occult blood.
    c. Listen for the presence of bowel sounds.
3. Renal
    a. Keep an accurate fluid intake and output record, including all of the blood or flush taken or given through the catheter.
    b. Test urine for occult blood (Multistix).
    c. Assess hourly urine output every 8 hours (should remain at least 1 cc/kg/hour).
4. Embolus
    a. Remove all air from the line.
    b. Never push clots or air through the catheter.

Maintenance of Continuous Blood Pressure Monitoring

References

1. Emery JL, Mithal A: The number of alveoli in the terminal respiratory unit of man during late intrauterine life of childhood. Arch Dis Child 35:544–560, 1960.
2. Kotas RV: Surface tension forces and liquid balance in the lung. In DW Thibeault, GA Gregory (eds), Neonatal Pulmonary Care, pp 35–53. Addison Wesley, Reading, MA, 1979.
3. Hallman M, Kulovich A, Kirkpatrick E: Phosphatidylinositol and phosphatidylglycerol in amniotic fluid: Indices of lung maturity. Am J. Obstet Gynecol 122:613–617, 1976.
4. Miller LK, Calenoff L, Boehm JJ, Reidy MJ: Respiratory distress in the new born. JAMA 243:1176–1179, 1980.
5. Herman S, Reynolds EOR: Methods for improving oxygenation in infants mechanically ventilated for severe hyaline membrane disease. Arch Dis Child 48:612–616, 1973.
6. Slota M: Pharmacologic paralysis. Critical Care Nurse 2(3):21–27, 1982.
7. Reynolds EOR, Taghizadeh A: Improved prognosis for hyaline membrane disease. Arch Dis Child 49:505–509, 1974.
8. Taghizadeh A, Reynolds EOR: Pathogenesis of bronchopulmonary dysplasia following hyaline membrane disease. Am J. Pathol 82:241–244, 1976.
9. Spahr RC, Klein AM, Brown DR, et al.: Hyaline membrane disease: A control study of inspiratory to expiratory ratio and its management by ventilator. Am J Dis Child 134:373–376, 1980.
10. Long JG, Philip AGS, Lucey JF: Excessive handling as a source of hypoxemia. Pediatrics 65:203–207, 1980.
11. Lamb JF, Ingraham CG, Johnson IA, Pitman RM: Essentials in Physiology. Blackwell Science Publications, London, 1980.
12. Emmanouilides GC: Persistence of fetal circulation. In DW Thibeault, GA Gregory (eds), Neonatal Pulmonary Care, pp 361–371. Addison Wesley, Menlow Park, NJ, 1979.
13. Kattwindel J: Apnea in the neonatal period. Pediatrics in Review 2:115–120, 1980.
14. Aranda JV, Grodin D, Sasynuik BI: Pharmacologic considerations in the therapy of neonatal apnea. Pediatr Clin North Am 28:113–129, 1981.
15. Etches PC, Scott B: Chest physiotherapy in the newborn: Effect on secretions removed. Pediatrics 62:713–715, 1978.

Appendices

Appendix 5.1
Gastric Aspiration for Shake Test

Purpose

To evaluate infants suspected of having respiratory distress related to lack of pulmonary surfactant.

Recommendation

To be obtained on all infants of <36 weeks' gestation.

Equipment

1. 5-cc syringe
2. No. 8 French catheter feeding tube

Procedure

1. Premeasure feeding tube for level of insertion and pass tube into stomach.
2. Gently aspirate at least 2 cc of gastric contents.
3. Cap syringe; quickly withdraw feeding tube.
4. Label and send specimen.

NOTE   Blood or meconium in the gastric aspirate specimen may cause spurious shake test results.

Appendix 5.2
Shake Test Procedure

1. Obtain approximately 1 cc gastric or amniotic fluid:
   a. Specimen must be free of blood or meconium.
   b. Collect specimen in a syringe or mucus trap.
2. To test fluid:
   a. In a plain glass test tube, pipette 1 to ½ cc fluid sample and an equal amount of 100% (isopropyl) alcohol.
   b. Shake the mixture in a stoppered tube for 15 seconds.
   c. Let specimen stand for 15 minutes (accurate time is critical).
3. Reading the results:
   a. No bubbles on surface of fluid: − (negative)
   b. Small bubbles, <⅓ diameter of tube: +1
   c. A single ring of bubbles ⅓ to completely around diameter of tube: +2
   d. A complete ring of bubbles with a second row in some places: +3
   e. A double row of bubbles completely around the tube: +4
4. Interpretation

Negative	No surfactant
+1	Inadequate surfactant
+2	Intermediate surfactant production
+3	Mature
+4	Fully mature

Appendix 5.3
Obtaining Peripheral Blood Gas Specimens

Purpose

To ascertain the blood gas status of the infant with compromised cardiorespiratory function who does not have an arterial catheter in place.

Procedure

1. Warm the infant's hand or foot for 15 minutes.
2. Measure the delivered FiO_2 with analyzer and use a technique that will keep it constant.
3. Assemble the following equipment:

   Lancet   Vaseline
   Blood gas tubes   Band-Aid
   Alcohol pad   Completed blood gas slip
   2×2 gauze pads

4. Call lab before starting to collect the specimen to notify them that it is going to be drawn.
5. Appropriate sites:
   a. Lower half of heel
   b. Lateral tip of finger
6. Using aseptic technique, wipe the site with alcohol and then dry it with a 2×2 gauze pad. Using the lancet, make a clean straight cut into the desired site; then apply a small amount of Vaseline.
7. Milk extremity lightly to avoid hemolysis, but enough to initiate a good blood flow.
8. Collect specimen by filling each tube three-quarters full and take it immediately to the lab. Record on gas slip the $TcpO_2$ reading immediately before and after the blood was drawn.
9. Draw other heel-stick specimens required (i.e., for Dextrostix, electrolytes, or Hct).
10. Wipe extremity dry and apply Band-Aid.
11. Any specimen that must wait in the lab should be placed on ice and sealed.
12. Chart amount of blood loss on data sheet (approximately 0.2 cc for the capillary blood gas).
13. Chart results of blood gas analysis on a blood gas flow sheet, with the *exact* time the specimen was drawn, and notify the physician of the results.

NOTE   Sites should be rotated whenever possible to avoid extensive bruising and/or unhealed wounds on a particular extremity. Also, hematomas underlying a blood-drawing site can alter the blood gas results.

Appendix 5.4
Nursing Care of an Infant with Respiratory Disease

Maximizing Oxygenation

Assessment

1. Blood gases
   a. Sample blood gas every 4 hours.
   b. Attach transcutaneous pO_2 ($TcpO_2$) monitor
2. Hemoglobin-carrying capacity
   a. Keep a careful record of blood intake and output: blood loss from lab sampling in excess of 5% of the infant's blood volume may significantly decrease oxygen-carrying capacity.
   b. Hct
   c. Blood pH
3. Use of $TcpO_2$ monitors
   a. Increase FiO_2 if $TcpO_2$ falls to <40 mm Hg; some infants require O_2 support when $TcpO_2$ reaches 50 mm Hg.
   b. Document changes in FiO_2 and the infant's state of activity or reaction to treatment.
   c. Change skin probe site every 3–4 hours; if skin becomes excessively reddened, change site as frequently as every hour.
   d. Recalibrate transcutaneous monitor every 8 hours
4. Examination
   a. Color: pink or cyanotic lips reflect degree of core oxygenation (acrocyanosis is less significant).
   b. Vital signs: apnea may occur secondary to hypoxia or hypercapnia; tachycardia may be an early response to hypoxia.
   c. Capillary filling: a decrease in skin perfusion will occur before it is reflected by a fall in blood pressure; capillary filling of the trunk normally requires <4 seconds.

Interventions

1. Delivery of appropriate FiO_2
   a. Analyze O_2 source every 8–12 hours; O_2 mixers on ventilators or nebulizer lose accuracy with constant use. Analyze the O_2 to ensure the desired FiO_2 is being delivered.
   b. Increase FiO_2 during vigorous treatments and/or when infant's $TcpO_2$ or blood gas reflects hypoxia.
   c. Decrease FiO_2 if $TcpO_2$ or blood gas reflects hyperoxia (>100 mm Hg); decrease the FiO_2 slowly (2–5%/5 minutes) to prevent a rebound hypoxia, the "flip-flop" phenomenon.
   d. Arrange continuous $TcpO_2$ monitoring for infants with an unstable oxygenation status.
2. Maintenance of a patent airway
   a. Oropharyngeal suction (see Appendix 5.14)
   b. ET suction (see Appendix 5.13)

c. Chest PT: vibration drainage (see Appendix 5.12)
d. Turn infant every 2 hours: dependent lobes of the lungs receive maximal perfusion through the effects of gravity, so turning the infant helps equalize these effects. The prone position maximizes oxygenation and can be done even when the infant is intubated.
3. Minimizing infant distress: data from $TcpO_2$ monitoring have demonstrated that neonates' oxygenation status may be dramatically affected by "routine" care, tests, and treatments.
   a. Eliminate routines that are not essential; scrutinize vital signs routines, chest PT, blood withdrawal schedules, etc., to minimize stress while ensuring safety and adequate care. Only lifesaving procedures are important enough to be done when an infant is experiencing a hypoxic episode.
   b. Provide sleep time: organize care to allow infant to sleep undisturbed for a minimum of 1 hour out of 3 hours.

Maximizing Ventilation

Assessment

1. Blood gases: normal pCO_2 range, 35–42 mm Hg.
2. Examination
   a. Respiratory rate
      1. Normal rate is 30–60 breaths/minute.
      2. Apnea: frequent episodes may cause CO_2 retention.
   b. Breath sounds
      1. Clarity: rales or rhonchi are abnormal.
      2. Depth
      3. Equality: loss of breath sounds on one side may indicate atelectasis, pneumothorax, or a misplaced tube.
   c. Effort: note presence or absence of retraction, grunting, and/or nasal flaring (see Silverman scoring, Table 2.4).

Interventions (see preceding section)

1. Maintain a patent airway: suction, and adjust head position.
2. Chest PT
3. Mechanical ventilation

Appendix 5.5
Retrolental Fibroplasia Protocol

Vitamin E Prophylaxis

1. All infants weighing less than 1800 grams, who receive oxygen for 24 hours or more should receive vitamin E.
2. Vitamin E 10–15 U every third day is recommended.
3. The route of vitamin E must be IM until the infant is taking gastric feedings, then vitamin E is given daily, with oral feedings at a dose of 10–15 U.

Ophthalmology Consultation

Ophthalmology consultation should be arranged for all infants who:

1. Had a birth weight less than 1500 grams;
2. Have been mechanically ventilated, including CPAP, for more than 24 hours;
3. Had an O_2 requirement (FiO_2) greater than 40% for more than 12 hours.

The need for follow-up exams should be determined after the initial examination.

Appendix 5.6
Respiratory Definitions

Acidosis A blood pH of less than 7.35 can be of either respiratory (CO_2) or metabolic acid origin.

Alveolar stability The tendency of an alveolus toward atelectasis, dependant upon the presence of sufficient surfactant to reduce surface tension.

Apnea A cessation of breathing for longer than 15 seconds, or an absence of respirations for any length of time which is accompanied by cyanosis and/or bradycardia.

Compliance The elasticity of an expandable material. Compliance (CV) is measured by determining the amount of pressure (P) it takes to deliver a known volume (V):

$$CV = \frac{V}{P}$$

Dead space That portion of the tidal volume *not* involved in gas exchange (i.e., the tidal volume in contact with the nose, throat, trachea, bronchus, etc.).

FiO2 The *f*raction of *i*nspired O_2; percentage of O_2 delivered.

Functional residual capacity (FRC) The amount of air remaining in the lung at the end of expiration in continuity with the airways.

Intermittent mandatory ventilation (IMV) A mode of positive pressure ventilation in which a set ventilatory rate is delivered, but the patient can also breath spontaneously between mechanical ventilations.

Minute volume The volume of gas inhaled (or exhaled) in a minute (the tidal volume times the respiratory rate)

Periodic breathing An irregular pattern of breathing seen commonly in premature infants. The pauses between breaths are not longer than 15 seconds, and all vital signs remain within normal limits.

Pulmonary vascular perfusion The amount of blood flow through the pulmonary vascular bed.

Respiratory distress syndrome (RDS; hyaline membrane disease) A pulmonary disease of immature lungs lacking sufficient surfactant and characterized by diffuse atelectasis.

Shunt The mixture of venous blood with arterial blood, consequently lowering the arterial pO_2. Can take place on either a cardiac or pulmonary level.

Surface tension The attractive force between two surfaces.

Tidal volume The volume of gas exchanged in a single breath.

Ventilation The exchange of gases within the alveolus. Measured by a comparison of the amount of CO_2 expired and the amount (or percentage) of alveolar CO_2. Hyperventilation is the state in which the expired CO_2 exceeds the alveolar CO_2, and hypoventilation is the inverse. Gas exchange is dependent upon the tidal volume and the difference in inspiratory and expiratory alveolar volume.

Ventilation/perfusion ratio A comparison of the ventilation of a segment of the lung to the perfusion of the same segment. When the ventilation-perfusion ratio is not equal to 1, alterations of blood gases will result.

Diffusion barrier: A thickening of the alveolar wall, interstitial space, or capillary wall that decreases the permeability of these structures to O_2. Various causes are edema, hypertrophy, mucus, immaturity, etc.

Appendix 5.7
Hand Ventilation

Purpose

For mechanical ventilation of infants who:

1. Are not intubated for bag/mask respiratory support.
2. Are intubated and require synchronized support, during ET suction, during arrest, or until a mechanical ventilator can be assembled.

Recommendations

1. Every infant who is intubated should have a bag and mask assembled at the bedside.
2. Any sick infant transported either within hospital or between hospitals should be accompanied by a mask and bag.
3. Extra sterile bags and masks should be available at all times for emergency use.

Procedure

Action

Preliminary measures

1. Clear the infant's airway (either ET tube or mouth, by suctioning).
2. Set the O_2 flow to 10 liters of oxygen-enriched air, if desired.

Bag Resuscitation

3. Attach the 100% O_2 tail or collar if 100% O_2 is desired. Remove the collar or tail if 40% O_2 is desired.

4. Gently compress the bag until the infant's chest rises and/or air flow through the lung can be heard with a stethoscope.
   a. If the pop-off valve can be heard during the compression, compress the bag more slowly and gently, and check to make sure a tight seal between the bag and airway has been achieved.
   b. Use of a pressure manometer in the line will allow the resuscitator to accurately control the amount of delivered pressure.
5. Continue as above until the infant no longer needs support or a ventilator is available.

Rationale

1. Ventilation will only be effective if the airway is clear.
2. The bag pressure pop-off valve is set to release at a liter flow of 10 liters/ minute.

3. If no O_2 is turned on, room air will be delivered. If 100% is used and the infant's heart is within normal limits and his color is pink, a decrease to 40% is recommended.

4. Only enough pressure to cause airflow through the lungs is needed to ventilate the infant. Rapid hard compression will increase the likelihood of excess pressures being delivered to the infant (and pneumothorax). The pop-off valve releases at 40 cm H_2O, which may be excessive for some infants.

Appendix 5.8
Drugs Commonly Used in Neonatal Respiratory Disease

Drug name	Dose/frequency	Route	Action	Side effects	Special precautions/instructions
Aminophylline (theophylline)	3–5 mg/kg: loading 4–6 mg/kg/24 h: maintenance	IV or oral	Transformed into caffeine (in neonates); cessation of apnea of prematurity	1. Tachycardia 2. Diuresis with increased sodium loss 3. Hypertension 4. Jitteriness (toxicity may cause seizures) 5. GI upset: distention and/or bleeding	1. Hold dose if resting HR[a] is greater than 180 beats/min 2. Monitor serum electrolytes and I & O 3. Take BP at least once a day 4. Observe for hyperreflexia, excess jitteriness, or seizures 5. Measure abdominal girths before meals twice daily and guaiac-test stools 6. Measure serum drug levels
Caffeine	20 mg/kg: loading 5 mg/kg/24 h: maintenance	IV or oral	Cessation of apnea	Same as Aminophylline	
Dopamine	5–20 μg/kg/min: continuous infusion	IV	1. Increased force of myocardium; (+) ionotrophy; increased pulse and systolic pressures 2. Decreased peripheral vascular perfusion 3. Renal vascular dilation	1. Hypertension: rise in diastolic pressures 2. Arrhythmias 3. Tissue necrosis when infiltrates tissue	1. Continuously monitor BP and ECG 2. Do not administer with bicarbonate; inactivated by alkaline solutions 3. Phentolamine (Regitine) is the antidote to prevent sloughing from dopamine infiltration
Epinephrine, racemic	1 : 100 solution, 0.08–0.1 cc in sterile normal saline:[b] every 4 h and as needed	Inhalant	Bronchodilator	1. Tachycardia 2. Arrhythmias 3. Flushing	1. Monitor HR before and after each dose 2. Hold dose if HR >200 beats/min after dose
Furosemide (Lasix)	1–3 mg/kg: every 8 h or as needed	IV, IM, or oral	Diuretic	1. Electrolyte disturbance (potassium or sodium) 2. Dehydration	1. Monitor serum electrolytes 2. Potentiates renal and ototoxicity of aminoglycosides
Mucomist	10–20% solution, 0.2–0.5 cc in sterile normal saline:[b] every 4 h or as needed	Inhalant	Liquification of respiratory secretions	1. Bronchospasm	1. Observe for wheezing or increased effort after treatment; keep racemic epinephrine available to treat severe bronchospasm

Drug	Dosage	Route	Action/Use	Side effects	Nursing considerations
Pancuronium (Pavulon)	0.04–0.10 mg/kg/dose as needed for movement	IV	Paralysis of voluntary muscles	1. Transient hypertension 2. Increased salivation 3. Transient rash and sweating	1. Monitor BP, either continuously if arterial line available, or every hour 2. Frequent oral suction 3. Paralyzation requires mechanical ventilation 4. Lost blink reflex: use artificial tears and eye pads if lids do not remain closed 5. Credé bladder gently to ensure emptying 6. Cold or aminoglycoside antibiotics can aggravate block
Sodium bicarbonate	1–2 mEq/kg	IV or oral	Buffer: correction of metabolic acidosis	1. Transient hyperosmolarity 2. Hypernatremia 3. High doses associated with intracranial bleeds	1. Dilute with equal amounts of water when given IV and give slowly. 2. Monitor serum sodium level; observe for dehydration
Tolazoline (Priscoline)	1–2 mg/kg IV over 15 min, then continuously 1–2 mg/kg/h	IV	Vasodilation of pulmonary vasculature	1. Flushing 2. Hypotensive shock (may lead to increased R → L shunt if peripheral BP not kept within normal limits) 3. GI hemorrhage	1. Infuse into scalp vein or vein in upper extremity; blood from superior vena cava is directed into the right ventricle and pulmonary artery to treat persistent fetal circulation
Vitamin E (α-tocopherol acetate)	10–15 mg every third day if IM or daily if oral	IM or oral	Lipid antioxidant; decreases incidence of retrolental fibroplasia		

[a] Abbreviations used: HR, heart rate; GI, gastrointestinal; I & O, intake and output; BP, blood pressure; ECG, electrocardiogram; R → L, right to left.

[b] Normal saline should be free of any preservative since this may irritate the respiratory tract.

Appendix 5.9
Emergency Thoracentesis

Purpose

To relieve acute symptoms associated with escape of air or fluid into the pleural cavity until a chest tube can be inserted.

Equipment

The following items should be assembled and kept at the bedside of any infant on ventilatory assistance or otherwise at risk for pneumothorax:

1. No. 23G ¾-inch butterfly needle
2. Three-way stopcock
3. 20-cc syringe
4. Betadine swab

Procedure

After a pneumothorax has been diagnosed, rapid decompression can be achieved by needle aspiration:

1. Prep skin with Betadine at the third intercostal space.
2. Assemble ¾-inch butterfly needle and closed three-way stopcock.
3. Insert needle at a 90° angle into identified area.
4. Attach 20-cc syringe to stopcock and aspirate air.
5. Use of stopcock allows air to be emptied from syringe without disconnecting it from the needle tubing.

Surgical placement of chest tube trochar can now proceed in a controlled manner. One person continues to aspirate the pneumothorax until chest tube is attached to water seal drainage.

Appendix 5.10
Maintenance of Chest Tube

Purpose

To continuously evacuate air and/or fluid from the pleural cavity.

Equipment

1. Pediatric underwater-seal chest drainage unit
2. Wall suction connector and suction connecting tubing
3. Tincture of benzoin
4. Wide adhesive tape
5. Two rubber-shod hemostats
6. Emergency thoracotomy set-up.

Procedure

Action

1. Restrain infant on procedure table; attach cardiorespiratory monitor.

2. Assist physician with insertion of chest tube, and dress site. Attach chest drainage unit to chest tube connector and increase suction until moderate bubbling appears in suction control chamber.

3. Secure all tubing connections with tape.
4. Obtain chest x-ray.

5. Check frequently for air leaks (underwater-seal chamber), at least three times/shift, and record in nursing notes (e.g., presence of bubbling in chamber).

6. Mark level of drainage collected on chest drainage unit at end of each shift and record this amount.

Rationale/Precautions

1. To prevent trauma to infant during procedure and provide adequate monitoring of infant's status.

2. Excess bubbling in the suction chamber will cause the water in this chamber to evaporate rapidly and frequent refilling will be required. NOTE: The amount of suction applied to the chest is regulated by the water level in the suction control chamber, so the ordered water level must be maintained to ensure that the appropriate amount of suction is applied to the chest.

3. To prevent accidental break in seal.

4. For placement of the catheter and overall visualization of lung fields.

5. Bubbling in the underwater-seal chamber indicates that air is being removed from the chest. If the bubbling stops suddenly, an obstruction of the chest tube should be suspected. A gradual reduction and the stoppage of bubbling over a period of days usually means that the pneumothorax has resolved.

6. Accurate output record of type and amount of drainage allows the physician to calculate the infant's blood volume status. (A loss of more than 5% blood volume or bright red or

Action

7. Milk chest tubes every hour. Report:
   a. Any sudden or unusual increase in distress or change in heart rate.
   b. Color change, especially acute or prolonged cyanosis.
   c. Bright red and/or pulsating bloody drainage.
8. Never clamp a chest tube without a specific order.

Rationale/Precautions

pulsating drainage should be reported immediately.)

7. Sudden deterioration in the infant may indicate that another or the reaccumulation of a pneumothorax has taken place. Hemorrhage or excess loss of serum through the chest tube may cause an infant to become hypovolemic, leading to shock.

8. Since most infants in the NICU have tension pneumothorax from air leak, clamping the tube will remove the escape for the air and the pneumothorax will reaccumulate until the air leak is healed. The tube may be clamped for several hours before it is removed to determine if air will reaccumulate or if the leak has healed.

Appendix 5.11
Oxygen Administration to Neonates

Delivery Room Resuscitation

When resuscitating an asphyxiated infant in the delivery room, a 100% O_2 bag should be used. Adjustment to a 40% O_2 bag should be made only when the infant's response to resuscitation warrants it. Blood gases should be drawn upon admission to the ICN if oxygen administration is still required.

Transcutaneous Monitoring of $TcpO_2$

The following guidelines should be used if the transcutaneous monitor is known to be well calibrated and securely fixed to the skin.

1. FiO_2 may be increased in increments of 5% every 30 seconds, if the monitor reads less than 40 torr, until the $TcpO_2$ is above 40 torr.
2. FiO_2 may be decreased slowly every 30 seconds if the $TcpO_2$ is above 90 torr.
3. The infant's color and clinical condition should be used as additional guards against inappropriate adjustments in FiO_2 based on faulty $TcpO_2$ reading or individual patient problems.
4. Oxygen changes made should be documented clearly, indicating length of change in O_2 requirements and infant's state. Blood for gas analysis should be drawn after the TCM reading has stabilized.

NOTE   A 15- to 45-second lag time occurs between arterial and transcutaneous pO_2 values. This argues for a 30-second interval between adjustments in FiO_2.

Monitored Resuscitation

1. Mechanically ventilated infants who require resuscitation or assistance with a bag should initially be bagged with an FiO_2 approximately equal to but not less than the FiO_2 set on the ventilator. Adjustments in FiO_2 should be made as warranted by the clinical conditions (i.e., persistent cyanosis).
2. When in doubt about ET tube patency or placement, the nurse may extubate the infant and bag with FiO_2 settings as above. The on-call physician must be paged immediately for reintubation.
3. When apnea and bradycardia spells require bagging, the FiO_2 given should be approximately equal to and not less than the environmental FiO_2 prior to the apnea/bradycardia episode.
4. A 100% O_2 bag may be used whenever the clinical condition of the infant demands it (i.e., insufficient response to a 40% O_2 bag).
5. The FiO_2 used during resuscitation should be charted in the nurse's notes and doctor's progress notes.

Continuously Delivered Oxygen

1. All O_2 must be analyzed every 8 hours to verify that the desired FiO_2 is being delivered.
2. Unless ordered otherwise, blood gases should be drawn no less than every 4 hours.
3. If available, a $TcpO_2$ monitor should be used on any infant receiving O_2.

Appendix 5.12
Chest Physiotherapy and Postural Drainage for Newborns

Purpose

1. To clear the lung and tracheobronchial tree of accumulating secretions.
2. To prevent formation of mucus plugs that block ET tubes.
3. To open atelectic areas of the lung.

Special Considerations

1. Vibration with a padded toothbrush is the preferred technique to clear small airways.
2. Clapping with a face mask or padded cup should be done with caution to prevent excess pressure being delivered to the chest. It is recommended for cases when an infant has large amounts of thick, tenacious secretions or debris in the lung, such as with meconium aspiration.
3. Duration of treatment depends upon the tolerance of the patient: one minute for each position, not to exceed 10 minutes total therapy to avoid fatiguing the infant. Increase FiO_2 5% if the $TcpO_2$ falls below resting levels during treatment.
4. The treatment should occur prior to feedings and oral medications to avoid the possibility of vomiting.

Procedure

1. Bilateral upper apical segments
   a. Baby sitting upright
   b. Therapy to upper anterior chest wall
2. Bilateral anterior apical segment
   a. Infant supine
   b. Elevated at 30° angle
   c. Therapy to upper anterior chest wall
3. Bilateral anterior upper lobe segments
   a. Infant supine
   b. No elevation
   c. Therapy to upper anterior chest wall
4. Right apical lateral segment and left apical posterior segment
   a. Infant on side
   b. Elevated at 30° angle
   c. Therapy to upper lateral chest wall
5. Bilateral posterior apical segments
   a. Infant rotated forward 15° from side
   b. Elevated at 30° angle
   c. Therapy to upper posterior chest wall
6. Right posterior upper lobe segment
   a. Infant on left side rotated forward 45°
   b. Bed flat
   c. Therapy to left middle back

7. Right middle segment and left lingua
   a. Infant rotated forward 45° from supine position
   b. Head down at 45° angle
   c. Therapy to lower anterior chest wall
8. Bilateral posterior segment
   a. Infant prone and flat
   b. Therapy to middle back
9. Bilateral anterior basal segments
   a. Infant supine
   b. Head down at 30° angle
   c. Therapy to lower anterior chest wall
10. Bilateral lateral basal segments
    a. Infant on side
    b. Head down at 30° angle
    c. Therapy to lower lateral chest wall
11. Bilateral posterior basal segments
    a. Infant prone
    b. Head down at 30° angle
    c. Therapy to lower back

Appendix 5.13
ET Suctioning

Purpose

1. To remove mucus and/or debris from the large airways.
2. To maintain a patent ET tube.
3. To obtain laboratory specimens for culture and BPD cytology.

Guidelines

1. Endotracheal tubes should be suctioned as necessary and as ordered.
2. Sterile technique must be observed.
3. All infants who have ET suctioning must be monitored with both a cardiac and respiratory monitor.
4. The ET tube should be cultured routinely.
5. Increase FiO_2 if $TcpO_2$'s are less than 40 during procedures.

Equipment

1. Sterile glove
2. Sterile suction catheter
3. Suction apparatus
4. Normal saline
5. 1-cc syringe
6. Hope bag and O_2
7. Stethoscope

Procedure

Action

1. Routine ET suctioning should be preceded by chest PT.

2. Listen to breath sounds before and after suctioning. Infant should be on cardiorespiratory monitor during procedure.

3. Instill 0.2–0.5 cc normal saline (NS) into ET tube and give 2–3 breaths with ventilator or bag. Usually 1 cc saline is sufficient during any suctioning procedure. If the se-

Rationale/Precautions

1. Chest PT enhances the movement of secretions and debris into large airways where suctioning is most effective

2. Improved breath sounds indicate the removal of obstruction by suctioning. Ventilation status can deteriorate during ET suctioning because of a displaced ET tube, bronchospasm, throwing a "plug," mechanical removal of too much thoracic air, etc., so the baseline status should be determined. Bradycardia from vagal stimulation and/or hypoxia can develop.

3. NS helps thin and loosen secretions. Blowing NS down the ET tube helps facilitate thinning secretions in the small airways. If a bag is used, the FiO_2 of the bag should equal the

Action

cretions are known to be very thin, saline is not necessary. If the consistency of the secretions is in question, do not put saline down the ET tube until passing the catheter a second time.

4. Put on sterile glove and remove catheter. Approximate distance from top of ET tube to ear and from ear to midsternum.

5. Using sterile technique, gently insert catheter into ET tube to the distance approximating the carina. At this point, or if resistance is felt, withdraw the catheter about 0.5–1 cm. Apply suction and remove catheter, rolling catheter between fingers as it is removed.

6. Do not allow the catheter to remain in ET tube longer than 10 seconds from beginning to end of procedure.

7. Give 3–4 rapid ventilations with respirator or bag. Then return infant to previous intermittent mandatory ventilation setting.

8. After infant's color, heart rate, and respiratory rate have returned to baseline, repeat suctioning procedure until only clear saline returns.

9. After clearing ET tube, suction nose and mouth (See Appendix 5.14).

10. *Caution:* Do not continue suctioning if infant has persistent bradycardia, cyanosis, or excess distress during suctioning. Bag infant, notify physician, and attempt suctioning again at later time.

Rationale/Precautions

FiO$_2$ the infant had been receiving through the ET tube prior to suctioning, so that excessive changes of pO$_2$ are not produced.

4. This distance should be the length of suction catheter needed to reach the carina (see "Intubation").

5. Pulling catheter back and rolling it help keep the tip from attaching to any trauma. The distance measured in item 4 should be equal to the point at which resistance felt. If resistance is felt sooner, the ET tube may be plugged.

6. Airway is effectively occluded by suction catheter and severe hypoxia can result if procedure is prolonged.

7. Rapid reexpansion of collapsed airways can help prevent prolonged hypoxia and excess respiratory effort.

8. Turn head to repeat suctioning, and change the angle of the catheter entering the trachea to help clear alternate sides.

9. Keep mouth clean to prevent infection and breakdown.

Appendix 5.14
Nasopharyngeal and Oropharyngeal Suction

Purpose

1. To maintain a patent airway.
2. To remove excessive secretions from the esophagus and the stomach.

NOTE   Culture any purulent secretions obtained.

Procedure

General instructions:

1. Wash hands prior to beginning procedure.
2. Have tracheal suction machine readily available if wall suction is not provided.
3. Keep suction catheter connected for immediate use.
4. Use sterile disposable catheter. Change catheter at least every 8 hours.
5. Keep sterile water in 4-oz bottle at the bedside to clean catheter tubing between suctionings. Change opened bottles every 8 hours.
6. Suctioning procedures should always be clean except when there is the history of recent trauma to the respiratory tract; this requires use of sterile technique.

The following adjustments in technique should be made for nasopharyngeal suctioning:

1. Use a bulb syringe initially to clear thick secretions.
2. Select an appropriate-size catheter. To suction pharynx, measure from nose to ear, and from ear to clavicle; if gastric suction is required, measure to tip of the xiphoid process.
3. Using a slight rotating motion, direct the catheter at a 90° angle to the face and pass it to the premeasured length through the nose or mouth.
4. When suctioning the nose, do not force catheter if unable to pass it easily into pharynx. Pull it back and reposition or try the next smaller size catheter. Use sterile lubricant on suction catheter to decrease friction irritation.
5. Report any evidence of obstructed nares.
6. Suction while pulling back on catheter and rotating slightly. Monitor heart rate with hand on chest if infant is not on a cardiac monitor and discontinue suctioning if heart rate drops.
7. If there are no untoward effects, repeat until the airway is clear.

Appendix 5.15
Tracheal Aspirate for Culture

Purpose

To screen infants with indwelling ET tubes for possible pulmonary infection. Tracheal culture specimen is obtained from each ET tube, every Monday, Wednesday, and Friday.

Procedure

Follow ET suctioning procedure (see Appendix 5.13) with these additions:

1. Have culturette and no. 10 blade ready.
2. Omit any normal saline instillation.
3. Pass catheter once only; then using sterile technique, cut off tip of catheter into culturette tube.
4. Send approximately 2 inches of catheter.
5. Remove cotton tip applicator from culturette before putting top on.
6. Break capsule of culture medium. Mark with infant's name and send to lab for culture and sensitivity analysis.

Appendix 5.16
Tracheal Aspirate for Cytology

Purpose

To obtain tracheal cells for diagnosis of BPD.

Equipment

1. Cork-top tube
2. Mucus trap
3. 0.5 cc saline
4. 2 cc 50% alcohol
5. Suction catheter
6. Sterile glove

Procedure

1. Instill 0.5 cc saline into ET tube.
2. Attach mucus trap to suction catheter and suction trachea following the ET suction procedure (Appendix 5.13).
3. Suction alcohol through catheter into mucus trap immediately. (The tracheal cells will autolyse and be destroyed if not immediately suspended in alcohol.) A 4 : 1 suspension is desired.
4. Aspirate cell washing and alcohol mixture from mucus trap and put into glass tube.
5. Label tube and send to pathology lab.

NOTE   A suspension of cells is desired—not mucus.

Appendix 5.17
Obtaining Umbilical Catheter Blood Gases

Purpose

To ascertain status of infant's cardiorespiratory system by arterial blood gas sampling.

Procedure

1. Wash hands thoroughly.
2. Assemble equipment as follows:
   a. Empty sterile 5-cc syringe
   b. Heparinized insulin syringe; after syringe has been coated, be sure to remove all remaining heparin.
   c. 2 × 2 sponges
   d. Fresh flush syringe
3. Using strict aseptic technique, close the stopcock and disconnect the flush syringe from the three-way stopcock. Cover all syringe tips to keep them sterile.
4. Wipe the stopcock with sterile gauze and saline if necessary.
5. Attach empty, sterile 5-cc syringe and discontinue IV flow by turning stopcock.
6. Draw back 2 cc of blood; then close the stopcock halfway to 45° angle. Maintaining sterility, disconnect syringe, cover the end, and put it aside.
7. Attach heparinized syringe, open the stopcock, and draw back 0.2 cc of blood.
8. Close the stopcock and disconnect the heparinized syringe; remove any air bubbles that may enter syringe and place the syringe aside.
9. Blood in the first syringe should be replaced slowly into infant.
10. Close the stopcock. Disconnect the 5-cc syringe and attach the flush syringe.
11. Open the stopcock and flush with ½ to 1 cc of dextrose (5%) in water. Record flush volume and the amount of blood withdrawn on data sheet.

6

Neonatal Jaundice

Betty Lou Glass

Management of a jaundiced infant can be quite complicated. There are guidelines found for all neonatal tests, but none can be relied upon in every circumstance. In dealing with hyperbilirubinemia, you must take each infant's age, birth weight, gestation, medical complications, and various laboratory values into consideration. Complete assessment of the patient's clinical condition becomes mandatory.

Pathologic versus Physiologic Jaundice

Jaundice is so common in newborns that the term "physiologic jaundice" has been developed. Jaundice is a result of bilirubin deposited in subcutaneous tissue, giving a yellow appearance. Assessment for hyperbilirubinemia can simply be made by blanching the skin of the forehead or cheek. If jaundice is observed nurses should obtain a bilirubin level and report the results. The diagnosis of physiologic jaundice is one of exclusion; see Table 6.1 for associated risk factors. Physiologic jaundice does not usually occur before the age of 48 hours and can only be considered "physiologic" if no disease process can be identified.

If the infant is term, asymptomatic, and feeding well, a total bilirubin level of 12% or less is defined as physiologic jaundice. An infant with physiologic jaundice usually requires no specific treatment unless the bilirubin level exceeds safe limits, in which case it is no longer "physiologic" but unexplained. Keeping the infant well hydrated may also limit the process. A serum bilirubin greater than 13% in any infant, term or premature, alerts caregivers to investigate the cause.

Physiologic elevations in bilirubin are the result of the complex biochemistry involved in the conversion of hemoglobin to bilirubin. The normal term infant has an increased red blood cell volume [hematocrit (Hct) 55–65%] at birth. During the first week of life, a large number of red blood cells (RBCs) are destroyed, fetal cells having a shorter life span than mature RBCs, and bilirubin is produced proportionately. Neither transport into hepatocytes nor conjugation enzymatic pathways are fully mature, even at term. Thus processing and metabolism of bilirubin is retarded in the face of increased bilirubin production.

Bilirubin Production and Metabolism

Unconjugated (indirect) bilirubin is derived from hemoglobin during the breakdown of RBCs. When catabolized, 1 gram of hemoglobin yields 35 mg of bilirubin. This

Table 6.1 Risk Factors Associated with
Hyperbilirubinemia

1. Polycythemia
   a. Chronic placental insufficiency
   b. Twin-to-twin transfusion
   c. Cord stripping
2. Enclosed hemorrhage
   a. Cephalohematoma
   b. Swallowed blood/gastrointestinal bleeding
   c. Intraventricular hemorrhage
   d. Pulmonary hemorrhage
3. Hemolytic processes
   a. Maternal-fetal incompatability (Rh or ABO)
   b. Genetic disorders
   c. Vitamin K deficiency
4. Increased enterohepatic recirculation
   a. Absent or reduced peristalsis
   b. Congenital intestinal obstruction
   c. No enteral feedings
5. Impaired hepatic function
   a. Immature enzyme systems
   b. Hepatitis (TORCH, HAA, other)[a]
   c. Breast milk inhibition
   d. Genetic disorders

[a] TORCH, toxoplasmosis, rubella, cytomegalovirus, and herpes; HAA, hepatitis-associated antigen.

occurs largely in the reticuloendothethial system (RES). Bilirubin is transported to the liver attached to albumin and then is actively transported into the liver cell (hepatocyte), where unconjugated bilirubin is converted to its water-soluble form: conjugated (direct) bilirubin. It is conjugated with glucuronic acid by the enzyme glucuronyl transferase. This enzyme's limited activity seems to be a central factor in physiologic jaundice. Impaired transfer of unconjugated bilirubin from the serum into the hepatocyte may be another limiting factor. Another source of unconjugated bilirubin is the enterohepatic circulation. Conjugated bilirubin can be "recycled" into the unconjugated form in the gastrointestinal tract and reabsorbed into the circulation (enterohepatic circulation). Nonhemoglobin pigments may also contribute their breakdown products (shunt bilirubin). Each of these aspects of bilirubin production and metabolism may contribute to the development of physiologic jaundice. Figure 6.1 diagrams bilirubin metabolism.

As mentioned above, unconjugated bilirubin going from the RES to the hepatic cell is bound to albumin. When the albumin binding site(s) are saturated, "free" or "unbound" unconjugated bilirubin may result. This unattached bilirubin becomes available to damage tissues, including the central nervous system (CNS). Indirect bilirubin concentrations indicate the amount of circulating biliruin but do not measure whether or not it is being safely transported. A rough estimate of binding is the "exchange index." This is calculated by multiplying total protein × 3.6, or serum albumin × 6.4. This value is the theoretical bilirubin level at which serum bilirubin exceeds albumin binding capacity and free bilirubin may occur. There are also laboratory tests that measure bilirubin-albumin binding capacity and can detect free bilirubin.

Irrespective of the cause, if bilirubin levels exceed the albumin capacity, free bilirubin may result. Free bilirubin may occur for three major reasons: 1) the amount of unconjugated bilirubin exceeds available albumin (high molar ratio); 2) certain compounds (including some drugs) compete for the same site, rendering the albumin unavailable for bilirubin binding; or 3) acidosis may interfere with binding.

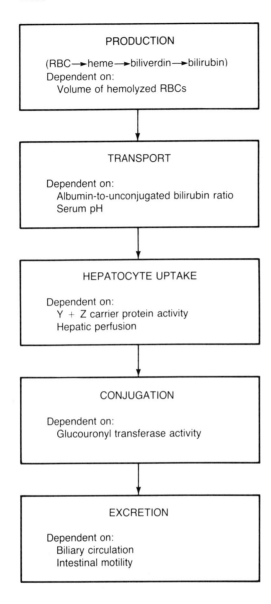

FIGURE 6.1 **Bilirubin metabolism.**

The entire subject of bilirubin encephalopathy is undergoing considerable scrutiny; for example, changes in serum osmolarity open the blood-brain barrier to allow bilirubin (even bound to albumin) to enter the CNS. This seems important in the pathogenesis of neural damage and downplays the role of albumin binding. Such controversies and confusion about pathophysiology should limit dogmatism about the therapeutic guidelines or "safe" levels of jaundice under all clinical circumstances.

Etiology of Hyperbilirubinemia

There are many causes and diseases involved in neonatal hyperbilirubinemia, but the basic differential is that they occur by two distinct mechanisms: overproduction and/or undersecretion of bilirubin.

Overproduction

Early appearance of jaundice (within 48 hours) is often due to hemolytic disease. Maternal-fetal blood group incompatibility is investigated to diagnose this process (see "Isoimmunization"). The infant who is severely bruised or ecchymotic because of trauma or breech delivery will experience jaundice from the breakdown of extravasated RBCs. This is seen usually on the second day. Polycythemia (Hct >70%), which can result from delayed clamping of the cord, maternal diabetes, placental insufficiency, or maternal-fetal or fetofetal transfusion, can also cause an overproduction of bilirubin. As this extra volume of RBCs is destroyed, an increased bilirubin load is presented to the liver. An extremely ruddy skin color is one sign of polycythemia. This observation should be verified with a central Hct because a high Hct obtained from a heelstick may only reflect poor perfusion of that extremity. Finally, increased enterohepatic circulation may occur with any form of intestinal obstruction. It is important for the nurse to observe and record the presence or absence of bowel sounds, bowel movements, postbirth increase in abdominal measurements, and bile-stained vomitus in any jaundiced neonate (see Chapter 8).

Undersecretion

There are two types of nonhemolytic jaundice: type I is caused by a reduction in glucuronyl transferase; type II is caused by deficient glucuronyl transferase activity. Phenobarbital is sometimes given to increase the enzyme activity of the less serious type II. Hypothyroidism can cause undersecretion. The hyperbilirubinemia of hypothyroidism usually lasts more than 10 days and is diagnosed by a low serum thyroxine value. The nurse may observe other signs of hypothyroidism, including acrocyanosis, an enlarged tongue, or hoarse cry.

In rare circumstances mother's milk has been found to inhibit the conjugation of bilirubin, but "breast milk jaundice" remains controversial. When breast milk is the suspected cause of hyperbilirubinemia, mothers require a lot of teaching and enthusiastic support, especially if breastfeeding is stopped. Based on current information and the variety of breast milk hyperbilirubinemia, most cases of neonatal jaundice that occur in breast-fed babies should not automatically lead to restrictions in breastfeeding.

The premature infant is at risk for neonatal hyperbilirubinemia for many reasons. One of the risk factors is extravascular hemolysis from bruising at birth or enclosed hemorrhage, particularly intraventricular hemorrhage. The preterm infant also often receives parenteral nourishment and may not have bowel movements, thus further decreasing the motility of his intestines. This enhances recirculation of conjugated bilirubin. Additionally, some drugs, possibly including free fatty acids from parenteral lipids, may compete for bilirubin-albumin binding; thus preterm infants requiring parenteral nutrition are at greater risk for CNS injury at lower serum bilirubin levels than are term infants. Serum proteins may be decreased in premature infants so that immaturity also increases the risk of kernicterus because of diminished albumin carrying capacity. Such factors are the reason guidelines about bilirubin therapy place the premature infant in a special risk category.

Mixed Jaundice

At certain times, hyperbilirubinemia is due to combined overproduction and undersecretion. Jaundice may also be caused by an elevated direct (conjugated) fraction. Elevated direct bilirubin levels indicate that hepatocyte excretion of conjugated bilirubin is obstructed. Congenital biliary obstruction and hepatitis are common causes of obstructive jaundice. The nurse's observation of the infant can assist the neonatologist in determining the cause of such "mixed" jaundice. Observations include skin color: a greenish cast indicates elevated direct bilirubin levels. Obtaining cultures and urine samples and assisting with lumbar punctures are part of the work-up necessary to determine if an infections process is the underlying cause. Intrauterine TORCH[1] infections, congenital syphilis, and hepatitis are some causes of congenital hepatitis and "combined" jaundice. Serological testing of the cord blood may help make the diagnosis. Careful observations of vital signs, clinical condition, and subtle physical findings (developing petechiae, apnea, etc.) are other clues.

Postnatal infections (sepsis) may also be heralded by elevated serum bilirubin levels. In some cases, jaundice may be the only early sign of infection. The hyperbilirubinemia of sepsis is often the mixed type, with elevations in both conjugated and unconjugated bilirubin. One should always be alert to the possibility of sepsis when an infant has an otherwise unexplained hyperbilirubinemia.

Isoimmunization

One major cause of pathologic neonatal jaudice is maternal-fetal blood group incompatibility, which results in erythroblastosis fetalis. Rh disease has been the prototype from which many lessons have been learned about neonatal jaundice. With the introduction of RhoGAM in the past decade, there has been a marked decrease in the number of sensitized Rh-negative mothers and affected infants. Rh incompatibility occurs when Rh-negative women carry Rh-positive fetuses and become (or already are) sensitized. The first infant is rarely affected unless the mother has had an Rh-positive blood transfusion or has aborted an Rh-positive fetus, either of which would cause antibody formation. Hemolytic anemia and severe hyperbilirubinemia pose great dangers to the fetus while in utero. The most severe consequence of this process is called hydrops fetalis, a life-threatening condition.

Most pregnant women have their blood typed. Those who are Rh-negtive should have antibody titers, particularly anti-D titers. If a rising titer is detected, amniotic fluid samples may be tested for increased levels of pigment. This level normally drops as pregnancy progresses. History of previous blood transfusions, previous pregnancies, serological tests, previously affected infants, and results of the amniocentesis alert the obstetrician to the presence and severity of erythroblastosis.

Another important hemolytic disease due to isoimmunization involves the A and B blood group factors. The mother forms antibodies against fetal blood cells that have passed the placenta and entered the maternal circulation. Antibodies of the immunoglobulin G class cross the placental barrier to the fetal circulation, attach to antigenic sites on fetal cells, and cause agglutination of fetal RBCs. The result is hemolysis.

ABO incompatibility is found with group A or B infants born to mothers of group O, or of group A or B if fetus is B or A, respectively. In general, ABO incompatibility is usually milder but less predictable in its clinical course than Rh disease. In ABO incompatibility, splenic and hepatic enlargement is uncommon, whereas infants with Rh incompatibility often have hepatosplenomegaly. Blood smears are useful tests for all hemolytic disturbances because bizarre, fragmented cells may be seen.

The Coombs test (direct and indirect), plus specific blood group tests are most valuable. A positive Coombs test and incompatible blood types between the mother

---

[1] Acronym for toxoplasmosis, rubella, cytomegalovirus, and herpes.

Table 6.2 Comparison of Rh and ABO Incompatability

	Rh incompatibility	ABO incompatibility
Mother	Negative	O, A, or B
Infant	Positive	A or B
First pregnancy affected	Rare	Often
Predictable severity in subsequent pregnancies	Usually	No
Stillbirth/hydrops	Frequent	Rare
Severe early anemia	$+++^a$	+
Incidence of late anemia	Common	+
Jaundice in first 24 hours	++	+
Hepatosplenomegaly	+++	+
Enucleated RBCs	+++	+
Reticulocytosis	++	+ to ++
Spherocytes	0	+
Direct Coombs test	+	+ to ++
Indirect Coombs test	Not necessary	+
Need for antenatal measures	Yes	No
Exchange transfusion frequency	~2/3	~1/10
Donor blood type	Rh-negative, group-specific when possible	Rh same as infant, group O *only*

^{a} +, occurs; ++, frequent; +++, ubiquitous.

and her baby are diagnostic of an isoimmune process. Hct and reticulocyte counts are useful in ABO and Rh incompatibility to document the disease's severity. Table 6.2 notes distinguishing features between the two diseases. Less commonly other blood groups may be involved (Kell, Duffy, etc.).

Depending on the severity of the infant's condition, exchange transfusion may be required to improve cardiovascular function, correct anemia, and remove sensitive RBCs, maternal antibodies, and bilirubin. Severe cases of hemolytic disease with pleural and pericardial effusions require positive pressure ventilation to ensure adequate ventilation until the infant is stabilized. This is the situation seen in hydrops fetalis.

Hydrops Fetalis

Hydrops fetalis is associated with profoundly lowered intrauterine serum proteins. This causes low colloid oncotic pressure and accumulation of fluid in all body spaces. These collections include massive ascites and pleural effusions. A hydropic infant has an enlarged liver and spleen, and may have petechiae and anasarca.

Erythroblastosis fetalis, chronic fetomaternal or twin-to-twin transfusion, plus other chronic anemias in utero can cause hydrops fetalis. Cardiac failure due to congenital heart disease or fetal arrhythmia, hypoproteinemia with renal disease, and congenital hepatitis are also precipitating factors to hydrops. Intrauterine infections such as syphilis, cytomegalovirus, and toxoplasmosis have been reported as causes. Several other factors, including maternal diabetes mellitus and parabiotic syndrome (multiple pregnancy) can also cause "hydrops."

The outlook for hydrops is improved by early diagnosis and aggressive perinatal management. It is successfully detected by ultrasound examination. All cases of polyhydramnios should be investigated for hydrops. The presence of hydrops is an indication for urgent delivery unless the fetus is previable or fatally malformed. The delivery room management of the hydropic neonate requires two skilled neonatal resuscitators and a coordinated team approach involving all perinatal caretakers. The

Table 6.3 Phototherapy and Exchange Transfusion Guidelines

	Bilirubin level (mg/100 ml)	<24 h old	24–48 h old	48–72 h old	>72 h old
Term infants	≥20	E[a,b]	E	E	E
	15–19	E	E	P	P
	10–14	P/E	I	I	I
	5–9	I	I	O	O
	<5		O	O	O
Preterm infants	≥20	E	E	E	E
	15–19	E	E	P/E	P/E
	10–14	P/E	I/P	I/P	I/P
	5–9	I/P	O	O	O
	<5	O	O	O	O

Adapted from Maisel MJ: Neonatal jaundice. In GB Avery (ed), Neonatology: Pathophysiology and Management of the Newborn, pp 473–544. Lippincott, Philadelphia, 1981; and from the American Academy of Pediatrics. Recommendations for Exchange Transfusions.

[a] Abbreviations used: E, consider exchange; P, consider phototherapy; I, investigate jaundice; O, observe.

[b] Use phototherapy after any exchange.

key to emergency management, after intubation and positive pressure ventilation, is to improve colloid oncotic pressure. This is accomplished by simultaneous paracentesis and isovolumetric replacement of whole blood. Following acute management, treatment of the hydropic neonate follows guidelines for the severely jaundiced and respiratorily compromised neonate. Two specific therapeutic modalities are available to lower serum bilirubin levels: phototherapy and exchange transfusion. Table 6.3 shows guidelines for initiating therapy; note the differences for preterm versus term infants.

Treatment

Phototherapy

Phototherapy is effective in treating hyperbilirubinemia. Complications can be minimized with proper precautions and observations. Inappropriate use may prolong the separation of parents and infant and causes undue hospitalization and expense. However, the use of phototherapy within specific guidelines is safe and effective. Nursing care of an infant under "bili lights" is aimed at minimizing the risks of treatment while maximizing its effectiveness.

Nursing Care

Eye Care   One of the most serious potential complications of bili lights is damage to the retina from exposure to bright lights. Eye shields are used routinely to cover the infant's eyes.

1. Place the naked infant beneath the bili lights. Use soft eye shields, securely but not tightly placed over the eyes. Be sure eyelids are closed when blindfold is applied.

2. Check the eyes several times per shift since purulent conjunctivitis may result from prolonged pressure or accumulation of discharge on the eyelids. The nurse should explain to the parents that the eye shields prevent retinal damage.
3. Clean the eyes every 8 hours, using sterile water and cotton balls to remove crusts. This can be taught to the mother to increase her involvement with the infant.
4. It is important to remove the eye patches when the parents are visiting and to encourage fondling and assistance with care of the jaundiced infant if the baby is allowed out of phototherapy. This allows parents to continue to explore their new infant despite the requirement of bili lights.

Skin Exposure to Light Blue light in the visible spectrum is absorbed by the unconjugated bilirubin molecule and converted to an easily transported form. Unconjugated bilirubin is deposited in subcutaneous skin, so exposure of jaundiced skin to bili lights causes this photosensitized oxidation process. This means that all the infant's skin must be directly exposed to the light to maximize the treatment.

1. Place the infant nude under the bili lights.
2. Turn and position the infant every 2 hours. If the baby has an umbilical catheter, place him in the lateral position with a small roll-prop to expose the back as much as possible.
3. The infant's skin is apt to become irritated during treatment, so it is necessary to keep the skin clean. The undiapered infant requires frequent bathing and linen changes. Light exposure to the genitalia does not cause problems and shielding seems unnecessary.

Monitoring Bilirubin Lights

1. The nurse should see that ordered laboratory values are obtained, documented, and reported to the physician.
2. Once lights are discontinued, bilirubin levels should be checked every 12 to 24 hours until stable to determine if rebound of hyperbilirubinemia occurs.

Prevention and Monitoring of Dehydration

1. Since a major untoward effect of phototherapy is increased insensible water loss (especially threatening to preterm infants), phototherapy infants may require an additional fluid intake of as much as 25 ml/kg/day.
2. Observe for dehydration signs such as poor skin turgor, sunken fontanelles, dry mucous membranes, scant urine, or thickened endotracheal secretions.
3. Measure urine specific gravity every 8 hours in term infants, every 4 hours in preterm infants. If the urine specific gravity is greater than 1.012, it should be considered a sign of dehydration in an infant less than 2 weeks old. The physician should be notified immediately.
4. Maintain adequate fluid intake and output records:
   a. If the infant is a slow eater, feed smaller amounts as frequently as every 2 hours.
   b. If an infant is receiving IV fluid, keep an accurate hourly record of fluid intake. Do not allow intake to fall behind the ordered rate.
   c. The urine output should remain between 1 and 3 cc/kg/hour. Maintain accurate output records (see Chapter 3).
   d. Weigh the infant. Significant weight loss should be reported to the physician promptly.
   e. Water feedings may be given between regular feedings to meet the increased fluid requirement in infants on "ad lib" oral intake.

5. Infants should be transferred from a radiant warming table to an isolette to *decrease* insensible water loss and to *increase* the effectiveness of the bili light by decreasing the distance between the light source and the infant. Banking two phototherapy lights on each side of the bed is useful when the infant remains on a radiant heated table.

Temperature Control

1. Frequent monitoring of temperature is required since some infants experience hypo-hyperthermic swings with thermal stress complications (see Chapter 2).
2. The nude infant is often exposed to drafts during care, so draft shields on heating tables should be used when possible. Porthole sleeves should be used on isolettes to decrease convective heat losses.
3. We have found that a large infant in an isolette can become hyperthermic, then tachypneic and tachycardic when extra mattresses put them closer to the light source. We do not advise using this technique for term infants and caution that closer observation of temperature be made if using this technique in preterm infants.

Additional Stimulation   A musical toy or radio provides auditory stimulation to compensate for loss of visual stimulation. Some mothers have made tape-recordings of words of encouragement and nursery rhymes to be played to the infant. The family and nurses are encouraged to touch the infant as well.

Function of Bili Lights

Unconjugated bilirubin absorbs visible blue light (not ultraviolet light). The energy absorbed from blue light acts to change bilirubin into photoisomers easily transferred by albumin to the liver and processed. Effective phototherapy requires adequate illumination of the exposed skin at a sufficiently short distance. Blue or special fluorescent lights with a narrow spectral band are more effective than white bulbs. The action of phototherapy appears to take place in the subcutaneous layer of the skin.

1. Check the irradiance and flux of the bili lights with a "bili meter" when lights are first initiated and then periodically throughout the therapy (effective wavelengths, 400–500 nm; flux, >5 W/em^2). Maintain a record of these readings at the bedside. If no progress is seen in serum bilirubin levels, change the lights.
2. Extra mattresses added to heating table platforms place an infant closer to light sources, but beware of hyperthermia.
3. A yellow plastic see-through drape may be placed over the isolette to protect personnel and parents because high-frequency (ultrablue) lights cause headaches and nausea.
4. Blue phototherapy light may mask cyanosis. Infants under these lights must occasionally be observed with the light off. If the infant has lung disease or frequent hypoxic episodes, a transcutaneous O_2 pressure (TcpO$_2$) monitor is recommended.

Explaining the phototherapy to the parents in "layman's terms" helps relieve some of the apprehension parents feel. Reporting current progress in the bilirubin level and other lab values can also help. To experienced personnel a parent's anxiety might seem disproportionate to the degree of sickness, but separation from one's infant creates anxiety even if the cause is transitory and not life threatening. Information can help during this period, but probably only being reunited with the infant removes anxiety altogether.

Exchange Transfusion

An exchange transfusion removes cells, bilirubin, and circulating maternal antibodies. The goal is to prevent kernicterus or bilirubin encephalopathy while preserving circulatory stability.

Fresh, whole, Rh-negative maternally compatible blood is used for the exchange transfusion. The ABO typing can be matched with either the infant's own or can be type O blood. The donor blood for ABO incompatibility must be type O and should not contain A or B antibodies. Rh typing should be compatible with the infant's. A crossmatch to the mother's serum further reduces the risks of transfusion reaction in both types of incompatibility. In addition, the blood should be either fresh or resuspended packed cells in fresh frozen plasma so that clotting factors are replaced.

Nursing responsibilities can be broken down as follows:

1. Order approximately twice the amount of the newborn's blood volume plus any additional blood needed to fill tubing. Blood volume estimate: 80–90 cc/kg body weight.
2. Assemble the blood-warming unit according to machine instructions. Prepare the sterile exchange transfusion tray. Have extra gloves and sterile drapes at hand. Calcium and albumin should be available.
3. Position and restrain the infant supine on a radiant heated table. The stomach must be emptied unless the infant has been without feedings for several hours. Vomiting can occur and suction must be set up.
4. Resuscitation equipment should be available, as well as atropine to reverse any vagal bradycardia.
5. A careful record of the amount of blood exchanged must be kept. With the first aliquot of blood "out," blood work should be obtained for pertinent lab tests. These tests always include bilirubin and Hct; other tests obtained will depend on the reason for exchange.

Two people must perform the procedure. Usually a physician or neonatal nurse practitioner is sterile and performs the exchange while a staff nurse circulates as recorder and observer. The person withdrawing blood must state clearly to the circulator/recorder each time an amount of blood is taken out or injected into the infant. The circulator then immediately records the amount of blood exchanged. This is a boring and tedious process, but the possibility of iatrogenic hypovolemia or volume overload is serious. Great care must be taken to avoid this complication.

Five to 10 cc increasing up to 10% of the infant's blood volume, can be removed with each pass. If the infant experiences tachycardia or bradycardia, hypoxia, or hypotension when blood is removed, smaller aliquots should be exchanged. The circulating nurse should continuously observe the heart and respiratory rate and blood pressure. This can be accomplished using a cardiac and respiratory monitor plus a continuous arterial pressure transducer or automatic cuff pressure device. The vital signs should be recorded every 15 minutes on the exchange sheet. A TcpO$_2$ monitor is also helpful in assessing the infant's response to the exchange. Dextrostix should also be obtained at 15- to 30-minutes intervals, especially if the infant's parenteral fluids have been stopped to do the exchange. In such cases a supplemental IV is a good technique to provide a source of calories and prevent hypoglycemia.

Observation for unusual symptoms or changes in vital signs is of utmost importance, especially during "out" phases. The transfusion may have to be discontinued, smaller aliquots of blood might be indicated, ventilation may need to be increased, or other supportive measures may need to be given during treatment. The exchange process is continued until two times the infant's estimated blood volume has been replaced. This method is called a double exchange, which theoretically removes 75% of the circulating bilirubin. At the completion of the procedure, postexchange blood work should be obtained and sent to the lab. Again Hct, bilirubin, and other tests are valuable.

Following completion of the exchange, the infant must be observed for spontaneous hemorrhage, respiratory compromise, hypocalcemia, hypoglycemia, fluid overload, hypovolemic shock, decreased urine output, or compromised circulation of lower extremities. Necrotizing enterocolitis (see Chapter 8) may also rarely follow exchange transfusion. The infant's vital signs, including blood pressure, should be monitored every 15 minutes during the first hour and hourly for the next 3 hours postexchange. Our policy is to wait 24 hours to resume feedings and observe for complications after an exchange transfusion. Follow-up laboratory tests in 4 hours will determine the need for additional exchanges.

It should be noted that exchange transfusion (complete or partial) is also used in some places for disseminated intravascular coagulopathy (DIC) and the "polycythemia/hyperviscosity syndrome." Neither situation has been demonstrated to benefit from the procedure, and the risks from the procedure are real.

Case Studies

Case 1

Mrs. J., a 21-year-old primigravida, delivered by cesarian section a 40-week-old meconium-stained male infant, weighing 7 lbs, 3 oz. The Code Pink team (neonatologist and nurse) attending the delivery quickly dried the slightly cyanotic infant and obtained a heart rate of 96 beats/minute. The infant was suctioned for a small amount of meconium-stained fluid from below the vocal cords and received free-flow oxygen. An Apgar score of 6 was given at 1 minute and 8 at 5 minutes. The infant was admitted to the intensive care nursery for observation and chest physiotherapy. Once stabilized, the neonate was transferred to the normal nursery at 12 hours of age.

On the second day of life, the nurse reported jaundiced skin. The total bilirubin level was 9.9 mg/dl. The parents were informed that their baby was jaundiced and were assured that the condition would be monitored closely, with lab values every 8 hours. The parents were quite anxious after the problems in the delivery room, despite a thorough discussion with the pediatrician. The news of their infant's jaundice increased their anxiety. The bilirubin level obtained 8 hours later was 12.9 mg/dl. Orders were written for phototherapy and sterile water feedings between breastfeedings. Eight hours later, despite the use of bili lights, the serum bilirubin level was 13 mg/dl.

During the night the staff nurse found Mrs. J. crying inconsolably because she had read about jaundice and the danger of brain damage (kernicterus). The mother expressed guilt because she felt that there was "something wrong with her breast milk, perhaps (she) was eating the wrong foods?" She also felt depressed because she could not hold the infant often, since phototherapy was in progress.

Nursing and medical staff reassured the parents that the infant was being closely monitored and was in no danger. They encouraged the mother to come into the nursery and breastfeed for each feeding. The primary nurse provided literature about physiologic jaundice and included the mother in the conference on the infant's care plan. The mother was encouraged to fondle the infant while he was under the bili lights. The mother wore tinted lens glasses and a yellow plastic cover was placed over the isolette to protect her eyes. Mrs. J. was taught how to do infant eye, cord, and skin care and was encouraged to perform this daily.

Mrs. J. seemed less anxious while she was assisting with the infant's care, but did express fear that the water feedings would "fill the baby up" and curb her baby's appetite for breast milk. The primary nurse explained the need for increased fluids during phototherapy to compensate for water lost through the skin. The eye shields were removed while the lights were turned off briefly each time the parents visited. The staff assured them that discontinuing phototherapy for short periods was not detrimental to their son's treatment. It was explained that intermittent phototherapy has been shown to be effective, and since the most rapid decrement in bilirubin occurs within the first few hours after each period of phototherapy, it was alright to stop the therapy during visits, feedings, and procedures.

Unfortunately, on day 4, the bilirubin level was at 13.5 mg/dl despite phototherapy. The Coombs tests had been negative. The complete blood count and blood smear results showed no evidence of hemolytic disease. Since further investigation revealed no evidence of infection, the pediatrician ordered that breast milk be discontinued and formula feedings be substituted.

The physician explained to the mother that most studies revealed that the average bilirubin levels in breast-fed infants were found to be similar to those of formula-fed infants, and in most surveys the incidence of hyperbilirubinemia (indirect bilirubin, 14 mg/100 ml) was not significantly higher in breast-fed infants. She further informed Mrs. J. that occasionally a high hormone level in the breast milk induces jaundice, and for this reason she felt it advisable to stop breastfeeding for 48 hours to see if the bilirubin level would decline. The mother had feelings of guilt, which she openly expressed to the nursing staff. To help Mrs. J. continue lactation, the nurses instructed her in the use of a breast pump. The primary nurse reinforced the information that breastfeedings had been stopped for a limited time only and that the problem would not recur even if her milk was identified as the source of the problem.

Twenty-four hours later the infant's bilirubin levels had fallen to 11.5 mg/dl, then to 10.9 mg/dl 12 hours later. Breast milk analysis revealed that pregnanediol concentration was within normal limits and breast milk was not the cause. The mother was relieved when informed about the low level of hormone in her milk.

At 6 days of age, the infant's bilirubin level was 9.3 mg/dl and the bili lights were discontinued. The mother was quite happy when told that breastfeeding could be resumed. There was only a slight rise in bilirubin level after breastfeeding started again and the lights were stopped. The parents were aware of each bilirubin test result and were delighted with the declining pattern for the next 24 hours. On the infant's seventh day of life, Mrs. J. and her infant were discharged together.

Case 2

Mrs. G. was a 25-year-old gravida 2, para 1, with a history of polyhydramnios and twin pregnancy. At the 35th week of pregnancy, she went into spontaneous labor. After 2½ hours of labor, twins were delivered vaginally by forceps extraction. Twin A was hydropic, presenting with massive ascites, generalized edema, and extreme pallor, and weighed 2680 grams, almost twice the weight of twin B. The infant was intubated and ventilated. The Apgar scores were 1 at 1 minute and 6 at 5 minutes. The cord blood revealed a pH of 7.18. Twin A was transferred to the intensive care unit on a ventilator with settings of FiO_2 100%, peak pressure 25 cm H_2O, positive end-expiratory pressure 5 cm H_2O, and intermittent mandatory ventilation of 30 breaths/minute. Twin B weighed 1360 grams, had an uncomplicated delivery, and was transported to the ICN in room air and placed in an isolette. He underwent the routine admission procedures for a small infant.

Twin A was placed on a radiant heating table on a Bournes B/P 200 ventilator. Arterial blood gas monitoring revealed metabolic acidosis. This was corrected with $NaHCO_3$ infusion. The central Hct was 42%. Chest and abdominal x-rays revealed good lung expansion but significant cardiomegaly. The lungs showed a reticulogranular pattern indicating respiratory distress syndrome. There was evidence of a fluid-filled abdomen. Peritoneal paracentesis was performed in the right lower flank and 36 cc of dark, straw-colored fluid was removed. Once stabilized, the infant required close observation for potential problems including fluid overload with cardiac failure.

Intravascular volume and perfusion were uncompromised and there was no blood group incompatability, anemia, or hemolysis. Immediate exchange transfusion was deferred. Weighing at 8-hour intervals and measurement of hourly urine output were started. Routine care for an intubated infant was given.

The reticulocyte count was 2.8%, and the peripheral smear was compatible with increased hematopoietic activity. The urine was found to have 3+ bilirubin. Serum blood was drawn, with the following results: total bilirubin, 10.2 mg/100 ml; albumin, 3.4 g/100 ml; total protein, 4.0 g/100 ml; blood type, O+; direct Coombs, negative. Examination of the infant revealed petechiae, and coagulation studies showed prothrombin time and partial thromboplastin time were increased. The fibrinogen was 50 mg/100 ml, and platelets were 83,000/mm^3. The infant was transfused with 25 cc fresh whole blood. Furosemide was given after transfusion. Phototherapy was started using two sets of high-intensity bili lights banked at 45° angles on either side of the heated table. Routine care for an infant under bili lights was instituted.

Mrs. G. came to the NICU in a wheelchair as soon as her condition permitted and asked to be allowed to stay with her babies. She immediately named the twins. She was shown simple care techniques to encourage this early involvement. She assisted with oral hygiene with support from the primary nurse. Lemon-glycerin "swabs" were used on Twin A's dry lips.

At 18 hours of age, the infant had an abdominal sonogram, and no malformations were seen. The etiology of the declining Hct was not readily explained except that blood loss was probably due either to a hemolytic process or DIC. The infant was steadily weaned down to an FiO_2 of 35%. Sterile dressings over the peritoneal tap site were changed frequently because of persistent drainage. Each dressing was weighed dry and then again at each dressing change, and the infant was found to be loosing 2–3 cc each hour from this site.

Because the fibrinogen and platelets were low, the infant was monitored for hemorrhage. At 20 hours of age, the infant experienced an acute fall in blood pressure. At the same time loud rhonchi were audible to auscultation and there was a precipitous fall in the $TcpO_2$. The endotracheal (ET) tube was suctioned and a large amount of bright-red blood was obtained. Repeated suctioning failed to clear the ET tube, and active bleeding persisted for approximately 15 minutes with an estimated blood loss of 15 cc. Fresh whole blood was given immediately. The ET tube was gently lavaged with saline to clear it. Care was taken to insert the suction catheter no farther than the length of the ET tube so that the pulmonary hemorrhage would not restart.

The abdomen was distended and a soft, red rubber tube was passed to decompress it. Blood was also found in the stomach. Low Gomco suction was started with antacid every 2 hours and IV cimetidine because of suspected gastric ulcer. Finally, an ultrasonogram revealed a fresh intraventricular hemorrhage. The following plan was instituted:

1. Chest physiotherapy was stopped to prevent dislocation of a pulmonary clot and subsequent hemorrhage.
2. Saline lavage of the ET tube was done every 2–3 hours with 0.5 cc at each pass of the catheter until clear fluid was obtained.
3. Daily head measurements for increasing size were instituted; unfortunately, extensive scalp edema made initial baseline measurements unreliable.
4. Intake and output of gastric fluid was recorded and replacement of this fluid was done every 8 hours IV.
5. The gastric pH was tested every 4 hours.
6. The abdominal girth was measured every 4 hours.

Antibiotics, started after initial evaluation, were continued because of the suspicion that infection might be the cause of DIC.

Day 2

At 1 PM hyperbilirubinemia (bilirubin, 19.8 mg/100 ml; negative free bilirubin) became apparent, and an exchange transfusion was done. Before exchange, 20 cc of albumin were given to increase binding capacity, which was measurably low.

The infant's pO_2 dropped after 150 cc of blood was exchanged, despite increasing the FiO_2 from 50% to 100% and increasing ventilator inspiratory pressure. The exchange was stopped at 260 cc total, although 400 cc was the original goal, since the infant did not tolerate the procedure (heart rate fell to 90 beats/minute, $TcpO_2$ to 30 torr). The infant was resuscitated and the exchange was terminated.

Bilirubin levels after the exchange were 15.1 mg/100 ml. Four hours later the bilirubin value had risen to 18.8 mg/100 ml, and the albumin was 3.35 mg/24 hours. The exchange index was 21.4, with a reserve albumin binding capacity of 2.5–5.0 mg/100 ml, but no free bilirubin was found.

Day 3

A second exchange transfusion was attempted. At 150 cc the $TcpO_2$ dropped and the infant needed ventilatory support. The exchange was stopped at 255 cc because of continued ventilation difficulty. Chest x-rays revealed clear lung fields and decreased heart size. Phototherapy was continued. There was no evidence of congestive heart failure, and coagulation studies revealed improving DIC. The parents were aware of the response to both exchanges and were given frequent reports by the physician and primary nurse. The social worker and chaplain gave invaluable support and comfort to both parents and their family during this time.

Day 4

Since the infant's clinical picture had improved, Intralipid and hyperalimentation were started. Twin A was stable on ET constant positive airway pressure (5 cm H_2O). The edematous infant was given meticulous skin care to prevent breakdown. Measures to decrease pressure on edematous tissue included the use of sheepskin mattress covers, alternating pressure mattresses, and frequent position changes. Slight elevation of lower extremities and passive range-of-motion exercises for all extremities were part of the daily nursing care.

Phototherapy was continued. An x-ray revealed free air below the diaphragm, possibly from paracentesis or gastric ulcer. Measurements of the infant's abdominal girth and testing gastric material for occult bleeding and pH were done every 4 hours. The girth remained stable, but the gastric drainage was heme-positive and acidic despite Cimetidine administration.

Day 6

A follow-up x-ray revealed that the stomach was decompressed and free air had abated. The total bilirubin was 9.8 mg/100 ml, and phototherapy was stopped. No congenital infections were identified by cord blood testing. The umbilical arterial catheter was removed, and Triple Dye was applied to the cord. Vitamin E oil was applied to raw areas on the skin caused by the generalized edema. The areas healed within a few days. Surgical consultations noted abnormal bowel on examination but advised no intervention at this time.

The head sonogram showed bilateral ventricular dilation with porencephalic cyst, hemorrhage, and hydrocephalus. The nursing staff measured the fontanelles and head circumference daily. The head of the bed was elevated at all times. Lumbar punctures were performed every other day and removed dark, "Coke"-colored cerebrospinal fluid. Despite this therapy to relieve pressure, ventricular size continued to increase.

Day 8

Laboratory tests showed that the DIC had resolved. The infant was stable on room air. Gavage feedings were started and tolerated well, without residuals or vomiting. The nursing staff documented frequently that the infant nipple-fed poorly, was lethargic, and was irritable when stimulated. The infant progressed from nipple feeding once a day to once a shift. The mother fed the infant every evening.

This intelligent, optimistic mother had a good support network with her sisters and husband. Daily reports were given by physicians and nurses by phone, and the mother visited each evening. A major primary nursing responsibility was to provide information, educate, or answer any questions that the parents had. Maternal-infant contact was fragmented and delayed because of the course of the infant's hospitalization.

Twin A eventually required the placement of a ventricular reservoir to relieve hydrocephalus. Against very high odds this hydropic premie did survive a massive, acute neonatal disorder, unfortunately at great risk for eventual neurological handicap. The family had a realistic picture of prognosis and participated in his serious early course.

Suggested Reading

Hutchison AA, Drew JH, Yu VYH, et al.: Nonimmunologic hydrops fetalis: A review of 61 cases. Obstet Gynecol 59:347–352, 1982.

Maisels MJ: Neonatal jaundice. In GB Avery (ed), Neonatology: Pathophysiology and Management of the Newborn, pp 473–544. Lippincott, Philadelphia, 1981.

Poland RL, Ostrea EM: Neonatal hyperbilirubinemia. In MH Klaus, AA Fanaroff (eds), Care of the High Risk Neonate, pp 243–266. Saunders, Philadelphia, 1979.

Seipien GM, Bernard MU, Chard MA, et al.: Comprehensive Pediatric Nursing. McGraw-Hill, New York, 1979.

Appendix

Appendix 6.1
Blood Warmer

Purpose

All exchange transfusion blood must be warmed to body temperature.

Equipment

1. Fresh blood from blood bank.
2. Blood warmer unit (Figure 6.2)[2]
3. Blood-warming bag with blood filter and tubing
4. IV pole with pressure device

[2] Blood warmer available from Fenwall Labs, Division of Travenol Laboratories, Inc., Deerfield, IL.

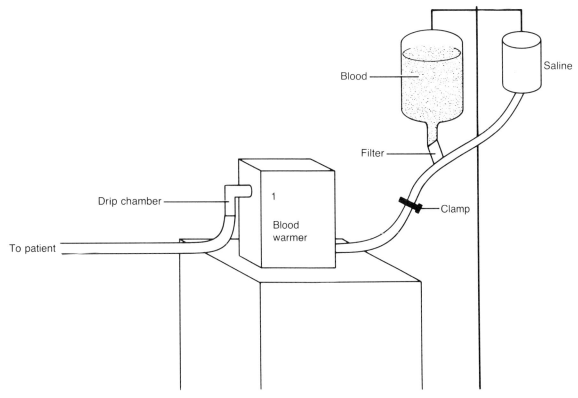

Figure 6.2 **Blood warmer unit.**

Procedure

1. With another nurse check identification information on the bag against the blood request form. Blood should be obtained immediately from blood bank when needed to ensure freshness of blood and clotting factors.
2. Put the blood filter into the blood bag. Fill the filter and tubing. Connect the Y piece of filter tubing to the saline.
3. Close the clamp on the blood filter after filling the tubing with blood.
4. Plug the blood warmer unit into the electric outlet. The temperature guage needle should enter the green scale, indicating a safe temperature range.
5. Open the door of the unit and secure the blood-warming bag on hang-pins, making sure that the bag is smooth and flat against the back panel. The blood warmer bag should be placed in the warmer unit so that the drip chamber is in the *upper* corner.
6. Close the door of the blood warmer unit and fasten the latch. *Do not reopen!*
7. Attach blood-filled tubing into female adapter at *bottom* of blood warming bag. (The blood flows upward into the blood-warming unit.)
8. With the blood warmer door closed, allow the blood to flow into the warming bag by opening the clamp and release chamber, allowing blood to run through the tubing until the complete length of tubing is filled.
   Do not open the blood warmer door!
9. Cover the patient end of the tubing with the needle cap to prevent contamination. Open the clamp to allow the blood to expel air from the tubing and needle. Close the clamp.
10. When ready to begin the transfusion, open the clamp on the patient end of the blood-warming bag and regulate the rate. For rapid infusion, attach the pressure infusor to the unit of blood and infuse at a pressure of 300 mm Hg.
11. Discard the blood-warming bag after single use.

7

Bacterial and Viral Infections and Their Complications

Doris Johnson
Parveen Chowdhry

Most infants adjust from intrauterine life with little difficulty. For some, however, birth is complicated by infections of various kinds and survival is jeopardized. Because infectious agents induce an array of illnesses in the newborn, we have limited discussion to those most prevalent or serious in the neonatal period. Two specific complications, septic shock and disseminated intravascular coagulation (DIC), are discussed in detail. Finally, a brief overview is presented about diagnosis and treatment, as well as nursing management.

Observation is an essential factor in detecting, treating, and preventing the spread of infection because the early stages of neonatal infection may present subtly. The newborn has two humoral defense mechanisms against infection. The first is passively acquired from the mother. The second is active and depends on the infant's own ability to synthesize specific antibodies. The low level of antibodies transmitted across the placenta, reduced globulin formation, less efficient phagocytosis, and the neonate's inability to concentrate these cells at sites of inflammation render all newborns susceptible to invasion by microorganisms.

Bacteria or viruses may gain access to the fetus by a number of routes. Basically, there are three ways in which infections may be acquired:

1. Before delivery, bacteria or viruses can enter via ruptured membranes (ascending infection), or from the maternal bloodstream across the placenta (hematogenous). This latter is the typical route for the TORCH[1] group of agents, as well as syphilis and *Listeria monocytogenes.*

2. During the birth process, direct contact with an organism in the birth canal, such as *Herpes simplex, Neisseria gonorrhoeae,* and group B Streptococcus, can lead to infection. Under normal circumstances colonization by some organisms occurs as a necessary process. However, when the normal defense of the skin or mucous membranes is compromised, when there are a great many microor-

---

[1] Toxoplasmosis, rubella, cytomegalovirus, and hepatitis.

179

ganisms, or when the microorganisms are highly virulent, subsequent infection may occur.

3. Postnatally, the infant may acquire infection from other infants or from contaminated materials or equipment. Hands may not only be the means of transmission, but also a significant reservoir for such bacteria as *Staphylococcus aureus* (1). It is crucial that all personnel who have any contact with the infant or infant's equipment wash their hands thoroughly between neonatal contacts.

Bacterial Infections

Bacterial infections tend to be severe in the neonate, progress rapidly, and are variable in their manifestation. A hallmark of the infamous syndrome of neonatal sepsis is overwhelming systemic spread of bacterial infection, often without any obvious focus, which rapidly compromises cardiovascular competency. Almost all infection can be modified by antibiotics. For these reasons rapid, accurate diagnosis is crucial for optimal outcome.

Most perinatal bacterial infections are caused by organisms found in the normal flora of the mother's genital or intestinal tract. Maternal history provides important clues about the possibility of neonatal bacterial infection. Pneumonia, meningitis, and/or sepsis is a risk for the infant born after premature (prelabor) rupture of membranes, when there has been a prolonged interval between amniotic membrane rupture and the delivery, when there has been a traumatic delivery after fetal hypoxemia, and/or in the presence of active maternal infection. Possible routes of infection in the newborn infant include skin, umbilical cord, airway, GI tract, or open lesions from trauma or congenital defects.

Escherichia coli

Escherichia coli is the most common gram-negative bacteria causing septicemia during the neonatal period. Its normal habitat is the lower intestinal tract. Under usual conditions *E. coli* does not cause any harm; however, it is known as "opportunist" and if given a chance will cause infection elsewhere in the body (2). One significant problem caused by this organism is gastroenteritis in hospital nurseries. Prevention is based on handwashing, isolation of infected infants, and discharge of clinically well, colonized infants. Treatment of infections caused by *E. coli* is based on sensitivity tests and administration of the appropriate antibiotics.

Staphylococcal Infections

There are two major species of this Gram-positive coccus: *Staphylococcus epidermidis* (coagulase negative) and *Staphylococcus aureus* (coagulase negative). *S. epidermidis* has low pathogenicity and is a normal inhabitant of the human skin. This organism may cause minor infections, but the incidence is low and they usually are not serious. Infants with indwelling vascular catheters, endotracheal tubes, and ventriculoperitoneal shunts have increased risk of infection with *S. epidermidis*.

Both *S. epidermidis* and *S. aureus* have two important characteristics: they are resistant to chemical disinfection and heat, and have the ability to acquire resistance to many chemotherapeutic agents. Particularly, the virulence of *S. aureus* depends on its ability to produce substances that are injurious to tissue and increase its spread. Such toxins cause tissue breakdown plus destruction of red blood cells and leukocytes, part of the body's defense against infection.

S. aureus colonization occurs in many infants within the first 5 days of hospitalization. Sources are the mother's oropharynx or perineal region or the oropharynxes of nursery personnel and other newborns. The skin, nose, throat, and umbilicus are frequent sites colonized. The bacteria on the skin are both transient and resident. The transient population may be removed by proper washing, but this will not affect the resident population. Hospital-acquired (nosocomial) staphylococcal infection has been attributed to contamination by carriers. Airborne transmission may play a significant role. Clinical manifestations of *S. aureus* infection include abscesses and pustular rashes. When *S. aureus* gains entrance to the neonatal bloodstream, abscess formation may occur in deep organs, including lungs, liver, and kidneys. It may cause pneumonia, meningitis, and, in particular, septic arthritis and osteomyelitis in the newborn.

If staphylococcal disease does occur in the nursery, the epidemology of infectious spread must be determined. Infants and personnel who have come in contact with the infected infant(s) should be cultured. Neonatal nasopharyngeal and umbilical cultures are appropriate, as are the anterior nares of nursery personnel. Precautionary measures instituted to control a nursery epidemic include:

1. Stressing and enforcing good handwashing technique
2. Isolation of colonized infants
3. Cohort nursing
4. Topical antimicrobial therapy for colonized infants
5. Triple Dye on umbilicus of all newborn admissions
6. Weekly baths with pHisoHex for colonized infants
7. Transfer of infants to clean isolettes every 7 days
8. After discharge of infants, requesting parents to observe for skin lesions and report them to their pediatrician.

It may become necessary to take some unusual and more stringent steps to control the spread of a staphylococcal infection in a nursery. Implementation should be discussed with staff and parents. Some possible steps are:

1. Restricting visitors to parents only
2. Limiting an infant's time out of the isolette to breastfeeding and only 15 minutes twice daily
3. Discontinuing use of a common family room for infant visiting

Treatment of staphylococcal infections varies with the location and extent of the infection. Frequently, Staphylococcus is resistant to penicillin, making methicillin the initial drug of choice. There is an emerging incidence of multiple antibiotic–resistant Staphylococcus. Vancomycin may be helpful for resistant strains.

Group B β-Hemolytic Streptococcus

Group B β-hemolytic *Streptococcus* (GBHS) is the most common gram-positive bacterium isolated from the blood of infants with septicemia. Five to 30% of pregnant women are asymptomatic carriers (3). GBHS causes two clearly defined syndromes, depending on time of onset. The early-onset syndrome is seen in the first few days of life. Sixty-five percent of reported cases involve premature infants (3). It can be acquired by the ascending route in utero or by contact with infected tissue during birth.

Early-onset GBHS infection may present suddenly and progresses rapidly. The primary focus is usually the lungs, although meningitis may be present in 30% of infected cases (4). Usual symptoms include respiratory distress, apnea, hypotension, shock, and generalized bleeding from DIC. DIC indicates a grave prognosis, with rapid deterioration and death likely despite appropriate antibiotic and supportive therapy. Diagnosis of GBHS sepsis is established by positive blood culture, although the organisms can be cultured from many sites, including the nasopharynx, skin, and external ear canal. Speck et al. (5) discussed interpretation of cultures and the five subgroups of the organism. A tracheal aspirate may help make a presumptive diagnosis by detecting gram-positive cocci in chains and many polymorphonuclear leukocytes (PMNs). The mortality rate seems related to gestational age: for preterm infants it is 70–80%, and for term infants, 33% (4).

The late-onset GBHS syndrome occurs between the first and third week of life but may be seen as late as 16 weeks of age. The onset is insidious; lethargy, poor feeding, and fever are the most frequent symptoms. The skin may also be affected by abscesses, cellulitis, or impetigo. Many infants present with meningitis as their predominant clinical manifestation. The prognosis for survival is better than for the early-onset type: the overall mortality rate is 10–15%. A significant percentage of survivors may have neurological sequelae. The drug of choice for group B Streptococcus is penicillin when the infecting organism has been identified before treatment. However, a combination of penicillin and aminoglycoside is recommended prior to sensitivity test results and possibly for a reported synergistic action with combined therapy.

Symptoms and Signs

The role of the nurse in infants at risk for infection is eloquently expressed by Speck et al. (5, p. 276):

> It is often the nurse who alerts the medical staff to the diagnosis by observing subtle changes in color, tone, activity or feeding difficulties in the infant. Unless an excellent working relationship between the nurse and physician exists, early diagnosis is impossible.

The symptoms of sepsis are not uniform, but suspect infection when there is a change in the infant's behavior or clinical signs. The following signs *most* often suggest the possibility of sepsis:

Skin changes (pallor, jaundice, or cyanosis)
Lethargy and irritability
GI disturbances: poor feeding, abdominal distention, gastric residuals, vomiting, and diarrhea
Temperature instability
Unexplained weight loss
Unexplained metabolic acidosis
Unexplained apneic episodes
Respiratory distress
Tachycardia or hypotension
Hypoglycemia (uncommon, but may be associated with sepsis)

Diagnosis

Immediately upon admission to ICU, the following tests may be performed on infants at risk for perinatally acquired sepsis: gastric aspirate and external ear canal for culture and smear, differential, white blood cell count, and minisedimentation rate. Further tests include blood culture, lumbar puncture, urine cultures, blood gases, and chest x-rays. Whether to start antibiotic therapy will depend on individual clinical circumstances, the judgment of the physicians, and laboratory tests.

In each case culture results are important for the specific diagnosis of sepsis. Treatment rests on the choice of antibiotics. This choice depends on isolating the infective agent and determining its sensitivity to the drugs. We recommend starting the initial dose of antibiotics IV to make sure therapeutic levels of antibiotics are promptly achieved and maintained adequately. Furthermore, since cardiovascular collapse can occur rapidly in the septic neonate, an IV in place provides an immediate route for colloid therapy.

Duration of antimicrobial therapy in diagnosed sepsis depends on the clinical status of the infant, the nature of the offending organism, and the systems involved. The usual duration is 7–10 days and at least until cultures are negative for 72 hours. Infections involving the central nervous system (CNS) may need IV therapy for 2 weeks or longer. Sterilization of the cerebrospinal fluid (CSF) is the goal.

It should be remembered that most antibiotics are irritating to tissue and risk toxic side effects. They must be well diluted severalfold and administered relatively slowly, over 15 to 20 minutes. Administration of antibiotics through either a central arterial or venous catheter is not recommended. Keep umbilical catheters reserved for blood drawing and blood pressure monitoring. Insert a supplemental peripheral IV for medication administration and hyperalimentation. Consult a standard neonatology text for antibiotics, dosages, and side effects. The initial choice of antibiotics is based on the likely organism in your hospital.

Viral Infections

Unlike bacteria, viruses can not survive long unless they are ultimately related to living cells. During their incubation period they migrate to cells that they then invade. Symptoms of disease do not appear until viral multiplication is advanced and target cells are being attacked. Usually, by the time a clinical diagnosis can be made, viruses have gained a foothold in the tissue and are replicating.

Specific treatment of most viral infections is ineffective. Normally, the disease is brought to a halt when the body produces a specific antibody against the infecting virus in sufficient amounts. The specific antibody does not enter the cell, but limits infection to those cells already invaded and aids disposal of extracellular viral agents.

TORCHS Infections

Viral infections may be transmitted across the placenta from mother to fetus. An exception is *Herpes simplex* virus, which is acquired either by the ascending route or by direct contact with maternal lesions. The chronic intrauterine infections are exemplified by the TORCHS-type infections; this acronym stands for toxoplasmosis, rubella, cytomegalovirus, herpes, and syphilis. Such infants may appear normal at birth. However, one of several consequences may befall the fetus or neonate as a result of such chronic congenital infections, most commonly death in utero or immediately after birth or survival with congenital malformation.

Commonly observed signs of the classic TORCHS syndrome are progressive (direct and indirect) jaundice, petechiae, hepatosplenomegaly, respiratory distress, and convulsions. Infants may have cataracts and microcephaly, and may be small for gestational age. Some have hearing loss appreciable in the neonatal period. Visual impairment can also be detected but often is a later finding. Rubella infants typically have evidence of peripheral pulmonic stenosis. Babies suspected of having TORCHS infections should be handled as if possibly contagious. Any potentially pregnant personnel or nonimmune caregiver should not have contact with these infants.

Herpes Virus

Unlike the other TORCHS infections, herpes virus (*Herpes simplex*) infection is usually not chronic and often presents as an acute, sepsis-like neonatal illness. There are two strains of herpes virus, type 1 and type 2. Type 1 virus is spread primarily via the oropharynx; type 2 virus is transmitted venereally. Those previously infected have circulating antibodies against the virus. The incubation period varies from 2 to 20 days, with a mean of 6 days (6). Neonates acquire the type 2 virus at or immediately preceding birth from exposure to infected genital secretions. Transplacental infection with herpes virus is uncommon. Cesarean section delivery is recommended for infants whose mothers have known active genital herpes and a history of intact membranes or membranes ruptured less than 4 hours.

The infected infant often appears normal at birth. The disease may remain localized to skin, eye, or CNS, or may progress to a generalized form. Small scattered vesicles may appear. The infant becomes lethargic, feeds poorly, and develops temperature instability, then rapidly develops jaundice, dyspnea, cyanosis, petechiae, and hepatosplenomegaly. The progression of clinical signs frequently terminates with apnea, DIC, thrombocytopenia, shock, or seizures and death. Those who recover may manifest severe CNS damage and blindness from retinal involvement.

When skin lesions are absent, presumptive diagnosis is difficult because histology and culture of virus from skin lesions provides the definitive diagnosis. Positive culture results can be obtained within 24 to 48 hours. Antiviral drugs such as cytosine arabinoside and adenine arabinoside have been used with limited success. Septic neonates may require supportive measures, depending on the type of infection and its severity. Attention to thermoregulation, reduction or discontinuation of oral feedings, and correction of metabolic acidosis, may all be required. Oxygen therapy may be administered to relieve cyanosis, with intermittent monitoring of arterial pO_2 (oxygen pressure) values. Depending upon the severity of the infection, anemia and/or shock can occur and need to be aggressively managed.

Nursing Management of the Infected Neonate

Rest is an important goal when nursing infected infants because they are easily fatigued. Every effort must be made to conserve the infant's energy while providing necessary care:

1. Be organized in caring for infants: collect all equipment before starting care, do what needs to be done, and let the infant rest.
2. Assess the infant's level of consciousness: alert, drowsy, etc.
3. Maintain a neutral thermal environment.
4. Ensure proper body alignment.
5. Administer gavage feeding if the infant tires easily.

Nursing care varies when or if other complications develop, many of which may be life threatening to an infant. The following list gives some ideas for care of infants suspected of or with confirmed infections. Remember, nursing management of an infant changes frequently and should be constantly reevaluated. Each individual who is responsible for nursing care of that infant should update the care plan according to changes in the infant's status.

1. Support infant-parent interaction during hospitalization:
    a. Encourage the parents to visit regularly.
    b. Encourage parent participation in the infant's care.
    c. Facilitate verbalization of concerns.
    d. Approach the parents in a positive manner when discussing topics related to health care.
    e. Teach the parents what they want to know first, then teach them what you have assessed that they need to know.
    f. Reinforce parenting skills.
2. Isolate the infant as ordered:
    a. Follow procedures for isolation (see Table 7.1 below).
    b. Provide visual and auditory stimulation to the infant.
3. Assist with or collect cultures as ordered.
4. Administer medications as ordered:
    a. Give only one antibiotic at a time.
    b. Infuse within 1 hour.
    c. Observe for side effects.
5. Maintain stable environmental temperature:
    a. Place the infant in an isolette or on a radiant warmer, or clothe warmly in an open crib.
    b. Monitor temperature frequently.
    c. Avoid situations that might predispose the infant to chilling.
6. Observe, record, and report:
    a. Response to therapy: antibiotics, blood products, etc.
    b. Alterations in vital signs.
    c. How the infant feeds, sleeps, eliminates, and responds to stimuli.
    d. Amount taken at each feeding and residuals before feeding.
    e. Intake and output.
    f. Daily weights.
7. Prevent aspiration of feedings:
    a. Elevate the head during feedings.
    b. Place the infant on his abdomen or side after feeding.
    c. Check placement of the feeding tube prior to feeding gavaging formula.
8. Prevent tissue breakdown:
    a. Change the infant's position every 1 to 2 hours.
    b. Massage the bony prominences every shift.
    c. Change diapers and clean the cord frequently.
    d. Use a sheepskin or air mattress.
9. Assess respiratory status frequently:
    a. Keep the airway patent by positioning the infant to prevent pooling of secretions.
    b. Relieve nasal congestion by suctioning and saline drops, if needed.
    c. Administer oxygen as needed to relieve a transcutaneous pO_2 less than 40 torr.
    d. Note any changes in respiratory effort and report quality and rate of respirations.
    e. Have equipment available to institute resuscitative measures if necessary.
10. Observe, record, and report signs of complications:

a. Meningitis: bulging anterior fontanelles, increasing irritability, seizures, lethargy, apnea, and uneven pupillary response.
b. Joint involvement: limited movement, local inflammation.
c. Shock: fall in blood pressure, rapid pulse, decrease in urinary output, imparied circulation of extremities.

11. Initiate discharge planning as the infant's condition stabilizes. Depending on the causative organism and extent of disease, parents should either be reassured that the disease has resolved or counseled about the infant's need for follow-up, as appropriate. Developmental follow-up is particularly important for the TORCHS infections.

Preventing Nosocomial Infection

The nurse is responsible for protecting the infant from his environment. The basis of this protection is through handwashing with an antiseptic detergent or soap. It is important that the nurse uses appropriate techniques and that she monitors other personnel and visitors, including parents, who may come into contact with the infant (see Appendices 7.1 and 7.2).

Hands should be washed up to the elbows for 2 to 3 minutes before entering the nursery. Betadine is a povidone-iodine wash preparation we use since it is both bacteriocidal and antiviral. Friction and thorough rinsing also enhance the removal of organisms. Personnel and visitors should be especially careful to wash their hands before feeding, after diaper change, before going from one infant to another, and after touching anything that is not clean. Clean scrub clothing or uniforms should be worn daily. When leaving the ICN, a lab coat should be used to cover the uniform. All other personnel must scrub their hands and should wear a cover gown over street clothes when handling any infant or equipment. Face masks can be worn when anyone has upper respiratory problems or cold sores, but masks must be changed frequently or they will act as a reservoir of infection. Anyone with a communicable disease is excluded from the nursery or from contact with the infant. The potential of communicable diseases exists whenever there is a fever of undetermined origin, acute respiratory or GI tract infections, open draining wound infections, or a history of exposure to a communicable disease. Each case must be handled individually.

Respiratory equipment, blood pressure apparatus, stethoscopes, and items shared among infants should be cleaned with an appropriate disinfectant between use. Cribs and isolettes should be cleaned between infants and weekly when infants are nursed in isolettes for long periods of time. Articles damaged by heat should be sterilized with a gas sterilizer. Toys should be made of readily disinfected materials and cleaned before being placed in an isolette. Stuffed animals can be wrapped in plastic wrap.

When caring for an infant suspected of infection, isolation technique is modified depending upon the mode of transmission. Tables 7.1 and 7.2 show our current guidelines. Isolette portholes left open allow transmission of pathogens into them, and isolettes prevent infection only if neighboring infants are kept in isolettes also. Strict sterile technique should be used for all diagnostic procedures. (See Appendix 7.3 for isolation policy and procedures.)

Complications of Infections

Any systemic infection, whether bacterial or viral, may lead to an acute cardiovascular decompensation in the newborn. Nursing management of these infants includes

Table 7.1 NICU Infection Precautions for Infection Exposure[a]

Infection exposure	Routine lab tests	Isolette	Gloves	Gown	Trash and linen (double bagging)	Other	Duration of precaution	Mode of transmission	Separation from mother	Comments
Infants receiving blood transfusions	Weekly urine for CMV[b] screen after 1 month of age	No	No	No	No	Isolette if confirmed			No	
Born out of asepsis	No	No	No	No	No	Routine pHisoHex bath		None	No	
Fever, maternal	No	No	No	No	No	Check maternal culture results			Only if mother is isolated	Precautions if obstetrician diagnoses a contagious process
Herpes, maternal	No	Yes	No	Yes	No	Teach mother importance of handwashing, even at home	While mother has lesions	Contact with contaminated secretions	Until mother can care for infant 24 h a day	The exposed infant may not return to the nursery after going to mother's room
PROM 24 or foul-smelling at birth	C&S of ear; gastric C&S with Wrights' stain	No	No	No	No	CBC and ESR at birth and at 24 h	24 h		No	
Pustules, neonatal	C&S of pustule	Yes	Yes	Yes	Yes		Until lesions negative	Contact	No	Treat pustules like *S. aureus* until ruled out
TORCHS screen	Cord blood	Yes	Follow precautions for suspected organism				Until results have been reported		No	

Based on center for Disease Control Guidelines: Infection, vol. 4, no. 4. Center for Disease Control, Atlanta, 1983.

[a] General policy:

1. Good handwashing is required between babies.
2. For uninfected infants to be protected against airborne infections, they must remain inside their isolettes, where they breathe filtered air. When they are out of their isolettes, they must be taken out of the area of the infected infant.
3. A physician's order is required:
   a. To initiate isolation;
   b. To take an isolated infant out of an isolette, even to be weighed.

[b] Abbreviations used: CMV, cytomegalovirus; PROM, prolonged rupture of membranes; C&S, culture and stain; CBC, complete blood count; ESR, erythrocyte sedimentation rate.

Table 7.2 NICU Infection Precautions for Active Infections[a]

Active infection	Routine lab tests	Isolette	Gloves	Gown	Trash linen (double bagging)	Other	Duration of precaution	Mode of transmission	Separation from mother	Comments
CMV[b], confirmed	No	Yes	Yes	Yes	Yes		Until discharged from hospital	Urine, stool, and respiratory	No	No pregnant personnel
Diarrhea	Stool C&S	Yes	Yes	Yes	Yes	Cohort nursing[c]	Until asymptomatic	Oral-fecal	No	
Gonorrhea		No	No	No	No			Discharge may be infective		
Hepatitis B: HB$_s$Ag(+) or HB$_e$Ag(+)	No	Yes	Yes	Yes	Yes	Needle, stool, and secretion precaution	Until discharged from hospital	Body fluids, urine, and stool	No	Hyperimmune globulin (Hbg) recommended; breastfeeding individualized
Hepatitis A	Antibody screen	Yes	Yes	Yes	Yes	Needle precaution	Individualized	Blood and body fluids	Only if mother acutely ill	
Hepatitis non-A or non-B	No	Yes	Yes	Yes	Yes	Needle precaution	Individualized	Transfusions; contact with blood or body fluids	While mother acutely ill	

						Special precautions	Duration of precautions	Spread by	Private room/isolation needed	Comments
Herpes simplex, neonatal	No	Yes	Yes	Yes	Yes		Until free of lesions	Shed from lesions	Only if mother isolated	No pregnant personnel
Listeria	No	Yes	If lesions present	Yes	Yes	No	As ordered	Contact	No	
Rubella, congenital	No	Yes	Yes	Yes	Yes	Mask if susceptible	Until discharge	Respiratory and contact	No	No pregnant personnel
Salmonella and Shigella	Stool C&S with Wright's stain	Yes	Yes	Yes	Yes	Cohort nursing[c]	Until C&S negative three times	Oral-fecal	No	
S. Aureus	No	Yes	No	Yes	Yes	Cohort nursing[c]	Until discharge	Contact or airborne	No	
Streptococcus, β-hemolytic	No	Yes	No	Yes	Yes		As ordered	Contact or respiratory	Only if the infant's has been isolated	
Syphilis	No	If lesions are present	If lesions are present	No	No		For 24 h after effective drug therapy	Veneral or contact with lesions	No	Spinal tap may be indicated
Toxoplasmosis	No	No	No	No	No		None needed	No		

Based on Center for Disease Control Guidelines: Infection, vol. 4, no. 4. Center for Disease Control, Atlanta, 1983.

[a] See Table 7.1, footnote a for general policy.

[b] Abbreviations used: CMV, cytomegalovirus; C&S, culture and stain; HB$_s$Ag, hepatitis B surface antigen; HB$_c$Ag, hepatitis B core antigen.

[c] Infants with same infection nursed by same nurse(s).

anticipation of this outcome. Cardiovascular collapse can be secondary to septic shock or follow acute hemorrage caused by DIC. Although these complications are infrequent, early recognition and treatment are essential if the infant is to survive.

Septic Shock

Sepsis is a generalized disease process resulting from invasion of the blood stream by microorganisms or secretory products of microorganisms. The basic mechanism of shock is an impaired ability to delivery adequate amounts of oxygen and nutrients to the tissues. If not recognized early it leads to circulatory collapse and death. When the underlying process is associated with sepsis, the result is septic shock. An excellent review on the subject is provided by Perkin and Levin (7, 8).

Pathophysiology

The precise manner in which microcirculatory failure occurs is unclear. The process seems to be complex and is likely to be the result of a multitude of factors. It is perhaps the result of interaction between the pathogens and/or their toxins with the products activated by the host's defense mechanism to ward off the infectious process (9). Septic shock may result from the direct effect of the organisms or their products on the cardiovascular system (10), or from an indirect effect of secondary products released from the tissues, such as kinins and the myocardial depressant factors (MDFs) (11). Other vasoactive substances released from damaged, ischemic, necrotic, or infected tissues, such as histamine, serotonin, prostaglandins, products of arachidonic acid (thromboxane), and endorphins, may also play significant roles (12). Lysosomes released from leukocytes may also contribute to the pathogenesis. Activation of complement factors by the endotoxin in gram-negative bacteria and teichoic acid in gram-positive bacteria results in activation of PMNs, which adhere to each other and to capillary endothelium (13). The activated PMNs also release lysosome enzymes, as described by Weissman et al. (14); this leads to endothelial cell cytotoxicity.

During the initial phase both pre- and postcapillary sphincter constriction occurs, leading to cellular hypoxia followed by a phase of excessive vasodilation. The combined effect is capillary leakage. Vasodilatation results from released vasoactive substances and histmaine, which cause increased vascular capacitance and lowered vascular resistance, resulting in relative hypovolemia. The net result is uneven blood distribution and relative or absolute hypovolemia progressing to circulatory failure.

Cells damaged by hypoperfusion are unable to maintain normal cellular metabolism. As a consequence, there is extracellular movement of potassium and intracellular accumulation of sodium and water resulting in swelling of the cell and further reduction in blood volume. Damage to capillary endothelial cells leads to extravasation of protein-rich fluid and potentiates hypovolemia. The circulatory failure ultimately leads to multiple organ system dysfunction and may be associated with the syndrome of DIC.

Diagnosis

Early diagnosis is crucial since the aim is to reverse the process before the extensive deterioration of vital organs has occurred. Symptoms include a falling blood pressure and evidence of impaired tissue perfusion, such as prolonged capillary filling time (greater than 5 seconds in the trunk), cold clammy skin, oliguria, and metabolic acidosis.

During the early phase of septic shock, the blood pressure may be normal or slightly elevated. Cardiac output is elevated, with bounding pulses and wide pulse pressure. Urine output is adequate, even increased. Capillary filling time may be normal. There may be metabolic acidosis, but respiratory alkalosis is commonly seen during the early phase, since hyperventilation often occurs.

Later phases manifest classic signs of shock such as hypotension, decreased pulses, decreased cardiac output, prolonged capillary filling time, narrow pulse pressure, oliguria, and lethargy. Associated with this phase are hypoxemia, metabolic acidosis, and elevation of blood lactate concentrations. Clinical evidence of bleeding from DIC may become evident.

Urine output in sepsis may be normal initially, despite relative hypovolemia. Falling urinary output reflects cardiac failure and hypoperfusion as septic shock advances. Metabolic acidosis is the classic acid-base disturbance in shock. This results from accumulation of lactate due to anaerobic metabolism. However, the final stage of shock is characterized by combined respiratory and metabolic acidosis, which signifies a poor prognosis. The administration of buffers or colloids may correct acid-base imbalance. Repeated sampling of serum pH and electrolytes is necessary if an overcorrection is to be detected early.

Blood Pressure Monitoring During the early stages of shock, observation of pulse pressure is helpful since it generally correlates with cardiac output. Indeed, lowered pulse pressure occurs before significant lowering of the systolic blood pressure is observed. In hypovolemia diastolic pressure may be elevated initially as the peripheral vascular resistance responds. In suspected shock the blood pressure needs to be monitored continuously. Table 2.6 shows normal blood pressure for weight at 12 hours of age. The most accurate blood pressure in newborn infants is obtained from direct, intra-arterial lines, usually in an umbilical artery. However, these can be inaccurate if improperly zeroed or if air bubbles or clots are present in the tubing or dome, dampening the pressure wave transmission. Peripheral arterial lines can also be used to do continuous intra-arterial blood pressure monitoring.

Every infected infant does not need catheterization. There are several techniques to measure blood pressure noninvasively. These include auscultation, palpation, Doppler monitoring, and flush method. All use a pressure cuff applied to an extremity. Each method is reasonably accurate, provided the infant's peripheral circulation is good. However, cuff blood pressure may be unreliable or inaccurate when an infant becomes hypotensive and peripheral perfusion is significantly compromised.

Management of Septic Shock Syndrome

Patients in septic shock are critically ill and need continuous monitoring, including heart rate, pO_2, apnea, and skin temperature monitoring. An intra-arterial catheter for continuous blood pressure monitoring, pulse wave monitoring, and frequent blood sampling is beneficial. Ventilatory support and oxygen are often indicated and should be employed based on the blood gases. Fluid intake and urine output need diligent recording. IV lines are necessary for fluid and drug administration. Central venous or pulmonary wedge pressure is sometimes useful to guide fluid and electrolyte therapy. Aggressive antibiotic therapy is critical, based on presumptions about possible organisms and their antibiotic sensitivities. The initial choice of antimicrobial agent used should provide a broad-spectrum coverage. As soon as the in vitro sensitivity pattern is available, antibiotic therapy may be modified.

Cardiovascular support is vital. Cardiac rhythm disturbances are common and may be due to a number of factors, such as electrolyte and acid-base abnormalities, hypovolemia, or drug side effects. Intracardiac catheters may lead to cardiac arrhythmia and need to be repositioned if this is detected (15). Hypovolemia is part of the septic shock syndrome. Urgent measures are indicated to correct it. The aim of fluid therapy is to provide circulatory volume and red cell mass to ensure adequate oxygen-carrying capacity. Overexpansion or too rapid expansion can produce volume overload.

The amount of fluid given must be carefully monitored in patients with septic shock to prevent pulmonary edema. However, increased fluids may be necessary to improve urine output. A central venous pressure line may be helpful when attempting to monitor the adequacy of the blood volume versus the cardiac output. The normal range for neonatal central venous pressure is 6–10 mm Hg. The use of colloid (plasma, albumin, fresh whole blood) is indicated in septic shock. The usual empirical dose is 10 mg/kg. If this does not effectively improve vital signs, a second infusion at the same dose may be necessary. When fluids and colloid therapy are ineffective in reversing shock, vasoactive agents may be needed. Alkali therapy is contraindicated in respiratory acidosis since bicarbonate contributes to hypercarbia when pulmonary status is compromised. Bicarbonate is only useful for metabolic acidosis.

Improvement in the circulating blood volume should result in adequate urine output. If oliguria persists in spite of adequate fluid replacement, diuretics may be tried, but their use is controversial. Dopamine sometimes improves renal blood flow (at least in lower doses) and it may help here. Major organ systems such as the liver, pancreas, and GI tract are involved in shock. Patients may develop stress gastric ulcer and paralytic ileus. Antacid therapy and/or cimetidine may be useful. The first sign of an ulcer can be bright red or coffee-ground gastric secretions. An additional complication is DIC, which may present with bleeding or thrombosis and is common in neonates with sepsis and septic shock.

Disseminated Intravascular Coagulation

Disseminated intravascular coagulation (DIC) is a process of inappropriate coagulation with the vascular system. It is frequently observed in association with sepsis as well as hypoxemia and acidosis. Commonly encountered clinical conditions during the neonatal period that increase the risk of DIC include perinatal asphyxia, respiratory distress syndrome, necrotizing enterocolitis, erythroblastosis, meconium aspiration, and sepsis. In sepsis it is likely that hypoxemia and acidosis act as triggering factors, leading to capillary endothelial damage, which in turn triggers the clotting cascade. In addition, thromboplastin or thromboplastin-like material may be released into the circulation from damaged or necrotic tissue to trigger DIC. Placental abnormalities such as abruption or infarction may also lead to DIC.

Pathogenesis and Clinical Presentation

Generalized intravascular coagulation leads to depletion of blood factors and platelets essential for normal hemostasis. These factors are consumed in DIC at a rapid rate and overwhelm the capacity of the organism to regenerate them. Along with rapid consumption, the fibrinolytic system is also activated, leading to production of fibrin split products, which inhibit conversion of fibrinogen to fibrin. When the clotting factors are depleted, the neonate can no longer maintain normal clotting function. At this point the infant may present with frank hemorrhage. More commonly, however, the first sign of DIC in a sick infant is bleeding from puncture sites or the umbilical stump. The neonate may also present with evidence of generalized petechiae or frank hemorrhage from any or all orifices: hematuria, or pulmonary, GI, or intracranial hemorrhage. The early stage of DIC, when the consumption of clotting factors is occurring, may be evidenced only by abnormal laboratory tests. These tests include falling platelet count and fibrinogen levels, and lengthening prothrombin time and partial thromboplastin time. Often DIC is grave and progresses rapidly to hypotension, shock, and death. Detailed reviews of the pathogenesis can be found in the texts by Oski and Naiman (16) and Gladen and Buchanan (17).

Diagnosis

In a sick premature neonate with suspected DIC, the laboratory test results most useful for diagnosis are a low platelet count, increased prothrombin time, and activated partial thromboplastin time. For these last two tests, abnormal values for neonates are more than double control values. A low fibrinogen concentration is also consistent with DIC. The blood smear may reveal bizarre red blood cell morphology, suggesting microangiopathy; this serves as a valuable clue. It is important to take into account the gestation age when evaluating laboratory tests. Premature infants have reduced levels of nearly all the clotting factors compared with levels in term infants and adults. The vascular fragility of premature infants is also enhanced when compared with term infants and adults: they bruise more easily.

Differential Diagnosis of the Bleeding Neonate In order to make an accurate diagnosis of DIC, it is important to know the clinical manifestations of other blood disorders in newborns. Neonates may have ecchymoses and petechiae as a result of birth trauma, without evidence of abnormal blood clotting tests. Some infants may have GI bleeding as a result of maternal blood swallowed at birth. Such maternal blood can be distinguished from fetal blood: a simple laboratory test, the Apt Test, can distinguish maternal from fetal hemoglobin.

Severe liver disease may present with bleeding since the liver is responsible for syntheses of most of the blood coagulation factors. Vitamin K, useful in preventing hemorrhagic disease of the newborn, is ineffective in stopping hemorrhage secondary to severe liver disease. In severe liver disease, component blood therapy is helpful.

Consumptive thrombocytopenia is observed in neonates with necrotizing enterocolitis, vascular thrombosis, infection, or vascular malformation. Neonates with congenital infection, usually from the TORCHS group, also may present with bleeding.

Immune thrombocytopenia may be categorized into two types; isoimmune or autoimmune. The isoimmune type is analogous to RH erythroblastosis. The maternal platelet count remains normal because the mother has formed antibodies against fetal platelets. Low neonatal versus normal maternal count provides a simple diagnostic criterion. The other blood clotting factors are normal. Treatment consists of transfusion with platelets of maternal origin (platelet pheresis). Autoimmune thrombocytopenia is associated with maternal disease in which antibodies are formed against common platelet antigen. This antibody causes thrombocytopenia in the mother, and upon transplacental passage, leads to thrombocytopenia in the fetus. Platelet counts are low in both mother and infant. The level of circulating maternal antiplatelet antibody correlates with the presence of neonatal thrombocytopenia. Prenatal maternal steroid therapy may benefit the fetus.

Evidence of bleeding following circumcision may be one clue to a hereditary deficiency of clotting factors in the newborn. Such disorders are all rare. Evaluation of various blood clotting factors responsible for the disorder confirm the diagnosis.

Hemorrhagic disease of the newborn clinically presents with bleeding from any site around 2 to 4 days of life. It is due to the absence of bowel flora and thus the impaired production of endogenous vitamin K precursors. Both prothrombin time and partial thromboplastin time are prolonged; platelet counts are normal. Treatment with vitamin K, 1 mg IV, is therapeutic within 4 to 6 hours. Prophylaxis with vitamin K has essentially eliminated this neonatal disease. Occasionally infants of mothers receiving Coumadin (one of the hydantoin group anticoagulants) may present with hemorrhagic disease. Infants on total parenteral nutrition should receive vitamin K (0.5 mg IM) each week until oral feedings are established.

Management of DIC

DIC is a serious problem of the sick neonate. Careful observation for any evidence of abnormal bleeding in the ill newborn is mandatory. Promptly informing the responsible physician and follow-up by appropriate lab tests will effect the best results. Management of DIC includes the following two steps:

1. Alleviation of the primary triggering mechanisms. This involves the recognition and treatment of the primary disorder (i.e., sepsis, hypoxia, erythroblastosis, etc.).
2. Correction of the hematological abnormalities. This may be achieved by using whole blood or blood component therapy. Exchange transfusion, although often used, is ineffective (18).
   a. Platelets may be life-saving in severe hemorrhage caused by platelet deficiencies.
   b. Fresh frozen plasma is an excellent source of labile and nonlabile clotting factors, but a poor source of platelets.

Success in management depends greatly on anticipation, early recognition, and aggressive treatment aimed at the initiating factors and preventing shock, which is frequently associated with this phenomenon.

Case Studies

Case 1: A Term Infant Who Had β-hemolytic Streptococcus Infection after Prolonged Rupture of Membranes

K. was a male infant with an estimated gestational age of 38 weeks and was delivered vaginally following 5 days rupture of membranes. The pregnancy had been normal, but the mother developed a fever 2 hours before delivery. Cervical cultures had been taken, and the mother was started on antibiotics before delivery. K. was born covered with purulent material and was foul smelling. Apgar scores were 3 and 5 at 1 and 5 minutes, respectively. Birth weight was 2530 grams. At birth severe respiratory distress was noted, which required intubation and ventilation in the delivery room. K. was transported to the ICN on the ventilator.

On admission the infant's respiratory rate was 48 breaths/minute, and his rectal temperature was 96.4°F; pulse rate, 138 beats/minute; and blood pressure 48 mm Hg in the right arm, using the Doppler method. His Silverman score was between 3 and 5 for nasal flaring and retractions of the intercostal spaces. Rales were audible throughout both lungs. A heated table was used to provide warmth and a Saran Wrap shield was used to prevent heat loss. Gastric secretions were sent for culture, Gram's stain, and the presence of PMNs. Gastric aspirate revealed 75–100 PMNs per high-powered field. A shake test was done to exclude respiratory distress syndrome as one cause for respiratory symptoms; the result was negative. Cultures were obtained from the blood, tracheal and gastric aspirates, external ear canal, and urine.

An umbilical arterical catheter was placed, along with a peripheral IV line. Chest x-ray revealed good lung expansion, no pneumonitis, and a normal cardiac silhouette. K. was started on penicillin and kanamycin shortly after the cultures were obtained. Metabolic acidosis was treated with bicarbonate. Vital signs, were checked hourly, including continuous blood pressure monitoring and intake and output; head circumference was measured every 4 hours. Laboratory findings included white blood cell count of 24,800/mm³, with 60% lymphocytes, 29% segmented neutrophils, 2% monocytes, and 9% band neutrophils; a microestimated sedimentation rate of 8 mm in 1 hour; and a normal platelet count.

At 6 hours of age, despite administration of massive doses of antibiotics and supporting blood pressure with volume expansion, K. continued to deteriorate. Dopamine drip was started. Respiratory failure required high peak pressures (45 cm) to achieve adequate oxygenation and correct CO_2 retention. K. developed bilateral pneumothoracies, and chest tubes were placed and monitored for drainage and patency.

Ongoing treatment included continuous bicarbonate by IV drip, plasma and blood transfusion, increased dopamine, and Priscoline to counteract the developing pulmonary hypertension. At 12 hours of age, there was evidence of renal failure. Pulmonary and intraventricular hemorrhage occurred and DIC was documented at this time. At 24 hours of age, K. suffered a cardiac arrest and died.

Three days later, group B Streptococcus was cultured from his admission blood and tracheal and gastric secretions. Because sepsis is so easily confused with other neonatal disorders, definitive diagnosis can only be established by laboratory tests. Specific aggressive but empirical antibiotic therapy must be given well before the diagnosis is made. Unfortunately, it may not produce an optimal outcome.

Case 2: Nosocomial Sepsis

A. was a female infant with a gestational age of 31 weeks and a birth weight of 1040 grams; she was delivered by cesarean section. The mother went into premature labor, and tocolytics failed to arrest the labor. A. was intubated at birth and had Apgar scores of 6 and 8. She was quickly weaned to room air. One week after extubation she only required nasal constant positive airway pressure and had mild CO_2 retention, which was resolved by an increased frequency of chest physiotherapy. She was started on hyperalimentation, and then began oral feedings, which were slowly increased as tolerated.

When A. was 8 weeks of age, the nurse caring for her observed increased irritability, grunting, nasal flaring, retraction of the intercostal spaces, stridor, and regurgitation of feedings. A. also developed episodes of apnea, bradycardia, and lethargy. This was associated with hypoxemia and residuals with feedings. Her respiratory rate was 92 breaths/minute, and she had an axillary temperature of 99°F, a pulse rate of 152 beats/minute, and blood pressure readings of 58 mm Hg in the right arm and 42 mm Hg in the left arm. A chest x-ray revealed left upper lobe atelectasis and pneumonia. Hourly checkings of vital signs, recording of intake and output, and monitoring of Silverman score were initiated. Oxygen therapy with continuous monitoring of $TcpO_2$ was started. There was frequent evaluation of blood gases. Chest physiotherapy was increased in frequency. Oral feedings were discontinued, and A. was started on IV therapy. She was intubated and mechanically ventilated.

Laboratory findings included a hemoglobin level of 13.7 grams/100 ml; a white blood count of 12,300/mm³, with 44% lymphocytes, 53% segmented neutrophils, and 5% band neutrophils; and a platelet count of 133,000/mm³. A gram stain of CSF revealed no organisms. Tracheal aspirate showed a few gram-positive diplococci and no PMNs. Tracheal aspirate culture eventually grew *S. aureus*. The spinal fluid was sterile. Initial treatment had included methicillin and gentamicin; following conformation of *S. aureus*, the gentamicin was discontinued.

The nurse's observation of subtle changes in A.'s appearance and behavior led to detection of the infection. Early recognition and diagnosis with institution of vigorous therapeutic measures are essential to increase the chance for survival and reduce the likelihood of permanent neurological damage.

References

1. Remington JS, Klien JO: Infectious Diseases of the Fetus and Newborn Infant. Saunders, Philadelphia, 1976.
2. Volk WA: Essentials of Medical Microbiology. Lippincott, New York, 1978.
3. McCracken GH: Bacterial and viral infections of the newborn. In G Avery (ed), Neonatology: Pathophysiology and Management of the Newborn, 2nd ed, pp 723–745. Lippincott, Philadelphia, 1981.
4. Sever JL, Larson JW, Grossman JH: Handbook of Perinatal Infections. Little, Brown & Co, Boston, 1979.
5. Speck W, Fanaroff A, Klaus M: Neonatal infections. In M Klaus, A Fanaroff (eds), Care of the High Risk Neonate, 2nd ed, pp 267–285. Saunders, Philadelphia, 1979.
6. Reynolds D, Stagno S, Alford C: Chronic congenital and perinatal infections. In G Avery (ed), Neonatology: Pathophysiology and Management of the Newborn, 2nd ed, pp 748–778, Lippincott, Philadelphia, 1981.
7. Perkin RM, Levin DL: Shock in the pediatric patient: Part I. J Pediatr 101:163, 1982.
8. Perkin RM, Levin DL: Shock in the pediatric patient: Part II. J Pediatr 101:319, 1982.
9. Duff JF: Cardiovascular and metabolic changes in shock and sepsis. Eur Surg Res 9:155, 1977.
10. Hierro FR, Palomegue A, Calvo M, Torralba A: Septic shock in pediatrics. Pediatrician 8:93, 1979.
11. Wiles JB, Cerra FB, Siegel JH, Border JR: The systemic septic response: Does the organism matter? Crit Care Med 8:55, 1980.
12. Siegel JH, Cerra FB, Coleman B, et al.: Physiological and metabolic correlations in human sepsis. Surgery 86:163, 1979.
13. Jacob HIS, Craddock PR, Hammerschmidt DE, Moldow CF: Complement-induced granulocyte aggregation: An unsuspected mechanism of disease. N Engl J Med 302:789, 1980.
14. Weissmann G, Smolen JE, Korchak HM: Release of inflammatory mediators from stimulated neutrophils. N Engl J Med 303:27, 1980.
15. Bachbinder N, Ganz W: Hemodynamic monitoring: Invasive techniques. Anesthesiology 45:146, 1976.
16. Oski FA, Naiman JL: Hematologic Problems in the Newborn. Saunders, Philadelphia, 1972.
17. Gladen BE, Buchanan GR: The bleeding neonate. Pediatrics 58:548, 1976.
18. Gross SJ, Filston HC, Anderson JC: Controlled study of treatment for disseminated intravascular coagulation in the neonate. J Pediatr 100:445, 1982.

Suggested Reading

American Academy of Pediatrics: Report of the Committee on Infectious Disease, 18th ed. American Academy of Pediatrics, Evanston, IL, 1977.

Broughton R, Krafka R, Baker CJ: Non-group D alpha-hemolytic streptococci as pathogens. J Pediatr 99:450, 1981.

Rhodes P, Puckett C: *Staphylococcus aureus* infections in the newborn. Perinatology/Neonatology 7:69–79, 1983.

Thibeault DW, Gregory GA: Neonatal Pulmonary Care. Addison-Wesley, Reading, MA, 1979.

Appendices

Appendix 7.1
Nursery Infection Control Policy

To prevent infection and cross-infection in the nursery, we ask that those entering the nursery and attending the babies adhere to the following requirements:

1. Nurses and doctors wear scrub suits in the nursery and long, white, buttoned coats outside the nursery.
2. Remove all watches, arm bands, and rings, with the exception of the wedding band.
3. Roll up long sleeves.
4. Wash hands, arms, and elbows with Betadine and water for 3 minutes, and use a plastic stick to clean the fingernails.
5. Wear a short-sleeved cover gown with the back closed.
6. Have nails a reasonable length and shape (rounded).
7. Have hair clean and secured away from the face and shoulders.
8. Wash hands between babies.
9. Consider each infant crib a separate and complete unit.
10. Consider the floor contaminated at all times.
11. Personnel health: an annual physical examination is mandatory, including tine test, serology, urinalysis, etc. Each person is expected to voluntarily report any symptom of illness and have it judged by the personnel health department.
12. All infants suspected of infection will be reported to the pediatrician. If isolation is indicated, the order will be written by the pediatrician. Infants to be isolated will be transferred to NICU. The order to discontinue isolation will be written by the neonatologist and/or pediatrician.
13. Cultures may be taken by a nurse when indicated.

Appendix 7.2
Clean Air Center and/or Laminar Flow Hood

Purpose

A laminar flow hood, equipped with a HEPA[2] filter, provides a clean air center. Laminar flow minimizes the possibility of airborne microbial contamination by providing air free of particles and airborne microorganisms. Effective air flow in the hood is approximately 90 feet/minute. Coughing or sneezing will disrupt the laminar air flow, introducing contaminants.

Procedure

1. Daily, and when spillage occurs, the work surface should be wiped with 70% ethyl or isopropyl alcohol. The Plexiglas surface should be cleaned with an aqueous solution of mild detergent.
2. The blower should be on continuously. If the blower is turned off, the hood should be recleaned and the blower operated for a minimum of 30 minutes before using the hood again.
3. Supplies utilized in the hood should be decontaminated by wiping the outer surface with 70% alcohol and/or by removing an outer wrap at the edge of the work bench as the item is introduced into the aseptic work area.
4. Supply items within the work bench should be limited to minimize cluttering the work area and provide adequate space for critical operations. A clean path of filtered air must be provided over the work site. Neither supplies nor movement of personnel should place a nonsterile item between the source of the clean air and the work site. The hands and arms should not be moved into the airstream behind the work site. All work should be performed at least 6 inches within the workbench to avoid drawing in contamination from the outside, and arms and hands should not be moved in and out of the work area any more than absolutely necessary.
5. Hands must be washed before drawing up fluids or medications. It should be noted that hands are clean but not sterile. Therefore, all procedures should be performed in a manner to minimize the risk of touch contamination. For example, the outside barrel of a syringe may be touched with the hands since it does not contact the solution, but the plunger and needle should not be touched.
6. All rubber stoppers of vials and bottles and the necks of ampuls should be cleaned with 70% alcohol prior to the introduction of the needle for the removal or addition of drugs.
7. Avoid spraying solutions onto the filter screen. When wet, the filter material becomes ineffective.
8. After each procedure, used syringes, bottles, vials, and other waste should be removed, but with a minimum of exit and reentry into the work area.
9. Monthly the laminar flow hood should be cultured and the filters changed. Records of these shall be kept in the NICU.
10. Twice a year the laminar flow hood requires inspection to ensure that federal standards are being met. Documentation of this inspection is kept by the pharmacy department.

[2] MEPA = high-efficiency particulate air.

Appendix 7.3
NICU Isolation: Policy and Procedure

Purpose

To prevent cross-contamination by infected infants.

Policy

1. Isolation is to be instituted and terminated by a doctor's order only.
2. Isolation for infants is to be done only in the NICU area.

Procedure

1. The infected infant is to be placed in an isolette in an area of the unit where all infants in close proximity are in isolettes.
2. Strict handwashing must be carried out both before and after handling a baby.
3. The infant may not be removed from the isolette except for a specific procedure (i.e., weighting, isolette changes, IVs, resuscitation). The person holding the infant must stay within a few feet of the infant's isolette and must wear an isolation gown. No other infants may be out of the isolettes while the isolated infant is out.
4. Trash should be kept in specially marked red isolation bags, separate from the other patients. Linen should be placed in a dissolvable bag (clear, with pink tag) to protect laundry personnel from direct contact with contaminated linen.
5. Disposable gloves should be worn whenever directly handling contaminated secretions (i.e., wounds, diarrhea, mucus, or lesions).
6. All linen and trash must be *double bagged* with red bags marked with isolation tape before disposal.
7. At the termination of isolation, *all* equipment used during isolation should be cleaned with Tergisyl or discarded, and the infant should be placed in a clean isolette or bed.

8

Surgical Nursing Care of the Neonate

Carmel Anne Cunningham
Mary T. Maholchic

The main focus of this chapter is the introduction and review of basic principles of neonatal surgical nursing. The chapter includes specific nursing care of abdominal and cardiac surgical patients as well as discussions about general, intraoperative, and postoperative nursing responsibilities. Basic pathophysiology of common congenital anomalies is discussed, but the reader is referred to pediatric surgery textbooks for more specific information (see Refs. 1–3 for examples).

The surgical neonate, while having many of the same needs as any newborn, requires intensive care and management with a different focus. Therefore, it is important to mention that early diagnosis, careful nursing assessment, and technical skill are vital. As always, the nurse is a key figure in patient and family care.

Intraoperative Anesthesia Considerations

The neonatal patient presents a challenge to pediatric anesthesiologists. Intraoperative anesthetic concerns include:

1. Hypothermia
2. Hypotension
3. Hypoglycemia
4. Infection
5. Metabolic acidosis
6. Retrolental fibroplasia secondary to high O_2 concentrations
7. Respiratory compromise

Certain complications are more prevalent during the different phases of anesthesia; these are categorized in Table 8.1. However, the chief concerns remain hypothermia, hypovolemia, hypoxia, and respiratory depression.

Preventive measures for hypothermia include transportation of infants in warmed transport isolettes, warming of operating rooms, use of an infrared heat lamp during the preparation for surgery, and use of stockinette over arms, legs, and head. Internal warming is necessary with warmed, humidified gas, plus warmed IV and rinsing solutions.

Table 8.1 Complications of Anesthesia

Phase of anesthesia	Complications

Induction	Drug reactions
	  Excitement
	  Hypotension
	  Nausea/vomiting
	Respiratory spasm
	  "Induction arrest"
	  Hypotension
	  Aspiration

Intraoperative	Airway patency Unstable cardiac reflexes Misjudged blood loss Hypothermia

Postoperative	Respiratory depression
	  Prematurity
	  Intraventricular hemorrhage
	  Failure of relaxant reversal
	    (due to acidosis)
	Hypothermia

Hypovolemia is controlled by the use of colloid replacement or glucose/electrolyte infusions in response to the losses of the infant. Losses are measured and replaced during the operation. Frequent monitoring of central venous pressure and arterial pressure assesses cardiovascular status and evaluates treatment.

Neonatal patients are routinely intubated for surgery. Often, as a result of prematurity or severity of anomaly, intubation has occurred preoperatively. It is imperative to frequently measure arterial blood gases to assess pH, arterial O_2, and arterial CO_2 throughout the procedure. Transcutaneous monitoring, if available, is useful.

General Postoperative Nursing Care

Assessment and interventions are aimed at the following potential and actual post-surgical problems:

1. Replacement of drainage losses
2. Third space consideration
3. Acute renal failure
4. Wound care
5. Dialysis
6. Sepsis
7. Parental support

Three of these issues are considered here in further detail.

Third Space Considerations

It is important for the nurse caring for infants who require surgery to recognize what is meant by the term *third space loss*. We refer to any loss of intravascular volume to

Table 8.2 Symptoms of third space loss

System	Findings
Cardiovascular	Blood pressure decreases Heart rate increases
Renal	Urine output decreases Urine specific gravity increases Weight increases
Respiratory	Tachypnea, respiratory distress
Skin	Edema (may be) present Decreased capillary filling time

interstitial compartments as third space loss. This normally occurs, for example, after the stress of bowel surgery. Third space fluid loss also can result from blood loss during the operative procedure, which creates vasoconstriction. If this blood is not immediately replaced, blood flow is shunted from other organs to maintain vascular volume. Hypoperfusion can cause capillary membrane damage. When vascular volume is restored, serum leakage occurs through damaged capillary membranes. Then hypoperfusion reoccurs followed again by vasoconstriction. The cycle continues and a shock state occurs. Each of these factors contributes to movement of fluid from the vascular to the interstitial compartment. Additionally, in gastrointestinal (GI) surgery, fluid is lost because of the ileus that occurs during and after surgery. This occurs because peristalsis, which allows fluid to drain to the tissues in the proximal intestine and be reabsorbed in the large bowel, ceases. Normal reabsorption is delayed until peristalsis resumes (2 to 4 days postoperatively) and pooling in the interstitial compartments occurs.

During the initial period of "third spacing," appropriate fluid must be administered to support the vascular volume. Calculated fluid requirements include normal maintenance, replacement of measured losses from nasogastric tube (NGT) or gastrostomy tube (GT) drainage, and estimated replacement of third space loss. Nursing responsibilities are important here. Monitoring urine output and specific gravity is vital. If the infant has an adequate blood volume and blood pressure, the urine output should be between 2 and 5 cc/kg/hour. Weight gain or edema are not good indicators of fluid overload in the initial postoperative period since third space loss occurs *within* the body. Central venous pressure monitoring may be necessary to more accurately measure vascular volume. Table 8.2 notes clinical findings when third space loss occurs. When this fluid shift resolves, urine output increases, and IV fluids should then be recalculated to prevent vascular overload. Inattention to fluid status during the development of third spacing will contribute to the hypovolemic cycle, and inattention as third spacing resolves can lead to fluid overload. This demonstrates the importance of carefully monitoring postoperative fluid status.

Acute Renal Failure

Although this is an uncommon complication of surgery in neonates, acute renal failure presents a real challenge to the health care team. It is therefore important to discuss the etiology, signs, symptoms, and treatment.

Acute renal failure is defined as a sudden and rapid deterioration or cessation of renal function sufficient to prevent normal homeostasis but with the potential for reversal (4). The most common causes in the general surgical neonate are hypoperfusion, transfusion reaction, dehydration (failure to adequately maintain vascular volume), or sepsis. Physiologically, the body compensates for hypovolemia by preserving blood flow to vital organs. Decreased blood pressure causes decreased venous return to the heart, thereby decreasing stroke volume. Epinephrine and norepinephrine levels rise, increasing heart rate and myocardial contractility, and causing peripheral vasoconstriction, which particularly involves the arterioles of the GI tract and kidneys. This, in turn, increases blood flow to the brain and heart. This response especially affects the kidney, which normally receives 25% of the cardiac output. Decreased renal blood flow reduces glomerular filtration and sodium excretion. Urine concentration increases and oliguria develops. Acute renal failure is reversible if the hypovolemia is reversed. Initial signs and symptoms are summarized in Table 8.3.

Initially the baby may be given a "fluid challenge" to assess the renal status and correct hypovolemia. Diuretics may also be administered to treat acute renal failure. When adequate vascular pressure can be demonstrated but oliguria persists then continued fluid load will cause renal damage and tubular necrosis. If oliguria persists, patient fluid management must be redesigned to replace only sensible and insensible losses in equal volumes. Such obligatory losses include urine output, insensible skin loss, GI losses (from NGT or GT), and losses from surgical drains. (Review Chapter 3 for appropriate calculations.) All fluids given, including blood products and medications, are counted as intake.

Nursing responsibilities cover four areas:

1. Renal
   a. Measure urine losses accurately.
   b. Measure urine specific gravity and dipstick test for microscopic blood, protein, sugar, and pH.
   c. Obtain urine lab tests as ordered.
2. Cardiovascular
   a. Measure blood pressure every hour.
   b. Measure central venous pressure every hour.
   c. Measure heart rate every hour.
3. Skin
   a. Assess skin turgor.
   b. Assess presence of edema.
4. Weigh infant twice a day.

In high-output failure, the damaged kidney is unable to concentrate urine or reabsorb sodium. Therefore, urine output increases markedly. Fluid replacement must be altered to meet these losses or dehydration can occur despite "good" urine output.

If renal failure becomes chronic, dialysis is instituted. There are two types: hemodialysis and peritoneal dialysis. Dialysis is indicated for patients with 1) severe hyperkalemia, 2) severe acidosis, and 3) intractable fluid overload, especially if

Table 8.3 Clinical Symptoms in Acute Renal Failure

	Symptoms
Cardiovascular	Blood pressure increases
	Central venous pressure decreases
Renal	Urine output decreases
	Specific gravity increases
	Urine sodium decreases
	Urine osmolality increases

pulmonary edema and hypertension are present. The reader is referred to renal physiology textbooks for further information.

Since sepsis is associated with acute renal failure, observe for its signs and symptoms:

1. Blood in stools or NG aspirate
2. Increasing abdominal circumference (AC)
3. Lethargy
4. Temperature instability
5. Wound and skin inflammation

Parental Support

Parental support is essential irrespective of the type of surgery planned. Preoperative teaching should be provided, using a combined team approach to discuss the disease, prepare the parents for potential outcomes of surgery, and describe the operation and immediate postoperative expectations. Postoperative teaching can include home care and daily nursing needs. This can be enhanced by including parents in physical care routines during the infant's hospitalization. Their skills and ability to deal with stress should be considered before beginning to teach them. These vary not only with the illness but also with every individual.

Be sure to take time to answer parents' questions, and provide them with an opportunity to give a return demonstration of skills before discharge. A coordinated team approach to discharge planning can facilitate the parents' optimal adjustment to caring for their infant at home.

Nursing Considerations for Abdominal Surgery

Preoperative Nursing Care

Certain signs and symptoms typically characterize an abdominal surgical problem. Careful nursing assessments in the following areas alert the team to consider further diagnostic evaluation.

General Nursing Assessments

Auscultation of Bowel Sounds   Normally, bowel sounds are present over the entire abdomen when normal peristalsis exists. The absence of bowel sounds suggests obstruction. If the intestines are only partially obstructed, auscultated bowel sounds become abnormal. They are described as irregular, loud, or high-pitched "tinkling" or "rushes."

Abdominal Circumference Measurements   Observe the infant for either increasing abdominal circumference, or the presence of a scaphoid or "flat, sunken" abdomen.

Testing Stools   Guaiac-positive stools preoperatively indicate the presence of blood in the bowel. Positive stools for reducing substances suggest abnormal absorption of sugars from oral intake.

Nursing Intervention

Nasogastric Tube Placement of an NGT that is large enough to effectively empty the stomach (usually a 10–12 French) can:

1. Decompress the stomach
2. Eliminate further trauma, obstruction, and perforation
3. Prevent aspiration that potentially may occur with vomiting
4. Relieve pressure on the diaphragm and aid ventilation

Elevation of the Head of the Bed This aids in preventing respiratory distress that can occur from increased pressure on the diaphragm by the distended stomach; it may also prevent aspiration.

Measurement of NG Losses Every 2 Hours

Placement of IV Line The placement of an IV line:

1. Maintains hydration
2. Maintains electrolyte balance
3. Maintains vascular volume; remember that fluid loss to the "third space" occurs when bowel inflammation is present
4. Replaces fluid losses from NGT

Thermoregulation Remember that hypothermia cases metabolic acidosis (see Chapter 2 for details).

Postoperative Abdominal Surgery Care

In addition to these concerns outlined under general postsurgical considerations, the following are special concerns following abdominal surgery:

1. Decompression of the stomach
2. Replacement of GI fluid losses
3. Gastrostomy care
4. Ileostomy/colostomy care
5. Wound care
6. Third space considerations

Some of these concerns are discussed further in this section.

Decompression of the Stomach

Stomach decompression may be achieved by an NGT or a surgically placed GT. Low, intermittent suction is usually preferred. Patency of the NGT or GT is essential to maintain gastric decompression. Effective decompression is paramount to avoid further trauma, and obstruction that can lead to perforation. It also prevents vomiting and thus reduces the risk of aspiration of regurgitated abdominal contents and reduces respiratory compromise that occurs secondary to pressure on the diaphragm.

Replacement of GI Fluid Losses

Replacement of GI losses is usually cubic centimeter for cubic centimeter with a specific electrolyte solution. If the losses are large, frequent serum electrolyte monitoring may be indicated.

Gastrostomy Care

The following are procedures for the care of an infant with a gastrostomy:

1. Cleanse the skin site every shift with hydrogen peroxide (H_2O_2).
2. Prevent accidental dislocation of the GT by securing it with tape or by attaching an infant nipple at the base of the tube.
3. Place mittens on infant's hands if necessary to prevent tube dislocation by infant movement.

Ileostomy/Colostomy Care

Ileostomy drainage is toxic to the skin because of its increased acidity and the presence of enzymes. Ileostomy/colostomy care should include:

1. Periostomy skin care
   a. Allow 48 hours for the ostomy to heal and to allow easy access to assess bowel/ostomy integrity. Note color of ostomy; a viable ostomy is pink. Apply Vaseline or xeroform gauze since dry dressings stick to bowel and cause irritation. Frequently change gauze to keep the wound and periostomal skin clean.
   b. Using Hollihesive/Stomahesive at the base of the stoma prevents skin contamination.
   c. A collection device is applied over Hollihesive, with a careful seal at the base allowing *no* skin to be uncovered or contaminated by drainage.
   d. Skin is cared for with soap, water, and pat drying and followed by application of the ostomy apparatus daily and as needed.
2. Measurement of ostomy losses; reabsorption of fluid occurs in the large intestine.
   a. Assess nutritional status
   b. Assess fluid and electrolyte balances.

Wound Care

The goals for surgical wound care are 1) prevention of sepsis, and 2) maintainance of skin integrity. To achieve these goals, change dressings that become saturated with drainage whenever necessary. If the drainage is purulent, then obtain a culture. If a large amount of drainage occurs, report this to the surgeon and institute weighing dressings dry, then wet, for fluid output calculation.

Gastroschisis and Omphalocele

Although gastroschisis and omphalocele are different congenital anomalies, surgical intervention and nursing responsibilities are similar and are therefore discussed together. Omphalocele is a herniation of the abdominal contents (which can include liver, spleen, bladder, and genitourinary organs, depending on the size of the defect) into the same semitransulucent sac from which the umbilical cord arises. Gastroschisis is a defect of the abdominal wall, always to the right of the umbilicus. In gastroschisis the bowel is thickened, often covered with a tough pseudomembrane and shortened because of a combination of amniotic irritation, strangulation by the

Table 8.4 Differences between Gastroschisis and Omphalocele

Factor	Omphalocele	Gastroschisis
Defect	2–15 cm	2–3 cm
Sac	Always (may rupture)	Never
Umbilicus	Top of sac	Left of defect
Contents	Bowel, liver, bladder, etc.	Bowel
Condition of bowel	Normal	Thick, inflamed
Length of bowel	Normal	Short
Nonrotation	Yes	Always
Alimentation	Normal	Delayed
Associated anomalies	50–65%	Uncommon

small opening and subsequent obstruction of the lymphatic and venous return. The severity of the constriction can cause fibrotic stenosis or overt atresia. Poor peristalsis and absorption by this inflamed bowel lengthens the postoperative course. Unless the sac has ruptured during delivery, in omphalocele the bowel is normal and alimentation can begin earlier.

Although they have a prolonged immediate postoperative course, babies with gastroschisis have a better long-term outcome than those with omphalocele because of the lower incidence of associated congenital anomalies. These other anomalies contribute to the 60% mortality rate of babies with omphalocele and compound their care. Table 8.4 lists the differences between gastroschisis and omphalocele.

Early, prenatal diagnosis with the use of ultrasound expedites the preoperative plan, since arrangements can be made for delivery at a center where surgery can be performed immediately after birth. The prognosis is excellent in children with no other associated congenital anomalies.

Preoperative Preparation

There are four important goals to be achieved while the infant is in the delivery/resuscitation suite of the regional center or in the referring hospital prior to transport: thermoregulation, GI decompression, fluid and electrolyte balance, and prevention of infection.

Thermoregulation Rapid and profound loss of heat occurs from large amounts of exposed intestine. Thus, it is important to:

1. Assess temperature immediately and hourly after delivery.
2. Place the infant under a warmer or in an isolette.
3. Place the infant in a sterile bowel bag [a plastic bag with a drawstring at the opening (Bowel Bag, Parke-Davis; E-Z Drape Sterile Isolation Bag, Deseret)] feet first to axillae. If a bowel bag is unavailable, wrap the abdomen in warmed saline towels, then cover with a dry towel and Saran Wrap.
4. Cover the head and extremities with a cap and blankets.

GI Decompression Place a 10 French NGT at intermittent suction to:

1. Decompress the stomach and intestines.
2. Prevent distension.
3. Prevent aspiration of regurgitated gastric contents.

Fluid and Electrolyte Balance The two principal steps to ensure fluid and electrolyte balance are:

1. IV line placement.
2. Infusion, at two times the maintenance volume, of a balanced electrolyte solution recommended to replace evaporative fluid losses and large extracellular loss that occur through exposed surfaces.

   Prevention of Infection   To prevent infection:

1. Use a bowel bag, previously described.
2. Administer antibiotic therapy.

Surgical Options

There are basically two surgical options for gastroschisis or omphalocele. The first is primary closure, performed on small defects only. It consists of the following steps:

1. Excision of the sac
2. Division of Ladd's bands (to prevent potential duodenal obstruction)
3. Stretching of the abdominal cavity manually to accommodate intestines in a congenitally small abdomen
4. Gastrostomy

The second option is a multistaged procedure, creating a bowel "pouch." This is accomplished by:

1. Excision of the sac
2. Division of Ladd's bands
3. Attachment of Silastic to the skin, creating the pouch. The intestines are gradually returned to the enlarging abdominal cavity over 5 to 14 days. The pouch is then removed in a second operation and the fascia and skin are closed.
4. Gastrostomy

Postoperative Nursing Considerations

Respiratory Care   Endotracheal (ET) ventilation is continued postoperatively since respiratory compromise occurs from increased intra-abdominal pressure elevating the diaphragm. The increased pressure is caused by returning the abdominal contents into the "too small" abdomen. High pressures are often necessary for ventilation. The nurse should:

1. Provide routine neonatal respiratory care.
2. Elevate the head of the bed.
3. Lift the baby (when necessary) in one motion, with care to keep the thorax higher than the abdomen.

Silastic "Pouch" Care   The major complication of gastroschisis is sepsis resulting from exposed gut and loss of skin integrity. The base of the pouch where the Silastic is sutured to the skin is wrapped in sterile gauze kept moistened with warmed 0.5% silver nitrate solution or Betadine applications. Silver nitrate stains the skin. Caretakers should assure parents that the staining is not permanent.

GI Care   In the immediate postoperative period, the following regimen is recommended:

1. Assess GI function
   a. Auscultate for bowel sounds.
   b. Measure GI losses.

  c. Measure AC every 2 hours.

  d. Maintain GT patency.

2. Implement nursing actions

  a. Replace GI losses by IV line.

  b. Irrigate GT with 3–5 cc normal saline every 2 hours.

  c. Set GT at low intermittent suction.

  d. Note frequency and character of stools.

3. Evaluate GI function

  a. Monitor to prevent distension and/or aspiration

  b. Monitor vascular volume.

  Nutrition in Gastroschisis/Omphalocele Patient Feeding by mouth is delayed because of the inflammation of the bowel and abdominal wall, as described initially. Hyperalimentation is implemented.

  Cardiac Assessments Increased abdominal pressure can cause compression of the vena cava, decreased venous return to the heart, and low cardiac output.

  Sepsis Broad-spectrum IV antibiotic therapy is continued.

  Complications Complications following repair include volvulus, adhesions, lactose intolerance, cramping, and sepsis. Signs and symptoms include vomiting, diarrhea, guaiac-positive stools, irritability, lethargy, and abdominal distension.

Long-Term Nursing Responsibilities

  Feeding Feeding by the oral route is begun when GI function is restored. This is assessed by decreased GT output, return of bowel sounds, and a reestablishment of stooling. A trial feeding can be given by using the GT as a feeding outlet. This is accomplished by elevating the GT with an empty syringe during feeding and for 2–3 hours after feeding. This allows for a backflow of formula up into the syringe if the intestines can not tolerate the feeding. This is a safety measure to ensure against further obstruction, vomiting, and aspiration. The syringe should be elevated only 10 cm higher than the baby. Syringes elevated to greater heights do not aid in venting since the pressure required for formula to pass retrograde through the GT would be excessive and hinder assessment of potential obstructions.

  Assessment of feeding tolerance is necessary. Observe the infant for:

1. Abdominal distension
2. Residual gastric aspirate (formula not digested by the next feeding time)
3. Vomiting
4. Diarrhea

Babies with gastroschisis have long-term irritability during feeding. This is due to cramping and diarrhea that occur when temporarily narrowed segments (still inflamed) partially obstruct and then release.

  Parent Education Parent education is also part of long-term nursing care. In parent teaching and support, it is important that parents understand that the feeding irritability is physiological and will resolve as bowel integrity improves. Parents need to be aware of the signs and symptoms of complications for home care.

Esophageal Atresia and Tracheoesophageal Fistula (TEF)

The incidence of esophageal atresia, with or without TEF, is 1 in 4000 live births. It is frequently associated with other conditions such as prematurity and cardiac, GI, renal, CNS, and skeletal problems. An early diagnosis of esophageal atresia is essential in order to avoid aspiration pneumonia and improve prognosis. The nurse plays a vital role by her assessments of respiratory symptoms at the time of birth.

There are four main types of TEF, illustrated in Figure 8.1. The most common, blind upper pouch with distal esophageal-tracheal connection, ocurs in 80–90% of all cases. It is described later.

Case Study

Baby J. was a 1500-gram infant of 35 weeks gestation and was born in a regional center. Apgar scores were 7 at 1 minute and 8 at 5 minutes. He was admitted to the full-term nursery where he was placed under the infant warmer in no acute distress. The obstetrician reported that polyhydramnios was noted when the membranes ruptured. During J.'s first 4 hours of life, the neonatal nurse observed excessive salivation, increasing respiratory distress, regurgitation of the initial feeding, and abdominal distension.

The nurse inserted an NGT (radiopaque-tipped no. 8 French catheter), and an x-ray was taken that revealed a tube coil in the esophageal pouch. The diagnosis of TEF was made. Nursing observations aided in early diagnosis, which is paramount in the prevention of aspiration pneumonia and in expediting surgical intervention. Other factors that effect or delay surgery are prematurity, distance between pouch and distal esophagus, and the presence of congenital anomalies.

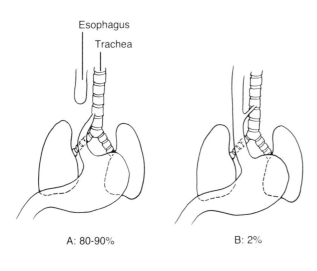

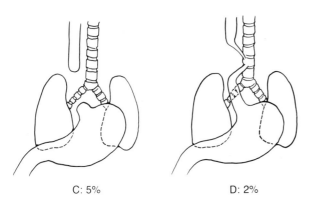

FIGURE 8.1   Combinations of esophageal atresias and/or fistulas. *A:* Blind upper pouch with tracheoesophageal fistula (80–90%). *B:* Tracheoesophageal fistula without esophageal atresia ("H-type" fistula) (2%). *C:* Esophageal atresia with no fistula connection to the trachea ("isolated esophageal atresia") (5%). *D:* Proximal pouch and distal esophagus connected by fistulas to the trachea ("K-type" fistula) (2%).

Preoperative Nursing Considerations in TEF

The following procedures are necessary prior to the operation:

1. Placement of a Replogle sump tube (Argyle Inc.) through nose or mouth, attached to constant suction to reduce accumulation of saliva in the pouch and prevent aspiration
2. Elevation of the bed to a 45° angle (this is imperative)
3. Measurement and replacement of saliva losses frm the Replogle tube

Surgical Options

Depending on the respiratory status and degree of other associated anomalies, definitive repair can be postponed until the patient is in condition to withstand anesthesia. A GT may be placed under local anesthesia for gastric decompression.

Primary anastomosis and division of the fistula is the operation of choice. The chest is entered through a right posterolateral incision. The fistula is cut and sewn. The proximal pouch is carefully dissected from the trachea and connected to the distal esophagus. Primary anastamosis can be performed in most cases; when the distance between the pouch and the distal esophagus is too great to perform a primary anastomosis, an esophagostomy is performed after the fistula is cut, and then the chest is closed. Later, a second operation is performed during which a colon interposition or gastric tube is used to create an "esophagus."

Postoperative Nursing Considerations

Respiratory Care As during the preoperative period, the head of the infant's bed should be elevated. Careful ET toilet should be done with the use of a "marked" catheter. At the time of surgery, the tube is measured from the mouth to the anastomosis and through the ET tube to the anastomosis and marked. Subsequent catheters should be carefully measured with the marked catheter, thereby avoiding recurrent fistula and/or anastomotic leak. Chest tube (CT) care entails:

1. Careful monitoring of fluid levels
2. Assessment of CT drainage (saliva in tube indicates anastomotic leak)
3. Measurement and description of fluid
4. Monitoring 24-hour volume of drainage from CT
5. Maintenance of CT patency by careful milking of the tubing
6. Daily chest films: anastomotic leaks present with air or fluid that is evident on x-ray film

Feedings A barium swallow radiogram should be done on the 10th postoperative day to establish if the anastomosis has healed. If no leak is seen, a clear liquid feeding regimen is begun. If a leak is seen, the child remains without feedings, and hyperalimentation is continued. Anastomotic leaks heal spontaneously in 1–2 weeks. The nurse should have suction available during the fluoroscopy because of the danger of aspiration.

If an esophagostomy ("spit fistula") has been performed, the following measures are instituted:

1. Careful skin care
2. Measurement of saliva losses

3. Sham feedings: the infant is fed by mouth while gastrostomy feeding is done. The oral feeding drains through the esophagostomy and is not nutritionally beneficial, but it aids in recognition of feeding with satiation and the establishment of sucking and swallowing reflexes.

Complications   The nurse should be alert to the following complications:

1. Anastomotic leak
2. Recurrent fistula
3. Atelectasis
4. Stricture
5. Gastroesophageal reflux

Diaphragmatic Hernia

A diaphragmatic hernia is a herniation of the abdominal contents through the diaphragm. The incidence is 1 in 4000 live births, occurring equally in males and females. It occurs on the left side 5 to 10 times more frequently; bilaterality is rare. There are five types of diaphragmatic hernia. Of these, Bochdalek hernia is the most common (occurring in 85% of all cases) and the most severe. The management and nursing care of this potentially lethal lesion is described below.

Presentation of symptoms varies proportionately to the degree of hypoplasia of the lung on the affected side. This degree of hypoplasia depends on the amount of abdominal contents that have herniated through the defect into the chest and at what time during gestation the hernia occurred. The prognosis is also dependent upon the degree of lung hypoplasia. The timing and the severity of the onset of symptoms are directly related to the degree of hypoplasia. Infants who are symptomatic in the first 24 hours of life have a mortality rate as high as 80%. The signs and symptoms of diaphragmatic hernia are listed in Table 8.5. When the diagnosis is made, actions must be taken for preoperative resuscitation and transport to a regional center, where continued resuscitation, surgery, and careful postoperative critical care can be done. These babies should be intubated prophylactically to increase lung volume, even if they are not yet in respiratory failure.

Table 8.5 Signs and Symptoms of Diaphragmatic Hernia

	Problem
Respiratory	Dyspnea Tachypnea Mixed acidoses Asphyxia
GI	Bowel sounds audible above the diaphragm Scaphoid abdomen
X-ray	Gasless abdomen by x-ray Mediastinal shift Mass-like pattern in left chest (affected side) with later changes; when air enters intestine, bowel loops are obvious in the chest
Cardiovascular	Dextrocardia Shift of the point of maximal impulse

Preoperative Preparation

There are four areas in which the nurse plays an important role prior to surgery: respiratory care, GI care, positioning, and drug therapy.

Respiratory Care   Assessment of respiratory status and correction of respiratory distress are the two primary goals. The latter usually requires:

1. Intubation
2. Mechanical ventilation
3. Frequent arterial blood gas sampling
4. Symptomatic treatment of ventilation and oxygenation disturbances

Observe for signs and symptoms of pneumothorax. Because of the need to correct hypoxia and respiratory acidosis, high ventilator pressures are often required. Hypoplastic lungs also rupture more easily. A change in the infant's condition may herald the development of a pneumothorax:

1. Increasing respiratory distress
2. Cyanosis
3. Mediastinal shift

GI Care   The principal goal is the relief of bowel dilatation, which causes mediastinal shifts toward the unaffected side. Shifting of the mediastinum causes obstruction of the vena cava. The increased pressure by the intestines also causes compression of the unaffected lung, thereby causing carbon dioxide retention. Relief is effected by insertion of a 12 French NGT set at low intermittent suction.

Positioning   In positioning the infant, one should:

1. Allow for maximum ventilation of unaffected lung by placing the infant with affected side down.
2. Decrease the already increased intrathoracic pressure by elevating the head of the bed.

Drug Therapy   Preoperative drug therapy has the following goals:

1. Paralysis of the infant and control of ventilation, thereby maximizing mechanical ventilation.
2. Control of metabolic acidoses (see Chapter 5).
3. Maintenance of vascular volume, using colloid and/or blood products.

Surgical Procedures

Surgical intervention is necessary. However, if the acidosis is severe, it is beneficial to correct it as best and as quickly as possible before the induction of anesthesia. Often this is difficult and attempts to do so may be unsuccessful until the pressure is relieved by removal of the intestines from the chest.

The child is placed in the supine position under a radiant warmer. After the induction of anesthesia, bilateral chest tubes may be inserted under direct vision to prevent tension pneumothorax from occurring during surgery or postoperatively. The bowel is rapidly removed from the chest. The surgeon will examine the ipsilateral lung and evaluate the degree of hypoplasia. Care is taken not to forcibly expand this lung. Expansion may take days or weeks. If the lung is not hypoplastic, the prognosis is improved. The diaphragmatic defect is visualized and repaired.

Next, the bowel is examined for malrotation (frequently occurring with this lesion, which may cause volvulus), corrected, and placed in the abdominal cavity. A gastrostomy is performed. Because the intestinal contents have not been in the abdomen during intrauterine life, the abdominal cavity is small. If the abdominal incision cannot be closed without tension, the skin alone is closed and a ventral hernia is created. In this case, the child is brought back to the operating room before the 10th postoperative day and the fascia is properly closed. After 10 days, the repair is made more difficult by adhesion of the intestines to the skin.

Postoperative Nursing Considerations

The major postoperative problems are respiratory, specifically hypoxia, retained carbon dioxide, and pneumothorax. See Chapter 5 for the standard nursing management of these problems.

Postoperative complications include poor respiratory function (causing persistent hypoxia), metabolic acidosis (causing tissue anoxia), pneumothorax, wound dehiscence, and infection. The cause of death in more than 50% of these infants is attributed to the hypoplasia of the lung.

Frequent communication with the parents of these infants is especially important because of the high mortality rate.

Intestinal Obstruction

Intestinal obstruction is a broad term and includes the majority of congenital abnormalities that require surgical intervention. Because specific preoperative and postoperative nursing care does not vary, the lesions are discussed together.

Obstructions, which can occur anywhere between the stomach and the anus, are divided into two groups: mechanical and functional. Table 8.6 distinguishes these two. Mechanical lesions are caused by an interruption of the intestine; thus complete activity of the bowel cannot occur. Functional obstruction occurs because of a physiological defect that prohibits peristalsis. Because reabsorption of fluid and complete evacuation of the bowel does not occur, there can be inflammation, ischemia, and perforation. These all contribute significantly to morbidity. The goal of the surgeon is to relieve the obstruction, and, when inflammation of the bowel has occurred, to exteriorize or vent the bowel proximal to the affected intestine and allow the bowel to heal.

The reader is referred to more comprehensive surgical texts for definition of the specific lesions. Table 8.7 distinguishes upper from lower GI obstructions, and Table 8.8 lists some common causes of obstruction.

Table 8.6 Classification of Intestinal Obstructions

Mechanical	Functional
Atresia and stenosis	NEC
Duodenal	Hirschsprung's disease
Jejunal	Meconium ileus
Ileal	Meconium plug
Colonic	Small left colon syndrome
Annular pancreas	
Webs	
Malrotation	
Early volvulus	
Imperforate anus	
Intussusception	
Hernia	

Table 8.7 Differences in Presentation of High versus Low GI Obstruction

High	Low
Polyhydramnios	Polyhydramnios (sometimes)
Scaphoid abdomen	Abdominal distention
Nonbilious vomiting	Bilious vomiting
"Double bubble" appearance on x-ray	Absence of passage of meconium in 24–48 hours

Table 8.8 Some Common Causes of Bowel Obstruction in the Newborn

Gastric outlet obstruction (e.g., pyloric stenosis)	Meconium ileus
Duodenal atresia	Meconium plug
Annular pancreas	Hirschsprung's disease
Malrotation of bowel	Imperforate anus
Ileal or jejunal atresia	NEC

Necrotizing Enterocolitis: A Special Neonatal Problem

A neonatal disease that often requires surgical intervention is necrotizing enterocolitis (NEC). It is an often fatal lesion of the intestinal tract. The increased incidence is related to improved methods of resuscitation and management of the smaller, sicker newborn. Risk factors associated with precipitating NEC include:

Asphyxia
Polycythemia/hyperviscosity
Exchange transfusions
Umbilical artery and vein catheters
Hypertonic feeding solutions
Patent ductus arteriosus (PDA)
Hypovolemia
Birth weight < 1500 grams
Prolonged rupture of membranes
Anemia
Sepsis
Congenital heart disease
Apneic spells
Respiratory distress syndrome
Cold stress

When asphyxia occurs, blood is shunted away from the mesenteric arteries to perfuse the heart and brain circulation. This selective circulatory ischemia can also be triggered by other problems such as maternal bleeding, neonatal anemia, PDA shunting, umbilical artery or vein catheterization, or exchange transfusion. The net result is decreased blood flow to the gut.

The following pathogenesis has been postulated for NEC. The intestinal mucosal cells, sensitive to ischemic insult, stop secreting protective mucus. This allows proteolytic autodigestion of the mucosa. Bacterial invasion into the intestinal wall from the lumen occurs as a result of the disruption of bowel wall integrity. Gas-forming organisms produce pneumatosis intestinalis. Sepsis results from bacterial seeding of the circulation. Lethargy and jaundice can also occur. The toxins and gas-forming organisms are sometimes absorbed by the lymphatic system of the portal venous system, reach the liver, and cause serious symptoms, even death. As a result abdominal distension, intramural air, and pneumatosis intestinalis develop, and

Table 8.9 NEC

Examination	Findings
Clinical	Blood in stools; diarrhea; vomiting; increased abdominal distension; increased residual; ileus with decreased or absent bowel sounds; progressive lethargy; jaundice; hypovolemia (decreased urine output); erythema of bowel wall; apnea
Laboratory	White blood cell count decreased; platelets decreased; decreased hematocrit; positive blood culture; metabolic acidosis
X-ray	Abnormal gas distribution; intramural air (air in bowel wall); portal or peritoneal air

perforation commonly follows. Bowel insult produces guaiac-positive or overtly bloody stools. Signs and symptoms of infants with NEC are found in Table 8.9.

Medical Management of NEC

As soon as the diagnosis of NEC is suspected, the following measures are instituted:

1. Nothing by mouth
2. NG tube set to straight drainage for decompression
3. Removal of any umbilical catheters
4. Peripheral IV fluid and electrolyte replacement done promptly
5. Total parenteral nutrition (TPN)
6. Broad-spectrum IV antibiotic therapy (when specific sensitivities are obtained, antibiotic therapy may be tailored)
7. Serial abdominal films (every shift) to monitor GI status and document occurrence of pneumoperitoneum

If improvement of the baby's clinical course occurs (distension reduction, resolution of pneumatosis intestinalis, reduced gastric residuals, and disappearance of blood in stools), the prognosis for recovery is good. The management is continued for 10–14 days. Feedings are begun slowly, advancing to full-strength formula and adequate calories.

In babies who show progression of the disease (continued distension, guaiac-positive stools, pneumatosis, decrease in platelet count, etc.), the regimen is continued for at least 3 weeks to allow for healing of the intestine. Central administration of TPN may be instituted.

Stricture of the scarred, healed intestine may also occur as a late problem. Observing for signs or symptoms of intestinal obstruction is important and should be taught to parents prior to discharge.

Surgical Intervention

The most clear-cut indication for surgery is pneumoperitoneum (free air), which implies bowel perforation. This concept is an important one. The decision to limit surgery to those babies with perforation is made because of the difficulty in determining the extent of necrotizing bowel and in assessing the bowel wall's integrity and its ability to heal. It is intraoperatively difficult to limit resection to just necrotic bowel when inflamed lengths of potentially "healable" bowel are present. Other absolute indications for surgery are:

1. Peritonitis
2. Sudden hyponatremia (indicating large third space loss in dead bowel)

3. Persistent metabolic acidosis
4. Disseminated intravascular coagulation
5. Persistent apnea, hypotension, and progressive clinical deterioration
6. Abdominal mass (indicates an intraperitoneal abscess following an undetected perforation, or infarcted loops of bowel)
7. Inflammatory changes in the abdominal wall (usually indicative of peritonitis)

The aim of the surgical procedure is removal of obviously necrotic or perforated segments of bowel. Preservation of the ileocecal valve (to avoid large fluid losses and malabsorption) is important. Extensive resection of "questionably" viable bowel is avoided in order to provide adequate length and avoid the "short-gut" malabsorption syndrome. Second-look operations are often indicated to reassess intestine that initially appears dark because of extensive interstitial hemorrhage rather than necrosis. Exteriorization of ends through separate stomas is the safest operative technique, since end-to-end anastomosis risks reperforation and spillage. The stomas provide good access to assess viability of remaining gut. Reanastomosis can occur 4 to 6 weeks postoperatively when the bowel is completely healed. A gastrostomy is performed for decompression during the intestinal healing period.

Open drainage of the peritoneal cavity through a lower quadrant incision has been used successfully in very tiny, sick babies. This can be done in the ICU and can be repeated if the condition does not improve. This procedure drains air, intestinal contents, and peritoneal fluid in babies who would not survive anesthesia. Closure has occurred spontaneously with no further procedure necessary to reestablish continuity. If stricture formation occurs, it can be repaired in a later operation.

Postoperative Management

The medical regimen is continued and ostomy care, as described earlier, is begun.

Early Detection and Prevention of NEC

The prognosis is improved when babies at risk for NEC are carefully observed prior to the development of signs and symptoms. In these babies, medical management can begin at the first sign of feeding intolerance. This approach is successful and decreases the need for operative therapy significantly. Mortality also is significantly decreased.

Prevention of NEC is the most desirable choice. Many centers have categorized infants at risk for developing NEC and instituted precautions to avoid NEC by delaying enteral nutrition and then using a slowly progressing feeding regimen. NEC can be prevented in high-risk babies by using prophylactic antibiotics (5). Although these measures involve exposing infants who may not develop the disease to antibiotics, it is certainly a justified alternative in the prevention of the incidence of such an acute threat to life (6).

Nursing Considerations for Neonatal Cardiac Surgery Patients

The development of the heart is a complex embryological process. Although true incidence is difficult to precisely ascertain, various sources have reported congenital heart defects in 8 of 1000 live births (7, 8). Affected infants who go untreated face a 50–60% mortality rate prior to their first birthday, with 30% of these dying in the neonatal period (7). Considering the devastating mortality, prompt, definitive diagnosis and specific surgical treatment are critical if these infants are to survive

As the surgical management of congenital heart disease becomes more complex, the need for highly skilled nursing care increases. To provide the best possible outcome, all involved with the care must understand, recognize, and anticipate pre- and postoperative problems associated with specific defects. The following discussion provides the nurse with a basis for that involvement. No attempts are made to analyze all forms of congenital heart disease in depth. Rather, basic information about life-threatening heart defects that require operative intervention is emphasized.

Preoperative Assessment

In addition to the general preoperative preparation afforded any neonatal surgical patient, there are specific clinical (Table 8.10) and laboratory assessments (Table 8.11) unique to the care of the infant awaiting repair or palliation of congenital heart defects. Frequently, preoperative deterioration in clinical status can be avoided or controlled by strict attention to subtle changes in the infant's clinical condition and implementation of appropriate nursing interventions. Identification and treatment of complicating factors such as congestive heart failure are critical. Surgery superimposed on an already unstable patient can increase mortality and morbidity, both intraoperatively and postoperatively (9).

Table 8.10 Preoperative Clinical Assessment of Infant

Respiratory
    Color
    Respiratory rate and pattern
    Signs of respiratory distress
    Chest expansion, symmetry; depth of respiration
    Breath sounds: symmetry, quality, abnormalities (rales, rhonchi, wheezes)

Cardiovascular
    Heart rate and rhythm
    Blood pressure
    Heart sounds, abnormal extra sounds, murmurs
    Thrills
    Pulses: pressure, symmetry, quality

GI
    Failure to thrive
    Slow feeding

Neurological
    Irritability
    Seizures
    Coma/lethargy

Fluid balance
    Edema/dehydration
    Urine output
    Body weight gain/loss
    Enlarged liver (>2 cm below the costal margin)

Miscellaneous
    Diaphoresis
    Body temperature
    Temperature of extremities

Table 8.11 Preoperative Laboratory Assessment of
Infant Status

Chest radiograph
   Pulmonary vascularity
   Lung expansion, aeration
   Heart size and contour
   Abnormal densities
   Tube and catheter placement

Arterial blood gases
   pO_2
   pCO_2
   pH
   O_2 saturation
   Base excess

Urinalysis
   Specific gravity
   Osmolality[a]
   Electrolytes[a]

Blood studies
   Elecrolytes
   Hematocrit
   Osmolality[a]

Coagulation studies

Electrocardiogram

Echocardiogram

Cardiac catheterization

   [a] Performed whenever the clinical condition
of the patient indicates the need for these assessments.

Lesions Characterized by an Increase in Pulmonary Blood Flow (See Table 8.12)

Acyanotic Lesions   The acyanotic heart defects that may require operative intervention in infancy include ventricular septal defect (VSD) and patent ductus arteriosus (PDA). Both lesions become clinically apparent because of shunting of blood from the left side of the heart to the right. In VSD, this occurs at the ventricular level, whereas in PDA the shunt is from the aorta to the pulmonary artery. How and when these infants become symptomatic depends upon the direction and volume of the shunt, which in turn is related to the size of the defect, pressures on the right and left side of the heart, and resistance to flow in the pulmonary and systemic circulations (10). It is not unusual for affected children to be asymptomatic at birth. High pulmonary vascular resistance at this time creates equal right and left ventricular pressures with resistance to pulmonary blood flow. Since there are no large pressure differences at the ventricular or ductal level, there is no appreciable left-to-right shunt and therefore no symptoms. When pulmonary vascular resistance decreases (normally during the first days to weeks of life), left ventricular pressure exceeds right ventricular pressure in these defects because resistance to blood flow in the systemic circulation becomes greater than that in the pulmonary circulation. When these normal gradients evolve, a left-to-right shunt develops and symptoms occur. Clinical presentation of both defects is variable and primarily determined by the volume of

Table 8.12 Categories of Congenital Heart Disease

Characterized by increase in pulmonary blood
    Acyanotic
        VSD
        PDA
    Cyanotic
        TAPVR
        Truncus arteriosus
        TGA

Characterized by decrease in pulmonary blood
    Hypoplastic right heart syndromes
        Tricuspid atresia
        Pulmonary atresia
    Combined defects: tetralogy of Fallot

Characterized by obstruction
    Acyanotic
        Pulmonary stenosis
        Aortic stenosis
        Coarctation of the aorta
    Hypoplastic left heart syndromes
        Aortic atresia
        Mitral atresia

the shunt. With small-volume shunts, affected children usually do well without the need for surgical intervention in infancy (11). However, if the left-to-right shunt is large, frequent respiratory infections, pneumonia, failure to thrive, and congestive heart failure may develop. Furthermore, significant pulmonary hypertension resulting from the high pulmonary blood flow can become a complicating factor in the management by causing a reversal of the shunt, cyanosis, and hypoxemia. The decision and timing of surgical intervention is dependent upon the severity of the presenting symptomatology and the potential for pulmonary hypertension to develop (12).

PDA   In preterm infants, the presence of a PDA may complicate recovery from hyaline membrane disease and necessitate medical and/or surgical intervention. Closure of the ductus arteriosus at birth is related to the maturity and clinical condition of the infant (12). Thus it is not surprising that this defect is less common in term than premature infants. In some symptomatic infants, pharmacological closure of the PDA can be accomplished by the administration of indomethacin, a prostaglandin synthetase inhibitor.[1] However, not all premature infants are candidates for a trial of indomethacin; hyperbilirubinemia, abnormal liver function, GI bleeding, CNS hemorrhage, renal insufficiency, and coagulopathy may preclude its use. If medical therapy is unsuccessful, the PDA can be surgically managed.

Cyanotic Lesions   Congenital heart defects that involve the combination of cyanosis and increased pulmonary blood flow usually indicate the presence of

[1] *Editors' note:* Those infants who do receive indomethacin must be monitored for adverse side effects including platelet dysfunction, transient renal failure, and gastric bleeding. Renal failure may be short lived but it still can be life threatening if fluid intake is not reduced while urine production is low. Weighing twice daily, recording of intake and output, measuring blood urea nitrogen levels, and frequent examination for fluid overload should be instituted following the administration of indomethacin. Additionally, indomethacin should be given with milk to help offset some of the GI irritation. Platelet counts may also be monitored to facilitate early detection of significant thrombocytopenia.

truncus arteriosus, total anomalous pulmonary venous return (TAPVR), or uncomplicated transposition of the great arteries (TGA). Truncus arteriosus and TAPVR are basically admixture lesions. Clinical presentation is variable and is determined by the degree of mixing of arterial and venous blood, as well as the volume of pulmonary blood flow. TGA involves separate pulmonary and systemic circulations created by the pulmonary artery arising from the left ventricle and the aorta arising from the right ventricle. Uncomplicated TGA is not associated with any other heart defects.

Truncus Arteriosus   Infants affected with truncus arteriosus have a large ventricular septal defect that allows complete mixing of oxygenated and unoxygenated blood. The admixed blood is pumped into the pulmonary and systemic circulations through a single arterial vessel that arises from the heart. If the pulmonary arteries, which originate from the single arterial vessel are large, pulmonary blood flow will be increased. In this instance, congestive heart failure and the risk of developing pulmonary hypertension are the primary complications, whereas cyanosis is minimal. When the pulmonary arteries are small, which sometimes occurs in variations of truncus arteriosus, pulmonary blood flow tends to be decreased. With this type of truncus arteriosus, congestive heart failure is not as much of a concern as is the severe cyanosis and hypoxia that result.

TAPVR   Just as with truncus arteriosus, there are variations of TAPVR that may present differently in the neonatal period. Regardless of the type of TAPVR, the basic defect that creates symptoms in the patient involves the delivery of the pulmonary venous return into the right atrium via an abnormal venous connection. This can occur by one of three possible routes: supracardiac, into the superior vena cava; cardiac, into the coronary sinus or right atrium; or subdiaphragmatic, into the portal vein. Since none of the pulmonary venous return enters the left ventricle, the maintenance of the systemic circulation is dependent upon a right-to-left shunt at the atrial level through a foramen ovale, or a coexisting atrial septal defect.

Two distinctly differing clinical pictures can be identified. If there is venous obstruction, caused by narrowing of the aberrant venous channel, pulmonary hypertension with decreased pulmonary blood flow may be evident. Pulmonary edema, congestive heart failure, poor peripheral pulses, hepatomegaly, cyanosis, respiratory distress, hypoxia, and acidosis all appear with early, rapid clinical deterioration in infancy when the obstruction is severe. With unobstructed TAPVR, variable degrees of cyanosis and congestive heart failure are present. Recurrent respiratory infections and failure to thrive are potential problems as in any cogenital heart defect with increased pulmonary blood flow.

Transposition   TGA may have a dramatic early presentation. Findings include cyanosis, tachypnea, and hypoxia. The severity and timing of presentation are related to the opportunity for mixing unoxygenated and oxygenated blood via the foramen ovale, PDA, or septal defects. If mixture of the separate circulations is minimal, tachypnea, profound cyanosis, hypoxia, and progressive metabolic acidosis become apparent soon after birth. Congestive heart failure and pulmonary hypertension can also be a part of the clinical features and complicate treatment.

Stabilization of these critically ill neonates is a vital part of the management plan. If survival depends on ductal flow, prostaglandin (PG) E_1 is commonly administered by continuous infusion through a scalp vein or an umbilical vein catheter to maintain patency of the ductus arteriosus while awaiting surgery. PGE_1 administration may be life saving for all duct-dependent lesions. It improves systemic and pulmonary circulation mixing, which in turn increases the arterial pO_2, allowing time for other stabilizing and supportive measures to be implemented. Close observation during PGE_1 administration is an essential part of nursing care so that potential side effects such as hypotension, hypoglycemia, apnea, and fever can be detected and controlled. Therapeutic effects of the drug, including an increase in pO_2 and the presence of a murmur (indicating a PDA), require documentation. Equally important to note is the absence of therapeutic effects since this may indicate interruption of the PGE_1 infusions or a need for dose adjustment.

Initial surgical management of TGA, as well as TAPVR, may include creation of an atrial septal defect using a Rashkind-Miller atrial balloon septostomy during the first cardiac catheterization. This palliative procedure allows for mixing of blood at the atrial level, with a concomitant rise in pO_2. Improvement in the clinical condition indicates successful palliation.

Lesions Characterized by a Decrease in Pulmonary Blood Flow

Table 8.12 lists anomalies associated with diminished blood flow to the lungs. These include pulmonary atresia, tricuspid atresia, and tetrology of Fallot. Cyanosis and hypoxia are variable features that become more intense as obstruction to pulmonary blood flow and right-to-left shunt increase.

An important consideration with these, as well as any other, cyanotic lesions is the potential for cerebral abscess, embolism, and thrombosis. Whenever there is right-to-left shunting of blood, bacterial or other emboli may gain access to the cerebral circulation from the systemic circuit. IV lines need to be filtered of any air or debris and must be maintained with strict asepsis to prevent potential neurological sequelae.

Hypoplastic Right Heart Syndromes   Although the anatomy of tricuspid and pulmonary atresia differ, they are discussed together since their physiology hemodynamics, and clinical and laboratory findings are similar. Symptoms are related to the presence of other cardiac defects. In isolated lesions congestive heart failure is not the primary problem. Rather, infants present early in the neonatal period with profound cyanosis and hypoxia. Untreated hypoxia leads to metabolic acidosis. Varying degrees of right ventricular hypoplasia may be present.

Blood flow to the lungs and ultimate systemic oxygen saturation are determined by the existence of a route for systemic venous return to reach the pulmonary circulation. Atresia of either valve, with an intact ventricular septum, dictates an obligatory right-to-left atrial shunt through the foramen ovale or atrial septal defect. A PDA is the only source of pulmonary blood flow. Closure of the ductus leads to catastrophic deterioration. Palliation with PGE_1 infusions and/or a Rashkind-Miller atrial balloon septostomy can be life saving.

Combined Defects   Tetralogy of Fallot constitutes a commonly occurring form of congenital heart disease. A ventricular septal defect with an aorta that overrides the ventricular septal defect, right ventricular hypertrophy, and varying degrees of pulmonary stenosis combine to form tetralogy of Fallot. Neurological sequelae, including cerebral injury secondary to episodes of severe hypoxia, and cerebral abscesses, emboli, or thrombosis resulting from the right-to-left ventricular shunt are potential complications in the preoperative patient.

Congestive heart failure is not a part of the clinical presentation. Predominant clinical findings include cyanosis and hypoxia that worsen as pulmonary blood flow decreases. In tetralogy of Fallot a combination of anatomical and physiological factors determines the amount of pulmonary blood flow and, therefore, the severity and onset of symptoms. Anatomically, a right ventricular outflow obstruction in the form of pulmonary stenosis prevents normal pulmonary blood flow. The pulmonary stenosis is usually infundibular in origin but can be valvular or supravalvular as well.

In general, severity of symptoms correlates with the severity of the pulmonary stenosis, which can range from mild to total atresia of the pulmonary valve. Infants who have severe pulmonary stenosis or atresia present early in the neonatal period with cyanosis and hypoxia. In these children a PDA is the major source of pulmonary blood flow. Again, PGE$_1$ infusions are indicated to maintain patency of the ductus until surgical palliation or repair can be performed.

A physiological event that influences pulmonary blood flow is the degree of pulmonary and systemic vascular resistance present at any given time. Whenever pulmonary vascular resistance is higher than systemic vascular resistance, pulmonary blood flow is decreased and right-to-left shunting occurs. Any situation, such as crying, bowel movement, exercise, or feeding, that increases pulmonary vascular resistance or decreases systemic vascular resistance can lead to acute episodes of profound hypoxia, dyspnea, and cyanosis. Another physiological consideration involves the sensitivity of the infundibular portion of the right ventricular outflow tract to endogenous release of catecholamines. Release of these substances in response to stress, emotion, or exercise can also cause constriction of an already stenotic portion of the infundibulum, resulting in life-threatening hypoxia. These episodes of rapid clinical deterioration are commonly referred to as "Tet" spells. Their occurrence is more common in patients with mild cyanosis. Without proper treatment, loss of consciousness, seizures, and death can result.

Lesions Characterized by Obstruction (See Table 8.12)

There are two categories of congenital heart disease that are classified as obstruction: acyanotic lesions such as pulmonary stenosis, aortic stenosis, and coarctation of the aorta; and hypoplastic left heart syndromes such as aortic and mitral valve atresia. Of these, only the acyanotic obstructive defects are discussed since there is no current surgery to successfully treat the hypoplastic left heart syndrome.

Pulmonary Stenosis   Pulmonary stenosis is a narrowing of the right ventricular outflow tract at the infundibular, valvular, or supravalvular level. In isolated lesions, stenosis is usually valvular from varying amounts of fusion of the valve leaflets. If the stenosis is mild, patients tend to be asymptomatic, although a murmur may be audible. As the severity of the obstruction increases, ventricular hypertrophy followed by right atrial hypertrophy, right-sided heart failure, and a right-to-left shunt at the atrial level through the foramen ovale develop. Severely affected infants are cyanotic and in congestive heart failure.

Aortic Stenosis   As with pulmonary stenosis, aortic stenosis is not isolated to one anatomical site. It is most frequently valvular but can also be subaortic or supravalvular. Regardless of the origin of the defect, the net result is the same. Left ventricular outflow is obstructed, the left ventricle hypertrophies, and cardiac output is decreased. Since the left ventricle is enlarged, it has an increased oxygen requirement, which can become even greater during periods of activity or exercise. If the demand for oxygen is not met, myocardial ischemia and infarcts can develop. Pulmonary edema can also become part of the clinical presentation as blood backs up from the obstructed left ventricle into the pulmonary circulation.

When the aortic stenosis is mild, a murmur may be the only finding. In severe forms, congestive heart failure can occur rapidly. Weak peripheral pulses, poor peripheral perfusion, a narrow pulse pressure, and cyanosis are increasingly evident with diminished cardiac output.

Coarctation of the Aorta   Coarctation is a narrowing of the aorta. In most instances, it occurs in the vicinity of a ductus arteriosus. Pressures in the aorta and left ventricle are high; distal to the defect, pressures are decreased. This alteration in hemodyanmics causes the characteristic findings of upper extremity hypertension and full pulses with decreased lower extremity blood pressure. Cool lower extremities also may be noted. When the work load on the left ventricle is high, congestive heart failure complicates the clinical course.

Recognition of coarctation of the aorta depends upon accurate determination of blood pressure in all four extremities plus documentation of higher readings in the upper extremities compared to the lower extremities. Thus it is critical to use appropriate-size blood pressure cuffs whenever blood pressures are taken.

Therapeutic intervention depends upon the clinical status of the patient. Congestive heart failure favorably responds to digitalization. Maintaining patency of the ductus arteriosus is a priority in some types of coarctation so that the systemic circulation is preserved. PGE_1 infusions are sometimes used until surgical correction can be performed.

Preoperative Planning and Interventions

Overall, the preoperative nursing care of the infant undergoing surgery for congenital heart disease is identical to that for any presurgical neonate. However, additional consideration needs to be given to detection and supportive care of specific problems unique to these infants because of their disease and the medical management that accompanies treatment. The following is a list of preoperative nursing procedures for the infant undergoing cardiac surgery:

1. Obtain baseline clinical and laboratory assessment:
   a. Perform complete assessment of infant's status (Table 8.10)
   b. Review laboratory studies (Table 8.11)
2. Observe for deterioration in clinical condition
3. Identify problems that the infant has the potential to develop and/or already is experiencing:
   a. Hypoxia
   b. Metabolic acidosis
   c. Congestive heart failure
   d. Side effects of medical therapy—indomethacin, digoxin and/or diuretics, PGE_1
   e. Effectiveness of nonsurgical palliative treatment (Rashkind-Miller atrial ballon septostomy)
4. Develop a preventive and/or supportive plan of nursing care:
   a. Hypoxia
      1) Assess for clinical signs: cyanosis, respiratory distress
      2) Assess arterial blood gases
      3) Monitor transcutaneous pO_2 continuously
      4) Alleviate respiratory distress
      5) Maintain ventilatory and/or oxygen therapy as indicated
   b. Metabolic acidosis
      1) Assess arterial blood gases
      2) Administer $NaHCO_3$ as ordered
   c. Congestive heart failure
      1) Assess for signs of congestive heart failure: tachypnea, tachycardia, hepatomegaly, cardiomegaly
      2) Maintain fluid and sodium restriction as indicated

3) Administer digoxin and/or diuretics as ordered
4) Assess therapeutic response to treatment
5) Weigh infant once or twice daily
   d. Medical therapy
1) Assess therapeutic response to treatment
2) Assess for side effects of medications
   e. Nonsurgical palliation (Rashkind-Miller atrial balloon septostomy)
1) Assess therapeutic response to treatment as demonstrated by a improvement in arterial pO_2 and a decrease in respiratory distress
2) Assess for improvement or deterioration in clinical status after the procedure
5. Reduce energy expenditure of the infant
   a. Gavage feeding
   b. Organize nursing care
   c. Neutral thermal environment

Postoperative Care

As with preoperative care, the postoperative cardiac neonate requires all nursing assessments and interventions given to any infant after surgery. In the following discussion, attention given is only to the nursing care unique to the infant whose surgery involves repair or palliation of congenital heart disease. Some nursing interventions listed are more applicable to the open heart surgery patient and in some instances can be related to the effects of cardiopulmonary bypass on the physiological state of the infant. Assessment of these infants involves both laboratory and clinical techniques. In general, assessment postoperatively is similar to preoperative assessment, with attention to detection of complications.

Cardiovascular System

Maintenance of adequate cardiac output and, therefore, circulation has paramount importance in the postoperative period if the heart is to recover. Inadequate perfusion ultimately leads to metabolic acidosis, which has a deleterious effect on myocardial metabolism and contractility. Much of the care provided postoperatively is directed toward assessment of cardiac output, with interventions designed to increase inadequate circulation.

Assessment
1. Direct blood pressure via arterial line
2. Pulses
3. Temperature
4. Capillary refill
5. Urine output (should exceed 1 ml/kg/hour)
6. Color
7. Width of pulse pressure (decreased pulse pressure may indicate tamponade or decreased cardiac output)
8. Right atrial or central venous pressures (open heart repair)
9. Left atrial pressures (open heart repair)
10. Auscultation of the heart
    a. Tamponade (distant muffled heart sounds)
    b. Presence or absence of murmurs/extra sounds
11. Heart rate (tachycardia common after cardiac surgery)

12. Assessment for arrhythmias
13. Assessment of neurological status (agitation may indicate cerebral hypoxia)
14. Hematocrit

Planning and Invervention

1. Perform assessments as outlined above.
2. Administer volume expanders as ordered to maintain cardiac output.
3. Administer ionotropic agents (e.g., dopamine) to increase cardiac output as indicated.

Respiratory System

Assessment

1. Arterial blood gases (hypoxia, respiratory acidosis)
2. Signs of respiratory distress
3. Auscultation of breath sounds
   a. Symmetry
   b. Rales, rhonchi, wheezes
4. Respiratory rate
5. Chest x-ray
6. Chest tube drainage: amount; type

Planning and Intervention

1. Perform assessments as outlined above.
2. Maintain normal oxygenation and ventilation through ventilatory support.
3. Provide chest physiotherapy for atelectasis.
4. Maintain chest tubes:
   a. Secure all connections
   b. Assess for patency
      1) Fluctuations of fluid in tubing
      2) Sudden deterioration in clinical status may mean obstruction of chest tube
   c. Milk chest tubes to prevent occlusion
   d. Assess for leaks in the system as indicated by constant, excessive bubbling in water-seal chamber of closed chest drainage system
   e. Assess for evacuation of pneumothorax by noting intermittent bubbling in water-seal chamber of closed chest drainage system

Renal System/Fluid Balance

Assessment

1. Signs of fluid overload
   a. Edema
   b. Pulmonary rales
   c. Tachypnea
   d. Gallop rhythm
   e. Hepatomegaly
   f. Increase in body weight
2. Signs of volume depletion
   a. Dehydration
      1) Decreased skin turgor
      2) Dry mucous membranes
      3) Sunken fontanelle

b. Decreased urine output (should be at least 1 ml/kg/hour)
c. Increased specific gravity
d. Increased osmolality
3. Urine electrolytes
4. Blood electrolytes (abnormalities common in postoperative open heart surgery patient)
5. Arterial blood gases (metabolic acidosis can occur after cardiopulmonary bypass)

Planning and Intervention
1. Perform assessments as outlined above.
2. Keep strict record of intake and output.
3. Weigh infant once or twice a day.
4. Maintain adequate fluid administration (especially important in polycythemia, where thrombosis can occur as a result of dehydration).
5. Limit fluids as indicated by condition of patient (e.g., congestive heart failure).
6. Include all IV fluids as intake (ordered fluids, as well as any flushes).
7. Check and measure postoperative chest drainage.
8. Add electrolyte supplements to or remove them from IV fluids, as indicated by blood electrolyte levels, to maintain electrolyte balance.
9. Administer $NaHCO_3$ to correct metabolic acidosis.

Hematological System

Assessment
1. Hematocrit: anemia may occur as a result of red blood cell hemolysis after cardiopulmonary bypass.
2. Coagulation profile: coagulation factors, including platelets, thrombin, and pro-thrombin, may be altered after cardiopulmonary bypass.
3. Assess for persistent bleeding, which can be secondary to inadequate reversal of heparinization of blood during cardiopulmonary bypass; altered coagulation; inadequate surgical hemostasis; or breakdown of suture lines.

Planning and Intervention
1. Perform assessments as outlined above.
2. Administer clotting factors as indicated.
3. Administer blood as indicated by decreased hematocrit.
4. Check test tube drainage for excessive blood loss.
5. Note continued bleeding from heelsticks that may indicate coagulation disorder.

Metabolic System

Assessment
1. Hypoglycemia/hyperglycemia
2. Increased serum bilirubin (secondary to increased red blood cell hemolysis after cardiopulmonary bypass)

Planning and Intervention
1. Use Dextrostixs to detect altered glucose states.
2. Treat hypoglycemia/hyperglycemia as indicated.
3. Perform routine care for phototherapy or exchange transfusion for elevated bilirubin levels as ordered.

Neurological System

Assessment Assess infant for potential neurological complications:
1. Seizures secondary to:
   a. Hypoxia
   b. Embolism/thrombosis (especially in lesions involving right-to-left shunts)
   c. Intracranial hemorrhage
   d. Metabolic derangements: hypoglycemia, hyponatremia, etc.
2. Paraplegia as a result of poor spinal cord perfusion during aortic cross-clamping necessary for coarctation repair
3. Phrenic nerve injury during PDA repair

Planning and Intervention
1. Prevent precipitating factors for seizures.
2. Assess for seizure activity.
3. Administer anticonvulsants as indicated.
4. Assess for paraplegia after coarctation repair.
5. Assess for diaphragmatic paralysis seen with phrenic nerve injury.
6. Maintain ventilatory support as needed to prevent hypoxia, hypercarbia, and acidosis.

Infections

Assessment Check for signs of sepsis:
1. Lethargy
2. Hyperthermia or hypothermia
3. Poor feeding
4. Jaundice

Planning and Intervention
1. Perform assessments as outlined above.
2. Assist with obtaining blood cultures, lumbar puncture, tracheal aspirates, and urine cultures if sepsis is suspected.
3. Administer prophylactic antibiotics.

Summary

The nursing care of a baby who requires surgery involves skill and patience. Certainly, taking care of any neonate requires skill, but recognition of a potential surgical problem as well as preoperative and postoperative nursing needs require increased nursing assessment, judgment, and knowledge. After surgery there are many potential communication problems. These can occur between the medical, surgical, and nursing teams and unfortunately can involve the parents. The nurse is a vital liaison and can provide much-needed continuity of care. The goal of neonatal nursing is to provide that continuity and to aim for a well-planned and optimum discharge to well-prepared parents.

Acknowledgments

Special thanks to Linda Lambert, R.N., M.S.; Janice Koch, R.N., B.S., N.N.P., Bonna Coulter, M.D.; and J. Laurance Hill, M.D. for their contributions of time, information, and guidance in preparation of this chapter.

References

1. Coran AG, Behrendt DM, Weintraub WH, Lee DC: Surgery of the Neonate. Little, Brown, Boston, 1978.
2. Holder TM, Ashcraft KW (eds): Pediatric Surgery. Saunders, Philadelphia, 1980.
3. Welch KJ (ed): Complications of Pediatric Surgery. Saunders, Philadelphia, 1982.
4. Grupe WE, Harmon WE: Acute renal insufficiency. In KJ Welch (ed), Complications of Pediatric Surgery, pp 54–64. Saunders, Philadelphia, 1982.
5. Grylack LG, Scanlon JW: A prospective controlled study of oral gentamicin in the prevention of necrotizing enterocolitis. Am J Dis Child 132:1192, 1978.
6. Amoury RAMD: Necrotizing enterocolitis. In TM Holder, KW Ashcraft (eds), Pediatric Surgery, pp 371–387. Saunders, Philadelphia, 1980.
7. Tyson KR: Congenital Heart Disease in Infants. Clinical Symposia, vol. 27, no. 3. CIBA Pharmaceutical Co, Summit, NJ, 1975.
8. Castaneda AR: Early and late results of corrective cardiac surgery during the first year of life. In W Bircks, J Ostermeyer, HD Schulte (eds), Cardiovascular Surgery, pp 381–389. Springer-Verlag, New York, 1981.
9. Litwak RS, Brown EG: Operative and postoperative care of the neonate and pediatric surgical patient. In RS Litwak, RA Jurado (eds), Care of the Cardiac Surgical Patient, pp 433–454. Appleton-Century-Crofts, Norwalk, CT, 1982.
10. Moller JH: Essentials of Pediatric Cardiology, 2nd ed. Davis, Philadelphia, 1978.
11. Stevenson JG: Acyanotic lesions with normal pulmonary blood flow. Pediatr Clin North Am 25:725–742, 1978.
12. Stevenson JG: Acyanotic lesions with increased pulmonary blood flow. Pediatr Clin North Am 25:743–758, 1978.

Suggested Reading

Babson SG, Benson RC: Management of High Risk Pregnancy and Intensive Care of the Neonate, 2nd ed. Mosby, St. Louis, 1975.

Bishop WS, Head JJ: Care of the infant with a stoma. Matern Child Nurs J 1:315–319, 1976.

Benzing G, Kaplan S: Late complications of cardiac surgery. Pediatr Clin North Am 18:1225–1241, 1971.

Danielson GK, Pluth JR, Smith HC, Schultz GL: 1979. Monitoring of the postoperative cardiac patient. In JW Eldridge, H Goldberg, GM Lemole (eds), Current Problems in Congenital Heart Disease, pp 165–175. SP Medical and Scientific Books, New York, 1979.

Farrow R, Ducan F: The Surgery of Childhood for Nurses. Williams & Wilkins, Baltimore, 1968.

Filston HC: Surgical Problems in Children. Mosby, St. Louis, 1982.

Hazel N: An infant who survived gastroschisis. Matern Child Nurs J 6:35–40, 1981.

Hollabough RS, Bolles ET: The management of gastroschisis. J Pediatr Surg 8:263–270, 1973.

Jones M, Stark V: Special problems of postoperative care in infancy and childhood. In MV Baimbridge (ed), Postoperative Cardiac Intensive Care, pp 200–227. Blackwell Scientific, Boston, 1981.

Kawabori I: Cyanotic heart defects with decreased pulmonary blood flow. Pediatr Clin of North Am 25:759–776, 1978.

Kawabori I: Cyanotic heart defects with increased pulmonary blood flow. Pediatr Clin of North Am 25:777–795, 1978.

Kieswetter WB: Imperforate anus. In TM Holder, KW Aschcraft (eds), Pediatric Surgery, pp 401–417. Saunders, Philadelphia, 1980.

King OM: Congenital heart disease. In OM King (ed), Care of the Cardiac Surgical Patient, pp 87–126. Mosby, St. Louis, 1975.

Langman J: Medical Embryology. Williams & Wilkins, Baltimore, 1979.

Loomis JC: Care of the pediatric patient following cardiovascular surgery. In AK Ream, RP Fogdall (eds), Acute Cardiovascular Management, Anesthesia and Intensive Care, pp 635–700. Lippincott, Philadelphia, 1982.

Pacifico AD, McKay R: Advances in the surgical management of congenital heart disease in infants and children. In DC McGoon (ed), Cardiac Surgery, pp 127–141. Davis, Philadelphia, 1982.

Philip A: Neonatology—A Practical Guide. Medical Examination Publishing, New York, 1977.

Raffensperger J, Primrose RB: Pediatric Surgery for Nurses. Little, Brown, Boston, 1968.

Rickham PP, Johnston JH: Neonatal Surgery. Appleton-Century-Crofts, New York, 1969.

Santulli TV: Meconium ileus. In TM Holder, KW Ashcraft (eds), Pediatric Surgery, p 356. Saunders, Philadelphia, 1980.

Smith RM: Anesthesia. In KJ Welch (ed), Complications of Pediatric Surgery, pp 3–11. Saunders, Philadelphia, 1982.

Srinivasan V, Subramanian S: Complications of cardiovascular surgery in infants. In PA DeVries, SR Shapiro (eds), Complications of Pediatric Surgery, pp 101–115. Wiley, New York, 1982.

Swyer PR: The Intensive Care of the Newly Born. Monographs in Pediatrics, vol. 6. S Karger, New York, 1975.

Index

A

Abdominal surgery, 204–217
  and decompression of stomach, 205–206
  in diaphragmatic hernia, 212–214
  in esophageal atresia and tracheo-esophageal fistula, 209–212
  in gastroschisis and omphalocele, 206–209
  gastrostomy care in, 206
  ileostomy/colostomy care in, 206
  in intestinal obstruction, 214–215
  in necrotizing enterocolitis, 215–217
  postoperative care in, 205–206
  preoperative care in, 204–205
  wound care in, 206
ABO incompatibility, 166–167
Accessory nerve, testing of, 96
Acid-base balance, 125–127
Acidosis, 28, 146
  metabolic, 126
  renal tubular, 48
  respiratory, 125, 126
  in septic shock, 191
Addiction to drugs, and withdrawal symptoms, 91–93, 103–104, 107–109
Admission
  for cesarean section and large babies, 37
  to intensive care nursery, criteria for, 21
  to normal nursery, 21–22
Age, gestational, 22
Air leak syndrome, 119–120
Airway pressure
  continuous positive (CPAP)
    application of, 122–123
    nasal, 133–135
  mean, increasing of, 122
Alcohol use, and fetal alcohol syndrome, 93
Alertness, assessment of, 94
Alveolar stability, 114, 146
Amino acids, in parenteral nutrition, 53
Aminophylline, in respiratory disease, 148
Anemia, 124–125
  after cardiopulmonary bypass, 227
Anesthesia
  complications of, 201
  nursing care in, 200–201
Antibiotic therapy, 183
Aorta, coarctation of, 224
Aortic stenosis, 223

Apgar scoring system, 20
  in hypoxic-ischemic encephalopathy, 83–84
Apnea, 129–131
Apt test, for maternal hemoglobin, 193
Ascites, in hydrops fetalis, 167
Asphyxia
  and development of CNS, 81–85
  management of, 85
  and necrotizing enterocolitis, 215
  and persistent fetal circulation, 128
  seizures from, 90, 104, 110–111
Aspirate, tracheal
  for culture, 159
  for cytology, 160
Aspiration
  gastric, for shake test, 140
  of meconium, 120
Assessment of neonate, 22–23
  Apgar scoring system in, 20
  elimination in, 23, 25
  in first 24 hours, 18–24
  fluid balance in, 49–51
  in heart disease, 218–219
    postoperative, 225–226
  neurologic function in, 22–23, 25, 94–96
  respiration in, 20, 22, 24–25
    after cardiac surgery, 226
  Silverman scoring in, 19, 20, 22
  vital signs in, 22, 23
Atelectasis, 115, 118
Atresia, esophageal, and tracheoesophageal fistula, 209–212
Atrial balloon septostomy, in cyanotic heart lesions, 222
Auditory nerve, testing of, 96
Autonomic nervous system, evaluation of, 96

B

Bacterial infections, 180–183
Balloon septostomy, atrial, in cyanotic heart lesions, 222
Bathing of neonates, 24, 42–43
Bicarbonate
  renal handling of, 48
  as therapy, 149
    in acidosis, 126
Bilirubin
  hyperbilirubinemia, 91
    see also Jaundice